Teen Health Series

Fitness Information For Teens, Third Edition

Fitness Information For Teens, Third Edition

Health Tips About Exercise And Active Lifestyles

Including Facts About Healthy Muscles And Bones, Starting And
Maintaining Fitness Plans, Aerobic Fitness, Stretching And Strength
Training, Sports Safety, And Suggestions For Team Athletes And
Individuals

Edited by Elizabeth Bellenir

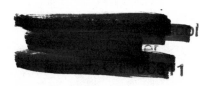

Omnigraphics

155 W. Congress, Suite 200
Detroit, MI 48226

Bibliographic Note

Because this page cannot legibly accommodate all the copyright notices, the Bibliographic Note portion of the Preface constitutes an extension of the copyright notice.

Edited by Elizabeth Bellenir

Teen Health Series

Karen Bellenir, *Managing Editor*
David A. Cooke, M.D., *Medical Consultant*
Elizabeth Collins, *Research and Permissions Coordinator*
Cherry Edwards, *Permissions Assistant*
EdIndex, *Services for Publishers, Indexers*

* * *

Omnigraphics, Inc.
Matthew P. Barbour, *Senior Vice President*
Kevin M. Hayes, *Operations Manager*

* * *

Peter E. Ruffner, *Publisher*
Copyright © 2013 Omnigraphics, Inc.
ISBN 978-0-7808-1267-3
E-ISBN 978-0-7808-1268-0

Table of Contents

Preface

Part One: Your Body And The Components Of Fitness

Chapter 1—What Is Fitness?..3

Chapter 2—Why Exercise Is Wise..9

Chapter 3—Meeting Your Muscles..19

Chapter 4—Bone Health...23

Chapter 5—Your Heart and Lungs..27

Chapter 6—Teen Nutrition...41

Chapter 7—Weighty Issues..57

Chapter 8—Mental Wellness...61

Chapter 9—Sleep Is Important For Fitness.............................65

Part Two: Making And Maintaining A Fitness Plan

Chapter 10—Tips For Getting Started On A Path
            To Fitness 71

Chapter 11—Fitness Self-Assessment.....................................75

Chapter 12—Fitness Guidelines For Children And
            Adolescents...81

Chapter 13—A Formula For Fitness 91

Chapter 14—When Is The Right Time To Work Out? 95

Chapter 15—Health Clubs And Fitness Friends....................99

Chapter 16—Selecting And Using A Fitness Facility..........103

Chapter 17—Exercise Caution Before Spending Money
            On Fitness Products...109

Chapter 18—A Physically Active Lifestyle............................113

Part Three: Exercise Fundamentals

Chapter 19—Kinds Of Exercise 125

Chapter 20—Cardiovascular (Cardio) Exercise 129

Chapter 21—Start Running.. 133

Chapter 22—Calisthenics 137

Chapter 23—Strength Training.. 145

Chapter 24—Stretching... 151

Chapter 25—Pilates And Yoga 155

Chapter 26—Measuring Exercise Intensity 163

Part Four: Activities For Team Athletes And Individuals

Chapter 27—Choosing The Right Sport For You 177

Chapter 28—Activities For Teens Who Don't Like Sports............... 183

Chapter 29—Baseball And Softball.. 187

Chapter 30—Basketball... 191

Chapter 31—Bicycling And Indoor Cycling.................................... 193

Chapter 32—Football... 197

Chapter 33—Frisbee.. 199

Chapter 34—Golf.. 201

Chapter 35—Gymnastics, Cheerleading, And Ballet....................... 205

Chapter 36—Martial Arts 211

Chapter 37—Skating: Inline Skates And Skateboards..................... 213

Chapter 38—Soccer 217

Chapter 39—Tennis, Table Tennis, And Volleyball.......................... 219

Chapter 40—Walking And Hiking.. 225

Chapter 41—Water Sports...229

Chapter 42—Winter Sports...241

Part Five: Sports Safety

Chapter 43—Fitness Safety Tips..251

Chapter 44—Safety Tips For Runners..................................257

Chapter 45—Helmets..263

Chapter 46—Clothes And Shoes For Workout
Comfort And Safety...269

Chapter 47—Increasing Activity Safely 273

Chapter 48—Tips For Exercising Safely In Adverse
Weather 281

Chapter 49—Understanding Hydration For Fitness..............289

Part Six: Overcoming Obstacles To Fitness

Chapter 50—Maintaining Fitness Motivation 297

Chapter 51—You Can Be Active At Any Size 303

Chapter 52—Sports Injuries...311

Chapter 53—Exercising While Recovering
From An Injury...319

Chapter 54—Exercise Suggestions For
People With Asthma..323

Chapter 55—Exercise Suggestions For
People With Diabetes 327

Chapter 56—Exercise Suggestions For
People With Physical Disabilities 333

Chapter 57—Compulsive Exercise: When Exercise
Turns Unhealthy 339

Chapter 58—Female Athlete Triad: Three Symptoms
That Mean Trouble 345

Chapter 59—Steroids And Other Performance Enhancers
Are Risky 349

Part Seven: If You Need More Information

Chapter 60—The President's Challenge 357

Chapter 61—Resources For More Information
About Fitness 361

Chapter 62—Resources For More Information About
Specific Sports And Activities 369

Index **375**

Preface

About This Book

When teens adopt healthy and active habits, the rewards can persist for a lifetime. According to the Centers for Disease Control and Prevention, the numerous benefits of physical fitness include weight control, stronger bones and muscles, and improved mental health and mood. In addition, by avoiding inactivity teens can help reduce the risks that cardiovascular disease, metabolic syndrome, type 2 diabetes, and some types of cancer will develop later in their lives.

Despite the benefits, however, many young people fail to meet guidelines for physical activity. A 2011 study reported that only 29% percent of high school students had participated in the recommended 60 minutes per day of physical activity on each of the seven days before the survey. Furthermore, 14% of high school students had not participated in 60 or more minutes of any kind of physical activity on any day during the seven days before the survey.

Fitness Information For Teens, Third Edition, offers teens a comprehensive, fact-based guide for living a healthy and active lifestyle. The book includes information about the developing body, the components of fitness, and making and maintaining a fitness plan. It discusses exercise fundamentals and activities for team athletes and individuals—whether beginners or experienced competitors. Sports safety concerns, nutrition challenges, and suggestions for overcoming obstacles concerning fitness and change are also addressed. The book concludes with information about the President's Challenge and directories of additional resources.

How To Use This Book

This book is divided into parts and chapters. Parts focus on broad areas of interest; chapters are devoted to single topics within a part.

Part One: Your Body And The Components Of Fitness begins with a definition of fitness, and it goes on to explain the importance of developing muscular strength, endurance, and flexibility. Additional chapters discuss other components of mental and physical fitness, including proper nutrition, weight management, and sleep requirements.

Part Two: Making And Maintaining A Fitness Plan provides guidance for taking the first steps on the path toward fitness and continuing on toward reachable goals. It offers suggestions for evaluating current fitness levels, identifying targets for improvement, and making progress toward the development of a physically active lifestyle.

Part Three: Exercise Fundamentals describes the basic categories of exercises, including aerobic exercise, muscle-strengthening exercise, bone-strengthening exercise, and exercises that help promote flexibility and balance. It also discusses how to measure exercise intensity, and it includes examples of various types of activities and their intensity levels.

Part Four: Activities For Team Athletes And Individuals provides facts about a wide range of team sports and individual activities that can be part of a well-rounded fitness program.

Part Five: Sports Safety discusses practical tips for preventing injuries. It reminds readers who participate in physical activities about the importance of following safety guidelines, including warming up and cooling down, using protective equipment such as helmets and appropriate footwear, taking precautions in adverse weather conditions, and avoiding dehydration.

Part Six: Overcoming Obstacles To Fitness describes the challenge of staying on course to meet fitness goals and offers suggestions for maintaining motivation. It explains commonly encountered barriers to fitness, including sports injuries and pre-existing conditions such as asthma, diabetes, or physical disabilities. It also discusses problems associated with compulsive exercise, female athlete triad, and the dangers of using steroids or other performance-enhancing substances.

Part Seven: If You Need More Information explains how the President's Challenge can help people set and reach fitness goals, and it offers directories of general fitness organizations and resources for more information about specific sports and activities.

Bibliographic Note

This volume contains documents and excerpts from publications issued by the following government agencies: Centers for Disease Control and Prevention (CDC); Federal Trade Commission (FTC); National Heart Lung and Blood Institute; National Institute of Arthritis and Musculoskeletal and Skin Diseases; National Institute of Diabetes and Digestive and Kidney Diseases; National Institute on Drug Abuse; National Institute on Mental Health; Office on Women's Health; President's Council on Fitness, Sports, and Nutrition; U.S. Consumer Product Safety Commission; U.S. Department of Health and Human Services; U.S. Department of Homeland Security; U.S. Department of Veterans Affairs; U.S. Food and Drug Administration; and the U.S. Public Health Service Commissioned Corps.

In addition, this volume contains copyrighted documents and articles produced by the following organizations: About.com; A.D.A.M., Inc.; American College of Sports Medicine;

American Council on Exercise; Ann and Robert H. Lurie Children's Hospital of Chicago; *Go Ask Alice!* (Trustees of Columbia University); iEmily.com; National Health Service (UK); National Women's Health Resource Center (HealthyWomen.org); Nemours Foundation; New York State Department of Health; President's Challenge; and the University of Michigan Health System.

The photograph on the front cover is © Doug Menuez/Thinkstock.

Full citation information is provided on the first page of each chapter. Every effort has been made to secure all necessary rights to reprint the copyrighted material. If any omissions have been made, please contact Omnigraphics to make corrections for future editions.

Acknowledgements

In addition to the organizations listed above, special thanks are due to Liz Collins, research and permissions coordinator; Karen Bellenir, managing editor; Lisa Bakewell, verification assistant; and WhimsyInk, prepress services provider.

About The Teen Health Series

At the request of librarians serving today's young adults, the *Teen Health Series* was developed as a specially focused set of volumes within Omnigraphics' *Health Reference Series*. Each volume deals comprehensively with a topic selected according to the needs and interests of people in middle school and high school.

Teens seeking preventive guidance, information about disease warning signs, medical statistics, and risk factors for health problems will find answers to their questions in the *Teen Health Series*. The *Series*, however, is not intended to serve as a tool for diagnosing illness, in prescribing treatments, or as a substitute for the physician/patient relationship. All people concerned about medical symptoms or the possibility of disease are encouraged to seek professional care from an appropriate health care provider.

If there is a topic you would like to see addressed in a future volume of the *Teen Health Series*, please write to:

Editor
Teen Health Series
Omnigraphics, Inc.
155 W. Congress, Suite 200
Detroit, MI 48226

A Note about Spelling and Style

Teen Health Series editors use *Stedman's Medical Dictionary* as an authority for questions related to the spelling of medical terms and the *Chicago Manual of Style* for questions related to grammatical structures, punctuation, and other editorial concerns. Consistent adherence is not always possible, however, because the individual volumes within the *Series* include many documents from a wide variety of different producers and copyright holders, and the editor's primary goal is to present material from each source as accurately as is possible following the terms specified by each document's producer. This sometimes means that information in different chapters or sections may follow other guidelines and alternate spelling authorities. For example, occasionally a copyright holder may require that eponymous terms be shown in possessive forms (Crohn's disease *vs.* Crohn disease) or that British spelling norms be retained (leukaemia *vs.* leukemia).

Locating Information within the Teen Health Series

The *Teen Health Series* contains a wealth of information about a wide variety of medical topics. As the *Series* continues to grow in size and scope, locating the precise information needed by a specific student may become more challenging. To address this concern, information about books within the *Teen Health Series* is included in *A Contents Guide to the Health Reference Series*. The *Contents Guide* presents an extensive list of more than 16,000 diseases, treatments, and other topics of general interest compiled from the Tables of Contents and major index headings from the books of the *Teen Health Series* and *Health Reference Series*. To access *A Contents Guide to the Health Reference Series*, visit www.healthreferenceseries.com.

Our Advisory Board

We would like to thank the following advisory board members for providing guidance to the development of this *Series*:

Dr. Lynda Baker, Associate Professor of Library and Information Science, Wayne State University, Detroit, MI

Nancy Bulgarelli, William Beaumont Hospital Library, Royal Oak, MI

Karen Imarisio, Bloomfield Township Public Library, Bloomfield Township, MI

Karen Morgan, Mardigian Library, University of Michigan-Dearborn, Dearborn, MI

Rosemary Orlando, St. Clair Shores Public Library, St. Clair Shores, MI

Medical Consultant

Medical consultation services are provided to the *Teen Health Series* editors by David A. Cooke, M.D. Dr. Cooke is a graduate of Brandeis University, and he received his M.D. degree from the University of Michigan. He completed residency training at the University of Wisconsin Hospital and Clinics. He is board-certified in internal medicine. Dr. Cooke currently works as part of the University of Michigan Health System and practices in Ann Arbor, MI. In his free time, he enjoys writing, science fiction, and spending time with his family.

Part One
Your Body And The Components Of Fitness

Chapter 1

What Is Fitness?

Defining Fitness

Physical fitness is to the human body what fine tuning is to an engine. It enables us to perform up to our potential. Fitness can be described as a condition that helps us look, feel and do our best. More specifically, it can be defined like this:

> "The ability to perform daily tasks vigorously and alertly, with energy left over for enjoying leisure-time activities and meeting emergency demands. It is the ability to endure, to bear up, to withstand stress, to carry on in circumstances where an unfit person could not continue, and is a major basis for good health and well-being."

Physical fitness involves the performance of the heart and lungs, and the muscles of the body. And, since what we do with our bodies also affects what we can do with our minds, fitness influences to some degree qualities such as mental alertness and emotional stability.

As you undertake your fitness program, it's important to remember that fitness is an individual quality that varies from person to person. It is influenced by age, sex, heredity, personal habits, exercise and eating practices. You can't do anything about the first three factors. However, it is within your power to change and improve the others where needed.

Knowing The Basics

Physical fitness is most easily understood by examining its components, or parts. There is widespread agreement that these four components are basic:

About This Chapter: Information in this chapter is excerpted from "Fitness Fundamentals: Guidelines for Personal Exercise Programs," President's Council on Fitness, Sports, and Nutrition (www.fitness.gov), February 8, 2012.

- **Cardiorespiratory Endurance:** The ability to deliver oxygen and nutrients to tissues, and to remove wastes, over sustained periods of time. Long runs and swims are among the methods employed in measuring this component.

- **Muscular Strength:** The ability of a muscle to exert force for a brief period of time. Upper-body strength, for example, can be measured by various weight-lifting exercises.

- **Muscular Endurance:** The ability of a muscle, or a group of muscles, to sustain repeated contractions or to continue applying force against a fixed object. Pushups are often used to test endurance of arm and shoulder muscles.

- **Flexibility:** The ability to move joints and use muscles through their full range of motion. The sit-and-reach test is a good measure of flexibility of the lower back and backs of the upper legs.

- **Body Composition** is often considered a component of fitness. It refers to the makeup of the body in terms of lean mass (muscle, bone, vital tissue and organs) and fat mass. An optimal ratio of fat to lean mass is an indication of fitness, and the right types of exercises will help you decrease body fat and increase or maintain muscle mass.

A Workout Schedule

How often, how long and how hard you exercise, and what kinds of exercises you do should be determined by what you are trying to accomplish. Your goals, your present fitness level, age, health, skills, interest and convenience are among the factors you should consider. For example, an athlete training for high-level competition would follow a different program than a person whose goals are good health and the ability to meet work and recreational needs.

Your exercise program should include something from each of the four basic fitness components described previously. Each workout should begin with a warm-up and end with a cool-down. As a general rule, space your workouts throughout the week and avoid consecutive days of hard exercise.

Here are the amounts of activity necessary for the average healthy person to maintain a minimum level of overall fitness. Included are some of the popular exercises for each category.

- **Warm-Up:** 5–10 minutes of exercise such as walking, slow jogging, knee lifts, arm circles, or trunk rotations. Low intensity movements that simulate movements to be used in the activity can also be included in the warm-up.

- **Muscular Strength:** A minimum of two 20-minute sessions per week that include exercises for all the major muscle groups. Lifting weights is the most effective way to increase strength.

- **Muscular Endurance:** At least three 30-minute sessions each week that include exercises such as calisthenics, push-ups, sit-ups, pull-ups, and weight training for all the major muscle groups.

- **Cardiorespiratory Endurance:** At least three 20-minute bouts of continuous aerobic (activity requiring oxygen) rhythmic exercise each week. Popular aerobic conditioning activities include brisk walking, jogging, swimming, cycling, rope-jumping, rowing, cross-country skiing, and some continuous action games like racquetball and handball.

- **Flexibility:** 10–12 minutes of daily stretching exercises performed slowly, without a bouncing motion. This can be included after a warm-up or during a cool-down.

- **Cool-Down:** A minimum of 5–10 minutes of slow walking, low-level exercise, combined with stretching.

A Matter Of Principle

The keys to selecting the right kinds of exercises for developing and maintaining each of the basic components of fitness are found in these principles:

- **Specificity:** Pick the right kind of activities to affect each component. Strength training results in specific strength changes. Also, train for the specific activity you're interested in. For example, optimal swimming performance is best achieved when the muscles involved in swimming are trained for the movements required. It does not necessarily follow that a good runner is a good swimmer.

- **Overload:** Work hard enough, at levels that are vigorous and long enough to overload your body above its resting level, to bring about improvement.

- **Regularity:** You can't hoard physical fitness. At least three balanced workouts a week are necessary to maintain a desirable level of fitness.

- **Progression:** Increase the intensity, frequency and/or duration of activity over periods of time in order to improve.

Some activities can be used to fulfill more than one of your basic exercise requirements. For example, in addition to increasing cardiorespiratory endurance, running builds muscular endurance in the legs, and swimming develops the arm, shoulder and chest muscles. If you select the proper activities, it is possible to fit parts of your muscular endurance workout into your cardiorespiratory workout and save time.

Measuring Your Heart Rate

Heart rate is widely accepted as a good method for measuring intensity during running, swimming, cycling, and other aerobic activities. Exercise that doesn't raise your heart rate to a certain level and keep it there for 20 minutes won't contribute significantly to cardiovascular fitness.

The heart rate you should maintain is called your target heart rate. There are several ways of arriving at this figure. One of the simplest is: maximum heart rate (220 - age) x 70%. Thus, the target heart rate for a 40 year-old would be 126.

10 Tips To Healthy Eating And Physical Activity For You

Start your day with breakfast: Breakfast fills your "empty tank" to get you going after a long night without food. And it can help you do better in school. Easy to prepare breakfasts include cold cereal with fruit and low-fat milk, whole-wheat toast with peanut butter, yogurt with fruit, whole-grain waffles, or even last night's pizza.

Get moving: It's easy to fit physical activities into your daily routine. Walk, bike, or jog to see friends. Take a 10-minute activity break every hour while you read, do homework, or watch TV. Climb stairs instead of taking an escalator or elevator. Try to do these things for a total of 30 minutes every day.

Snack smart: Snacks are a great way to refuel. Choose snacks from different food groups—a glass of low-fat milk and a few graham crackers, an apple or celery sticks with peanut butter and raisins, or some dry cereal. If you eat smart at other meals, cookies, chips, and candy are OK for occasional snacking.

Work up a sweat: Vigorous work-outs—when you're breathing hard and sweating—help your heart pump better, give you more energy, and help you look and feel best. Start with a warm-up that stretches your muscles. Include 20 minutes of aerobic activity, such as running, jogging, or dancing. Follow-up with activities that help make you stronger such as push-ups or lifting weights. Then cool-down with more stretching and deep breathing.

Balance your food choices: Don't eat too much of any one thing. You don't have to give up foods like hamburgers, french fries and ice cream to eat healthy. You just have to be smart about how often and how much of them you eat. Your body needs nutrients like protein, carbohydrates, fat and many different vitamins and minerals such as vitamins C and A, iron and calcium from a variety of foods. Balancing food choices and checking out the Nutrition Facts Panel on food labels will help you get all these nutrients.

Some methods for figuring the target rate take individual differences into consideration. Here is one of them:

- Subtract age from 220 to find maximum heart rate.

- Subtract resting heart rate (see below) from maximum heart rate to determine heart rate reserve.

- Take 70% of heart rate reserve to determine heart rate raise.

- Add heart rate raise to resting heart rate to find target rate.

Resting heart rate should be determined by taking your pulse after sitting quietly for five minutes. When checking heart rate during a workout, take your pulse within five seconds after

Get fit with friends or family: Being active is much more fun with friends or family. Encourage others to join you and plan one special physical activity event, like a bike ride or hiking, with a group each week.

Eat more whole grains, fruits, and vegetables: These foods give you carbohydrates for energy, plus vitamins, minerals and fiber. Besides, they taste good! Try breads such as whole-wheat, bagels, and pita. Spaghetti and oatmeal are also in the grain group. Bananas, strawberries, and melons are some great tasting fruits. Try vegetables raw on a sandwich or in a salad.

Join in physical activities at school: Whether you take a physical education class or do other physical activities at school, such as intramural sports, structured activities are a sure way to feel good, look good and stay physically fit.

Foods aren't good or bad: A healthy eating style is like a puzzle with many parts. Each part—or food—is different. Some foods may have more fat, sugar or salt while others may have more vitamins or fiber. There is a place for all these foods. What makes a diet good or bad is how foods fit together. Balancing your choices is important. Fit in a higher-fat food, like pepperoni pizza, at dinner by choosing lower-fat foods at other meals. And don't forget about moderation. If two pieces of pizza fill you up, you don't need a third.

Make healthy eating and physical activities fun: Take advantage of physical activities you and your friends enjoy doing together and eat the foods you like. Be adventurous—try new sports, games and other activities as well as new foods. You'll grow stronger, play longer, and look and feel better. Set realistic goals—don't try changing too much at once.

Source: "10 Tips To Healthy Eating and Physical Activity For You" President's Council on Fitness, Sports, and Nutrition (www.fitness.gov), January 5, 2012.

interrupting exercise because it starts to go down once you stop moving. Count pulse for 10 seconds and multiply by six to get the per-minute rate.

Controlling Your Weight

The key to weight control is keeping energy intake (food) and energy output (physical activity) in balance. When you consume only as many calories as your body needs, your weight will usually remain constant. If you take in more calories than your body needs, you will put on excess fat. If you expend more energy than you take in you will burn excess fat.

Exercise plays an important role in weight control by increasing energy output, calling on stored calories for extra fuel. Recent studies show that not only does exercise increase metabolism during a workout, but it causes your metabolism to stay increased for a period of time after exercising, allowing you to burn more calories.

How much exercise is needed to make a difference in your weight depends on the amount and type of activity, and on how much you eat. Aerobic exercise burns body fat. A medium-sized adult would have to walk more than 30 miles to burn up 3,500 calories, the equivalent of one pound of fat. Although that may seem like a lot, you don't have to walk the 30 miles all at once. Walking a mile a day for 30 days will achieve the same result, providing you don't increase your food intake to negate the effects of walking.

If you consume 100 calories a day more than your body needs, you will gain approximately 10 pounds in a year. You could take that weight off, or keep it off, by doing 30 minutes of moderate exercise daily. The combination of exercise and diet offers the most flexible and effective approach to weight control.

Since muscle tissue weighs more than fat tissue, and exercise develops muscle to a certain degree, your bathroom scale won't necessarily tell you whether or not you are "fat." Well-muscled individuals, with relatively little body fat, invariably are "overweight" according to standard weight charts. If you are doing a regular program of strength training, your muscles will increase in weight, and possibly your overall weight will increase. Body composition is a better indicator of your condition than body weight.

Lack of physical activity causes muscles to get soft, and if food intake is not decreased, added body weight is almost always fat. Once-active people, who continue to eat as they always have after settling into sedentary lifestyles, tend to suffer from creeping obesity.

Chapter 2

Why Exercise Is Wise

All Americans should be regularly physically active to improve overall health and fitness and to prevent many adverse health outcomes. The benefits of physical activity occur in generally healthy people, in people at risk of developing chronic diseases, and in people with current chronic conditions or disabilities.

Physical activity affects many health conditions, and the specific amounts and types of activity that benefit each condition vary. One consistent finding from research studies is that once the health benefits from physical activity begin to accrue, additional amounts of activity provide additional benefits.

Although some health benefits seem to begin with as little as 60 minutes (one hour) a week, research shows that a total amount of 150 minutes (2 hours and 30 minutes) a week of moderate-intensity aerobic activity, such as brisk walking, consistently reduces the risk of many chronic diseases and other adverse health outcomes.

Examining The Relationship Between Physical Activity and Health

In many studies covering a wide range of issues, researchers have focused on exercise, as well as on the more broadly defined concept of physical activity. Exercise is a form of physical activity that is planned, structured, repetitive, and performed with the goal of improving health or fitness. So, although all exercise is physical activity, not all physical activity is exercise.

About This Chapter: Excerpted from *2008 Physical Activity Guidelines for Americans*, U.S. Department of Health and Human Services (www.health.gov/paguidelines), 2008.

Studies have examined the role of physical activity in many groups—men and women, children, teens, adults, older adults, people with disabilities, and women during pregnancy and the postpartum period. These studies have also prompted questions as to what type and how much physical activity is needed for various health benefits. To answer this question, investigators have studied three main kinds of physical activity: aerobic, muscle-strengthening, and bone-strengthening. Investigators have also studied balance and flexibility activities.

Aerobic Activity

In this kind of physical activity (also called an endurance activity or cardio activity), the body's large muscles move in a rhythmic manner for a sustained period of time. Brisk walking, running, bicycling, jumping rope, and swimming are all examples.

Aerobic activity causes a person's heart to beat faster than usual. Aerobic physical activity has three components:

- Intensity, or how hard a person works to do the activity. The intensities most often examined are moderate intensity (equivalent in effort to brisk walking) and vigorous intensity (equivalent in effort to running or jogging).

- Frequency, or how often a person does aerobic activity

- Duration, or how long a person does an activity in any one session

Although these components make up a physical activity profile, research has shown that the total amount of physical activity (minutes of moderate-intensity physical activity, for example) is more important for achieving health benefits than is any one component (frequency, intensity, or duration).

Muscle-Strengthening Activity

This kind of activity, which includes resistance training and lifting weights, causes the body's muscles to work or hold against an applied force or weight. These activities often involve relatively heavy objects, such as weights, which are lifted multiple times to train various muscle groups. Muscle-strengthening activity can also be done by using elastic bands or body weight for resistance (climbing a tree or doing push-ups, for example).

Muscle-strengthening activity also has three components:

- Intensity, or how much weight or force is used relative to how much a person is able to lift

- Frequency, or how often a person does muscle-strengthening activity

- Repetitions, or how many times a person lifts a weight (analogous to duration for aerobic activity)

The effects of muscle-strengthening activity are limited to the muscles doing the work. It's important to work all the major muscle groups of the body: the legs, hips, back, abdomen, chest, shoulders, and arms.

Bone-Strengthening Activity

This kind of activity (sometimes called weight-bearing or weight-loading activity) produces a force on the bones that promotes bone growth and strength. This force is commonly produced by impact with the ground. Examples of bone-strengthening activity include jumping jacks, running, brisk walking, and weight-lifting exercises. As these examples illustrate, bone-strengthening activities can also be aerobic and muscle strengthening.

The Health Benefits Of Physical Activity

Studies clearly demonstrate that participating in regular physical activity provides many health benefits. The health benefits of physical activity are seen in children and adolescents, young and middle-aged adults, older adults, women and men, people of different races and ethnicities, and people with disabilities and chronic conditions. The health benefits of physical activity are generally independent of body weight. People of all sizes and shapes gain health and fitness benefits by being habitually physically active. The benefits of physical activity also outweigh the risk of injury and sudden heart attacks, two concerns that prevent many people from becoming physically active.

Students Do Best When They Are Physically Fit

The California Department of Education matched standardized reading and math scores with scores from state physical fitness tests of fifth-, seventh-, and ninth- grade students. The state officials found that higher math and reading scores were associated with higher fitness scores at each grade level.

Source: Excerpted from *BodyWorks: A Toolkit for Healthy Teens and Strong Families*, Office on Women's Health, U.S. Department of Health and Human Services, 2006. Reviewed by David A. Cooke, MD, FACP, May 2012.

Beneficial Effects Of Increasing Physical Activity

Overload is the physical stress placed on the body when physical activity is greater in amount or intensity than usual. The body's structures and functions respond and adapt to these stresses. For example, aerobic physical activity places a stress on the cardiorespiratory system and muscles, requiring the lungs to move more air and the heart to pump more blood and deliver it to the working muscles. This increase in demand increases the efficiency and capacity of the lungs, heart, circulatory system, and exercising muscles. In the same way, muscle-strengthening and bone-strengthening activities overload muscles and bones, making them stronger.

Progression is closely tied to overload. Once a person reaches a certain fitness level, he or she progresses to higher levels of physical activity by continued overload and adaptation. Small, progressive changes in overload help the body adapt to the additional stresses while minimizing the risk of injury.

Specificity means that the benefits of physical activity are specific to the body systems that are doing the work. For example, aerobic physical activity largely benefits the body's cardiovascular system.

Source: U.S. Department of Health and Human Services (www.health.gov/paguidelines), 2008.

Reducing Risk Of Premature Death

Strong scientific evidence shows that physical activity reduces the risk of premature death (dying earlier than the average age of death for a specific population group) from the leading causes of death, such as heart disease and some cancers, as well as from other causes of death. This effect is remarkable in two ways:

- First, only a few lifestyle choices have as large an effect on mortality as physical activity. It has been estimated that people who are physically active for approximately seven hours a week have a 40 percent lower risk of dying early than those who are active for less than 30 minutes a week.

- Second, it is not necessary to do high amounts of activity or vigorous-intensity activity to reduce the risk of premature death. Studies show substantially lower risk when people do 150 minutes of at least moderate-intensity aerobic physical activity a week.

Cardiorespiratory Health

The benefits of physical activity on cardiorespiratory health are some of the most extensively documented of all the health benefits. Cardiorespiratory health involves the health of the heart, lungs, and blood vessels.

Heart diseases and stroke are two of the leading causes of death in the United States. Risk factors that increase the likelihood of cardiovascular diseases include smoking, high blood pressure (called hypertension), type 2 diabetes, and high levels of certain blood lipids (such as low-density lipoprotein, or LDL, cholesterol). Low cardiorespiratory fitness also is a risk factor for heart disease.

People who do moderate- or vigorous-intensity aerobic physical activity have a significantly lower risk of cardiovascular disease than do inactive people. Significant reductions in risk of cardiovascular disease occur at activity levels equivalent to 150 minutes a week of moderate-intensity physical activity. Even greater benefits are seen with 200 minutes (three hours and 20 minutes) a week. The evidence is strong that greater amounts of physical activity result in even further reductions in the risk of cardiovascular disease.

Adverse Events

Some people hesitate to become active or increase their level of physical activity because they fear getting injured or having a heart attack. Studies of generally healthy people clearly show that moderate-intensity physical activity, such as brisk walking, has a low risk of such adverse events.

The risk of musculoskeletal injury increases with the total amount of physical activity. For example, a person who regularly runs 40 miles a week has a higher risk of injury than a person who runs 10 miles each week. However, people who are physically active may have fewer injuries from other causes, such as motor vehicle collisions or work-related injuries. Depending on the type and amount of activity that physically active people do, their overall injury rate may be lower than the overall injury rate for inactive people.

Participation in contact or collision sports, such as soccer or football, has a higher risk of injury than participation in non-contact physical activity, such as swimming or walking. However, when performing the same activity, people who are less fit are more likely to be injured than people who are fitter.

Cardiac events, such as a heart attack or sudden death during physical activity, are rare. However, the risk of such cardiac events does increase when a person suddenly becomes much more active than usual. The greatest risk occurs when an adult who is usually inactive engages in vigorous-intensity activity (such as shoveling snow). People who are regularly physically active have the lowest risk of cardiac events both while being active and overall.

The bottom line is that the health benefits of physical activity far outweigh the risks of adverse events for almost everyone.

Source: U.S. Department of Health and Human Services (www.health.gov/paguidelines), 2008.

Metabolic Health

Regular physical activity strongly reduces the risk of developing type 2 diabetes as well as the metabolic syndrome. The metabolic syndrome is defined as a condition in which people have some combination of high blood pressure, a large waistline (abdominal obesity), an adverse blood lipid profile (low levels of high-density lipoprotein [HDL] cholesterol, raised triglycerides), and impaired glucose tolerance.

People who regularly engage in at least moderate-intensity aerobic activity have a significantly lower risk of developing type 2 diabetes than do inactive people. Although some experts debate the usefulness of defining the metabolic syndrome, good evidence exists that physical activity reduces the risk of having this condition, as defined in various ways. Lower rates of these conditions are seen with 120 to 150 minutes (two hours to two hours and 30 minutes) a week of at least moderate-intensity aerobic activity. As with cardiovascular health, additional levels of physical activity seem to lower risk even further. In addition, physical activity helps control blood glucose levels in persons who already have type 2 diabetes.

Physical activity also improves metabolic health in youth. Studies find this effect when young people participate in at least three days of vigorous aerobic activity a week. More physical activity is associated with improved metabolic health, but research has yet to determine the exact amount of improvement.

Obesity And Energy Balance

Overweight and obesity occur when fewer calories are expended than are taken in through food and beverages. Physical activity and caloric intake both must be considered when trying to control body weight.

Because of this role in energy balance, physical activity is a critical factor in determining whether a person can maintain a healthy body weight, lose excess body weight, or maintain successful weight loss. People vary a great deal in how much physical activity they need to achieve and maintain a healthy weight. Some need more physical activity than others to maintain a healthy body weight, to lose weight, or to keep weight off once it has been lost.

Strong scientific evidence shows that physical activity helps people maintain a stable weight over time. However, the optimal amount of physical activity needed to maintain weight is unclear. People vary greatly in how much physical activity results in weight stability. Many people need more than the equivalent of 150 minutes of moderate-intensity activity a week to maintain their weight.

Over short periods of time, such as a year, research shows that it is possible to achieve weight stability by doing the equivalent of 150 to 300 minutes (five hours) a week of moderate-intensity walking at about a four mile-an-hour pace. Muscle-strengthening activities may help promote weight maintenance, although not to the same degree as aerobic activity.

People who want to lose a substantial amount of weight (more than five percent of body weight) and people who are trying to keep a significant amount of weight off once it has been lost need a high amount of physical activity unless they also reduce their caloric intake. Many people need to do more than 300 minutes of moderate-intensity activity a week to meet weight-control goals.

Regular physical activity also helps control the percentage of body fat in children and adolescents. Exercise training studies with overweight and obese youth have shown that they can reduce their body fatness by participating in physical activity that is at least moderate intensity on three to five days a week, for 30 to 60 minutes each time.

Musculoskeletal Health

Bones, muscles, and joints support the body and help it move. Healthy bones, joints, and muscles are critical to the ability to do daily activities without physical limitations.

Preserving bone, joint, and muscle health is essential. Studies show that the frequent decline in bone density that happens during aging can be slowed with regular physical activity. These effects are seen in people who participate in aerobic, muscle-strengthening, and bone-strengthening physical activity programs of moderate or vigorous intensity. The range of total physical activity for these benefits varies widely. Important changes seem to begin at 90 minutes a week and continue up to 300 minutes a week.

Building strong, healthy bones is important for children and adolescents. Along with having a healthy diet that includes adequate calcium and vitamin D, physical activity is critical for bone development. Bone-strengthening physical activity done three or more days a week increases bone-mineral content and bone density in youth.

Very high levels of physical activity, however, may have extra risks. People who participate in very high levels of physical activity, such as elite or professional athletes, have a higher risk of hip and knee osteoarthritis, mostly due to the risk of injury involved in competing in some sports.

Progressive muscle-strengthening activities increase or preserve muscle mass, strength, and power. Higher amounts (through greater frequency or higher weights) improve muscle function to a greater degree.

Reducing Cancer Risk

Physically active people have a significantly lower risk of colon cancer than do inactive people, and physically active women have a significantly lower risk of breast cancer. Research shows that a wide range of moderate-intensity physical activity—between 210 and 420 minutes a week (three hours and 30 minutes to seven hours)—is needed to significantly reduce the risk of colon and breast cancer; currently, 150 minutes a week does not appear to provide

Stress-Defeating Effects Of Exercise Traced To Emotional Brain Circuit

Evidence in both humans and animals points to emotional benefits from exercise, both physical and mental. Now, in recent experiments with mice, scientists have traced the stress-buffering effect of activity to a brain circuit known to be involved in emotional regulation as well as mood disorders and medication effects. The finding is a clue to understanding the neurological roots of resilience, key to developing new means of prevention and treatment for stress-related illness.

Background

In ongoing research, scientists at the National Institute of Mental Health (NIMH) have used a mouse model that mirrors particularly well the impact of social stress on mood in humans. Male mice are intensely aggressive when housed together; if these mice are placed in conditions that result in defeat by another mouse, they will behave in a way that mimics depression, much like a human might. Previous research demonstrated that mice housed in an environment with plenty of opportunities for exercise and exploration are relatively unfazed by bullying; they are resilient compared to mice housed in more Spartan surroundings. The benefits from activity and stimulation depend on the growth of new neurons in the brain in mice. A next step was to pinpoint where in the brain changes were taking place in response to exercise that resulted in stress resilience.

This Study

Before any mice were exposed to social defeat, all the mice in the study were housed for three weeks in either impoverished housing, with nothing but wood chip bedding; standard housing with a cardboard tube and place for a nest; or "enriched housing," with running wheels and tubes of various shapes and sizes to explore. After three weeks, half of the mice in each type of housing were then placed for two more weeks in close quarters with another mouse, but prevented from fighting by a barrier to prevent injury.

a major benefit. It also appears that greater amounts of physical activity lower risks of these cancers even further, although exactly how much lower is not clear.

Although not definitive, some research suggests that the risk of endometrial cancer in women and lung cancers in men and women also may be lower among those who are regularly active compared to those who are inactive.

Finally, cancer survivors have a better quality of life and improved physical fitness if they are physically active, compared to survivors who are inactive.

Mice that had been housed in the impoverished or standard housing, and that had been subject to social defeat, reacted to standard behavioral tests in a way that suggests depression; they were measurably passive and cautious, for example, avoiding light-filled spaces and preferring the safety of darkness. Bullied mice that had been housed in enriched environments behaved just like mice that had not experienced social defeat. As in earlier studies, the enriched environment seemed to protect them from the effects of social stress.

The NIMH investigators carrying out this study, Michael Lehmann and Miles Herkenham, then looked within the brain to see what exercise was changing to protect against stress. They focused on a functional circuit of brain centers known to be involved in emotional processing. In mice that had been housed in an enriched environment, levels of a protein that signals the activity level of neurons were increased in cells in the infralimbic cortex (ILC), a part of this circuit. Parts of the brain closely wired to and "downstream" from the ILC, that is, receiving activating signals from it, showed similar elevated activity. If the ILC was inactivated at the beginning of the experiment, environmental enrichment failed to have a positive effect. But if it was inactivated after the first three weeks of housing, environmental enrichment worked; the parts of the brain that receive signals from the ILC remained activated and the mice were stress resilient. The ILC was, in effect, a gateway for the positive activity in these "downstream" parts of the brain. Once these centers were activated by the ILC, it didn't matter if the ILC was still online.

Enrichment had the opposite effect on a part of the brain that is an important trigger for the body's stress response system. So enrichment seemed to enhance positive behavior, while at the same time, dampened activity in an area linked with an increased stress response.

Reference

Lehmann, M.I., and Herkenham, M. Environmental enrichment confers stress resiliency to social defeat through an infralimbic cortex-dependent neuroanatomical pathway. *Journal of Neuroscience* 31:6159-6173, 2011.

Source: Excerpted from "Stress-Defeating Effects of Exercise Traced to Emotional Brain Circuit," *Science Update*, National Institute of Mental Health, June 9, 2011.

Mental Health

Physically active adults have lower risk of depression and cognitive decline (declines in thinking, learning, and judgment skills). Physical activity also may improve the quality of sleep. Whether physical activity reduces distress or anxiety is currently unclear.

Mental health benefits have been found in people who do aerobic or a combination of aerobic and muscle-strengthening activities three to five days a week for 30 to 60 minutes at a time. Some research has shown that even lower levels of physical activity also may provide some benefits.

Regular physical activity appears to reduce symptoms of anxiety and depression for children and adolescents. Whether physical activity improves self-esteem is not clear.

Chapter 3

Meeting Your Muscles

Your Muscles

Did you know you have more than 600 muscles in your body? They do everything from pumping blood throughout your body to helping you lift your heavy backpack. You control some of your muscles, while others—like your heart—do their jobs without you thinking about them at all.

Muscles are all made of the same material, a type of elastic tissue (sort of like the material in a rubber band). Thousands, or even tens of thousands, of small fibers make up each muscle.

You have three different types of muscles in your body: smooth muscle, cardiac (say: kar-dee-ak) muscle, and skeletal (say: skel-uh-tul) muscle.

Smooth Muscles

Smooth muscles—sometimes also called involuntary muscles—are usually in sheets, or layers, with one layer of muscle behind the other. You can't control this type of muscle. Your brain and body tell these muscles what to do without you even thinking about it. You can't use your smooth muscles to make a muscle in your arm or jump into the air.

But smooth muscles are at work all over your body. In your stomach and digestive system, they contract (tighten up) and relax to allow food to make its journey through the body. Your

About This Chapter: "Your Muscles," August 2009, reprinted with permission from www.kidshealth.org. This information was provided by KidsHealth®, one of the largest resources online for medically reviewed health information written for parents, kids, and teens. For more articles like this, visit www.KidsHealth.org or www.TeensHealth.org. Copyright © 1995-2012 The Nemours Foundation. All rights reserved.

smooth muscles come in handy if you're sick and you need to throw up. The muscles push the food back out of the stomach so it comes up through the esophagus (say: ih-sah-fuh-gus) and out of the mouth.

Smooth muscles are also found in your bladder. When they're relaxed, they allow you to hold in urine (pee) until you can get to the bathroom. Then they contract so that you can push the urine out. These muscles are also in a woman's uterus, which is where a baby develops. There they help to push the baby out of the mother's body when it's time to be born.

You'll find smooth muscles at work behind the scenes in your eyes, too. These muscles keep the eyes focused.

A Hearty Muscle

The muscle that makes up the heart is called cardiac muscle. It is also known as the myo-cardium (say: my-uh-kar-dee-um). The thick muscles of the heart contract to pump blood out and then relax to let blood back in after it has circulated through the body.

Just like smooth muscle, cardiac muscle works all by itself with no help from you. A special group of cells within the heart are known as the pacemaker of the heart because it controls the heartbeat.

Skeletal Muscle

Now, let's talk about the kind of muscle you think of when we say "muscle"—the ones that show how strong you are and let you boot a soccer ball into the goal. These are your skeletal muscles—sometimes called striated (say: stry-ay-tud) muscle because the light and dark parts of the muscle fibers make them look striped (striated is a fancy word meaning striped).

Skeletal muscles are voluntary muscles, which means you can control what they do. Your leg won't bend to kick the soccer ball unless you want it to. These muscles help to make up the musculoskeletal (say: mus-kyuh-low-skel-uh-tul) system—the combination of your muscles and your skeleton, or bones.

Together, the skeletal muscles work with your bones to give your body power and strength. In most cases, a skeletal muscle is attached to one end of a bone. It stretches all the way across a joint (the place where two bones meet) and then attaches again to another bone.

Skeletal muscles are held to the bones with the help of tendons (say: ten-dunz). Tendons are cords made of tough tissue, and they work as special connector pieces between bone and muscle. The tendons are attached so well that when you contract one of your muscles, the tendon and bone move along with it.

Skeletal muscles come in many different sizes and shapes to allow them to do many types of jobs. Some of your biggest and most powerful muscles are in your back, near your spine. These muscles help keep you upright and standing tall.

They also give your body the power it needs to lift and push things. Muscles in your neck and the top part of your back aren't as large, but they are capable of some pretty amazing things: Try rotating your head around, back and forth, and up and down to feel the power of the muscles in your neck. These muscles also hold your head high.

Face Muscles

You may not think of it as a muscular body part, but your face has plenty of muscles. You can check them out next time you look in the mirror. Facial muscles don't all attach directly to bone like they do in the rest of the body. Instead, many of them attach under the skin. This allows you to contract your facial muscles just a tiny bit and make dozens of different kinds of faces. Even the smallest movement can turn a smile into a frown. You can raise your eyebrow to look surprised or wiggle your nose.

And while you're looking at your face, don't pass over your tongue—a muscle that's attached only at one end! Your tongue is actually made of a group of muscles that work together to allow you to talk and help you chew food. Stick out your tongue and wiggle it around to see those muscles at work.

Major Muscles

Because there are so many skeletal muscles in your body, we can't list them all here. But here are a few of the major ones:

In each of your shoulders is a deltoid (say: del-toyd) muscle. Your deltoid muscles help you move your shoulders every which way—from swinging a softball bat to shrugging your shoulders when you're not sure of an answer.

The pectoralis (say: pek-tuh-rah-lus) muscles are found on each side of your upper chest. These are usually called pectorals (say: pek-tuh-rulz), or pecs, for short. When many boys hit puberty, their pectoral muscles become larger. Many athletes and bodybuilders have large pecs, too.

Below these pectorals, down under your ribcage, are your rectus abdominus (say: rek-tus ab-dahm-uh-nus) muscles, or abdominals (say: ab-dahm-uh-nulz). They're often called abs for short.

When you make a muscle in your arm, you tense your biceps (say: bye-seps) muscle. When you contract your biceps muscle, you can actually see it push up under your skin.

Your quadriceps (say: kwad-ruh-seps), or quads, are the muscles on the front of your thighs. Many people who run, bike, or play sports develop large, strong quads.

And when it's time for you to take a seat? You'll be sitting on your gluteus maximus (say: gloot-ee-us mak-suh-mus), the muscle that's under the skin and fat in your behind!

To Strengthen Your Muscles

Muscle-strengthening activities involve having muscles work or hold against a force or some weight. Activities like push-ups, sit-ups, lunges, squats, lifting weights, and working with resistance bands do this—and so do a good game of tug-of-war, gymnastics, swinging on the monkey bars, and climbing a tree!

Source: Excerpted from "Get Motivated: Strengthening Muscles and Bones," reprinted with permission from www .presidentschallege.org. © 2012 The President's Challenge.

Chapter 4

Bone Health

Vital at every age for healthy bones, exercise is important for treating and preventing osteoporosis. Not only does exercise improve your bone health, it also increases muscle strength, coordination, and balance, and it leads to better overall health.

Why Exercise?

Like muscle, bone is living tissue that responds to exercise by becoming stronger. Young women and men who exercise regularly generally achieve greater peak bone mass (maximum bone density and strength) than those who do not. For most people, bone mass peaks during the third decade of life. After that time, people can begin to lose bone. Exercising allows them to maintain muscle strength, coordination, and balance, which in turn helps to prevent falls and related fractures.

The Best Bone Building Exercise

The best exercise for your bones is the weight-bearing kind, which forces you to work against gravity. Some examples of weight-bearing exercises include weight training, walking, hiking, jogging, climbing stairs, tennis, and dancing. Examples of exercises that are not weight-bearing include swimming and bicycling. Although these activities help build and maintain strong muscles and have excellent cardiovascular benefits, they are not the best way to exercise your bones.

About This Chapter: From "Exercise for Your Bone Health," National Institute of Arthritis and Musculoskeletal and Skin Diseases (www.niams.nih.gov), January 2009.

Exercise Tips

If you have health problems—such as heart trouble, high blood pressure, diabetes, or obesity—check with your doctor before you begin a regular exercise program.

Listen to your body. When starting an exercise routine, you may have some muscle soreness and discomfort at the beginning, but this should not be painful or last more than 48 hours. If it does, you may be working too hard and need to ease up. Stop exercising if you have any chest pain or discomfort, and see your doctor before your next exercise session.

If you have osteoporosis, ask your doctor which activities are safe for you. If you have low bone mass, experts recommend that you protect your spine by avoiding exercises or activities that flex, bend, or twist it. Furthermore, you should avoid high-impact exercise to lower the risk of breaking a bone. You also might want to consult with an exercise specialist to learn the

Exercise Is Medicine

Once thought of as a disease of "little old ladies," osteoporosis is now considered by many researchers as a pediatric disorder that manifests itself in old age. Peak bone mass and strength, which girls achieve in their 20s, predicts future fracture risk. In other words, the greater the bone mass and strength at the time girls reach their peak, the lower their chance of sustaining an osteoporotic fracture as they grow older. Research has also shown that the rate at which we accrue bone mineral is highest during late childhood and early adolescence. This is why it is critical to promote bone-healthy behaviors in children and teens.

Studies comparing athletes from different sports have shown the highest bone mineral density values in athletes participating in sports associated with high impact forces, such as in gymnastics, volleyball, and basketball, and in sports that require variable loads, or odd-impact loads to the skeleton, such as in soccer, tennis, and European handball. In addition to impact loading from jumping and sprinting activities, bone also adapts favorably to high joint reaction forces from vigorous muscular contractions, such as in weightlifting or resistance training. These types of activities should be considered when planning exercise programs for children and teens.

In addition to the type of exercise to optimize bone mass and strength, several randomized, controlled exercise interventions have also provided insight into the frequency and duration of exercise needed to build bone in young girls. Although an exact exercise prescription for bone health is not known, knowledge gained from these intervention studies can help practitioners plan community exercise programs to promote bone health in children and teens.

Several elementary school-based programs in which jumping and running games were added to physical education classes for approximately 10–30 minutes three days per week during the proper progression of activity, how to stretch and strengthen muscles safely, and how to correct poor posture habits. An exercise specialist should have a degree in exercise physiology, physical education, physical therapy, or a similar specialty. Be sure to ask if he or she is familiar with the special needs of people with osteoporosis.

A Complete Osteoporosis Program

Remember, exercise is only one part of an osteoporosis prevention program. Like a diet rich in calcium and vitamin D, exercise helps strengthen bones at any age. But proper exercise and diet may not be enough to stop bone loss caused by medical conditions or lifestyle choices such as tobacco use and excessive alcohol consumption. It is important to speak with your doctor about your bone health.

school year have shown significantly greater gains in bone mineral at the hip and lumbar spine in pre- and early pubescent girls compared to girls who participated in regular P.E. activities.[1–3] From these studies we can conclude that brief sessions of vigorous impact exercise three days per week can promote bone health throughout the developmental years. Young girls need to learn and practice these bone-healthy behaviors to optimize their bone mass and strength in adulthood and decrease their risk of osteoporosis in old age.

Additional information on bone health:

- ACSM's Position Stand on Physical Activity and Bone Health: http://journals.lww.com/acsm-msse/Fulltext/2004/11000/Physical_Activity_and_Bone_Health.24.aspx
- National Osteoporosis Foundation: http://www.nof.org/prevention/exercise.htm

1. Fuchs, R. K., J. J. Bauer, and C. M. Snow. Jumping improves hip and lumbar spine bone mass in prepubescent children: a randomized controlled trial. *J Bone Miner Res*. 16:148–156, 2001.
2. MacKelvie, K. J., K. M. Khan, M. A. Petit, P. A. Janssen, and H. A. McKay. A school-based exercise intervention elicits substantial bone health benefits: a 2-year randomized controlled trial in girls. *Pediatrics*. 112:e447, 2003.
3. McKay, H. A., M. A. Petit, R. W. Schutz, J. C. Prior, S. I. Barr, and K. M. Khan. Augmented trochanteric bone mineral density after modified physical education classes: a randomized school-based exercise intervention study in prepubescent and early pubescent children. *J Pediatr*. 136:156–162, 2000.

Source: "'Exercise is Medicine' for Building Strong Bones in Adolescent Girls," by Jeanne Nichols, Ph.D., FACSM, October 4, 2011. © 2011 American College of Sports Medicine. Reprinted with permission. For additional information, visit www.acsm.org.

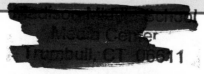

Strengthening Bones

Bone-strengthening activities make bones grow and get stronger through an impact (often with the ground) or tension force that promotes bone growth and strength. Activities like running, brisk walking, tennis, basketball, and volleyball are great for your bones, as are hopping, skipping, and jumping. Many bone-strengthening activities may also help strengthen your muscles.

You don't need to join a gym to get your bones and muscles stronger. Planned exercises (using weights, bands, or your body weight) and activities such as heavy gardening—with all that digging and shoveling—work, too.

Try and choose activities and exercises that work the major muscle groups of your body—legs, hips, back, chest, stomach, shoulders, and arms. Exercises for each muscle should be repeated 8 to 12 times per session. As with all exercise, if you haven't been active in a while, start slowly and build up.

Source: Excerpted from "Strengthening Muscles and Bones," reprinted with permission from www.presidentschallege .org. © 2012 The President's Challenge.

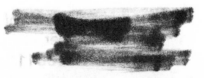

Chapter 5

Your Heart and Lungs

What Is The Heart?

Your heart is a muscular organ that pumps blood to your body. Your heart is at the center of your circulatory system. This system consists of a network of blood vessels, such as arteries, veins, and capillaries. These blood vessels carry blood to and from all areas of your body.

An electrical system controls your heart and uses electrical signals to contract the heart's walls. When the walls contract, blood is pumped into your circulatory system. Inlet and outlet valves in your heart chambers ensure that blood flows in the right direction.

Your heart is vital to your health and nearly everything that goes on in your body. Without the heart's pumping action, blood can't move throughout your body.

Your blood carries the oxygen and nutrients that your organs need to work well. Blood also carries carbon dioxide (a waste product) to your lungs so you can breathe it out.

A healthy heart supplies your body with the right amount of blood at the rate needed to work well. If disease or injury weakens your heart, your body's organs won't receive enough blood to work normally.

Anatomy Of The Heart

Your heart is located under your ribcage in the center of your chest between your right and left lungs. Its muscular walls beat, or contract, pumping blood to all parts of your body.

About This Chapter: Information in this chapter is reprinted from "What Is the Heart," November 2011, and "What Are the Lungs," June 2006, both from the National Heart Lung and Blood Institute (www.nhlbi.nih.gov). Images are reprinted with permission from *The Inner Man*, © 2008 Leonard Dank.

The size of your heart can vary depending on your age, size, and the condition of your heart. A normal, healthy, adult heart usually is the size of an average clenched adult fist. Some diseases can cause the heart to enlarge.

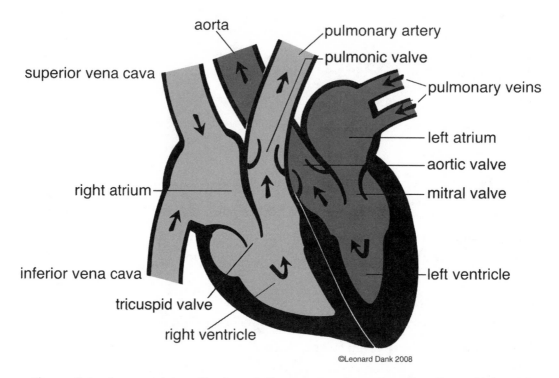

©Leonard Dank 2008

Figure 5.1. A normal, healthy heart. The arrows show the direction of blood flow. (Source: © 2008 Leonard Dank)

Figure 5.1 illustrates a normal, healthy, human heart and the pathway of blood through the heart. The heart is the muscle. It has four chambers. The heart's upper chambers are the right and left atria. The heart's lower chambers are the right and left ventricles. Some of the main blood vessels (arteries and veins) that make up your circulatory system are directly connected to the heart.

The superior vena cava and inferior vena cava (the plural form of the word cava is *cavae*) are on to the left of the heart muscle as you look at the picture. These veins are the largest veins in your body. After your body's organs and tissues have used the oxygen in your blood, the vena cavae carry the oxygen-poor blood back to the right atrium of your heart. The superior vena cava carries oxygen-poor blood from the upper parts of your body, including your head, chest, arms, and neck. The inferior vena cava carries oxygen-poor blood from the lower parts of your body.

The oxygen-poor blood from the vena cavae flows into your heart's right atrium and then to the right ventricle. From the right ventricle, the blood is pumped through the pulmonary arteries (in the center of the figure) to your lungs.

Once in the lungs, the blood travels through many small, thin blood vessels called capillaries. There, the blood picks up more oxygen and transfers carbon dioxide to the lungs—a process called gas exchange.

Oxygen-rich blood from your lungs passes through the pulmonary veins (shown to the right of the left atrium in Figure 5.1). The blood enters the left atrium and is pumped into the left ventricle. From the left ventricle, the oxygen-rich blood is pumped to the rest of your body through the aorta. The aorta is the main artery that carries oxygen-rich blood to your body.

Like all of your organs, your heart needs oxygen-rich blood. As blood is pumped out of your heart's left ventricle, some of it flows into the coronary arteries. Your coronary arteries are located on your heart's surface at the beginning of the aorta. They carry oxygen-rich blood to all parts of your heart.

Other Components Of Your Heart

The Septum: An internal wall of tissue divides the right and left sides of your heart. This wall is called the septum. The area of the septum that divides the atria is called the atrial or interatrial septum. The area of the septum that divides the ventricles is called the ventricular or interventricular septum.

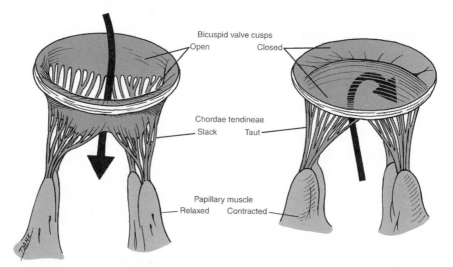

Figure 5.2. Heart valve action (mitral). (Source: © 2008 Leonard Dank)

Heart Valves: Your heart has four kinds of valves to regulate blood flow. They are the aortic valve, the tricuspid valve, the pulmonary valve, and the mitral valve.

For the heart to work well, your blood must flow in only one direction. Your heart's valves make this possible. Both of your heart's ventricles have an "in" (inlet) valve from the atria and an "out" (outlet) valve leading to your arteries.

Healthy valves open and close in exact coordination with the pumping action of your heart's atria and ventricles. Each valve has a set of flaps called leaflets or cusps that seal or open the valve. This allows blood to pass through the chambers and into your arteries without backing up or flowing backward. Figure 5.2 shows how heart valve action works.

Heart Contraction And Blood Flow

Heartbeat

Almost everyone has heard the real or recorded sound of a heartbeat. When your heart beats, it makes a "lub-DUB" sound. Between the time you hear "lub" and "DUB," blood is pumped through your heart and circulatory system.

A heartbeat may seem like a simple, repeated event. However, it's a complex series of very precise and coordinated events. These events take place inside and around your heart.

Each side of your heart uses an inlet valve to help move blood between the atrium and ventricle. The tricuspid valve does this between the right atrium and ventricle. The mitral valve does this between the left atrium and ventricle. The "lub" is the sound of the tricuspid and mitral valves closing.

Each of your heart's ventricles also has an outlet valve. The right ventricle uses the pulmonary valve to help move blood into the pulmonary arteries. The left ventricle uses the aortic valve to do the same for the aorta. The "DUB" is the sound of the aortic and pulmonary valves closing.

Each heartbeat has two basic parts: diastole and systole.

During diastole, the atria and ventricles of your heart relax and begin to fill with blood. At the end of diastole, your heart's atria contract (atrial systole) and pump blood into the ventricles.

The atria then begin to relax. Next, your heart's ventricles contract (ventricular systole) and pump blood out of your heart.

Pumping Action

Your heart uses its four valves to ensure your blood flows in only one direction. Healthy valves open and close in coordination with the pumping action of your heart's atria and ventricles.

Each valve has a set of flaps called leaflets or cusps that seal or open the valve. The cusps allow pumped blood to pass through the chambers and into your blood vessels without backing up or flowing backward.

Oxygen-poor blood from the vena cavae fills your heart's right atrium. The atrium contracts (atrial systole). The tricuspid valve located between the right atrium and ventricle opens for a short time and then shuts. This allows blood to enter the right ventricle without flowing back into the right atrium.

When your heart's right ventricle fills with blood, it contracts (ventricular systole). The pulmonary valve located between your right ventricle and pulmonary artery opens and closes quickly.

This allows blood to enter into your pulmonary arteries without flowing back into the right ventricle. This is important because the right ventricle begins to refill with more blood through the tricuspid valve. Blood travels through the pulmonary arteries to your lungs to pick up oxygen.

Oxygen-rich blood returns from the lungs to your heart's left atrium through the pulmonary veins. As your heart's left atrium fills with blood, it contracts. This event is called atrial systole.

The mitral valve located between the left atrium and left ventricle opens and closes quickly. This allows blood to pass from the left atrium into the left ventricle without flowing backward.

As the left ventricle fills with blood, it contracts. This event is called ventricular systole. The aortic valve located between the left ventricle and aorta opens and closes quickly. This allows blood to flow into the aorta. The aorta is the main artery that carries blood from your heart to the rest of your body.

The aortic valve closes quickly to prevent blood from flowing back into the left ventricle, which already is filling up with new blood.

Taking Your Pulse

When your heart pumps blood through your arteries, it creates a pulse that you can feel on the arteries close to the skin's surface. For example, you can feel the pulse on the artery inside of your wrist, below your thumb.

You can count how many times your heart beats by taking your pulse. You will need a watch with a second hand.

To find your pulse, gently place your index and middle fingers on the artery located on the inner wrist of either arm, below your thumb. You should feel a pulsing or tapping against your fingers.

Watch the second hand and count the number of pulses you feel in 30 seconds. Double that number to find out your heart rate or pulse for one minute.

The usual resting pulse for an adult is 60 to 100 beats per minute. To find your resting pulse, count your pulse after you have been sitting or resting quietly for at least 10 minutes.

Circulation And Blood Vessels

Your heart and blood vessels make up your overall blood circulatory system. Your blood circulatory system is made up of four subsystems.

Arterial Circulation

Arterial circulation is the part of your circulatory system that involves arteries, like the aorta and pulmonary arteries. Arteries are blood vessels that carry blood away from your heart. (The exception is the coronary arteries, which supply your heart muscle with oxygen-rich blood.)

Healthy arteries are strong and elastic (stretchy). They become narrow between heartbeats, and they help keep your blood pressure consistent. This helps blood move through your body.

Arteries branch into smaller blood vessels called arterioles. Arteries and arterioles have strong, flexible walls that allow them to adjust the amount and rate of blood flowing to parts of your body.

Venous Circulation

Venous circulation is the part of your circulatory system that involves veins, like the vena cavae and pulmonary veins. Veins are blood vessels that carry blood to your heart.

Veins have thinner walls than arteries. Veins can widen as the amount of blood passing through them increases.

Capillary Circulation

Capillary circulation is the part of your circulatory system where oxygen, nutrients, and waste pass between your blood and parts of your body.

Capillaries are very small blood vessels. They connect the arterial and venous circulatory subsystems.

The importance of capillaries lies in their very thin walls. Oxygen and nutrients in your blood can pass through the walls of the capillaries to the parts of your body that need them to work normally.

Capillaries' thin walls also allow waste products like carbon dioxide to pass from your body's organs and tissues into the blood, where it's taken away to your lungs.

Pulmonary Circulation

Pulmonary circulation is the movement of blood from the heart to the lungs and back to the heart again. Pulmonary circulation includes both arterial and venous circulation.

Oxygen-poor blood is pumped to the lungs from the heart (arterial circulation). Oxygen-rich blood moves from the lungs to the heart through the pulmonary veins (venous circulation).

Pulmonary circulation also includes capillary circulation. Oxygen you breathe in from the air passes through your lungs into your blood through the many capillaries in the lungs. Oxygen-rich blood moves through your pulmonary veins to the left side of your heart and out of the aorta to the rest of your body.

Capillaries in the lungs also remove carbon dioxide from your blood so that your lungs can breathe the carbon dioxide out into the air.

Your Heart's Electrical System

Your heart's electrical system controls all the events that occur when your heart pumps blood. The electrical system also is called the cardiac conduction system. If you've ever seen the heart test called an EKG (electrocardiogram), you've seen a graphical picture of the heart's electrical activity.

Your heart's electrical system is made up of three main parts:

- The sinoatrial (SA) node, located in the right atrium of your heart
- The atrioventricular (AV) node, located on the interatrial septum close to the tricuspid valve
- The His-Purkinje system, located along the walls of your heart's ventricles

A heartbeat is a complex series of events. These events take place inside and around your heart. A heartbeat is a single cycle in which your heart's chambers relax and contract to pump blood. This cycle includes the opening and closing of the inlet and outlet valves of the right and left ventricles of your heart.

Each heartbeat has two basic parts: diastole and systole. During diastole, the atria and ventricles of your heart relax and begin to fill with blood.

At the end of diastole, your heart's atria contract (atrial systole) and pump blood into the ventricles. The atria then begin to relax. Your heart's ventricles then contract (ventricular systole), pumping blood out of your heart.

Each beat of your heart is set in motion by an electrical signal from within your heart muscle. In a normal, healthy heart, each beat begins with a signal from the SA node. This is why the SA node sometimes is called your heart's natural pacemaker. Your pulse, or heart rate, is the number of signals the SA node produces per minute.

The signal is generated as the vena cavae fill your heart's right atrium with blood from other parts of your body. The signal spreads across the cells of your heart's right and left atria.

This signal causes the atria to contract. This action pushes blood through the open valves from the atria into both ventricles.

The signal arrives at the AV node near the ventricles. It slows for an instant to allow your heart's right and left ventricles to fill with blood. The signal is released and moves along a pathway called the bundle of His, which is located in the walls of your heart's ventricles.

From the bundle of His, the signal fibers divide into left and right bundle branches through the Purkinje fibers. These fibers connect directly to the cells in the walls of your heart's left and right ventricles.

The signal spreads across the cells of your ventricle walls, and both ventricles contract. However, this doesn't happen at exactly the same moment.

The left ventricle contracts an instant before the right ventricle. This pushes blood through the pulmonary valve (for the right ventricle) to your lungs, and through the aortic valve (for the left ventricle) to the rest of your body.

As the signal passes, the walls of the ventricles relax and await the next signal.

This process continues over and over as the atria refill with blood and more electrical signals come from the SA node.

Heart Disease

Your heart is made up of many parts working together to pump blood. In a healthy heart, all the parts work well so that your heart pumps blood normally. As a result, all parts of your body that depend on the heart to deliver blood also stay healthy.

Heart disease can disrupt a heart's normal electrical system and pumping functions. Diseases and conditions of the heart's muscle make it hard for your heart to properly pump blood.

Damaged or diseased blood vessels make the heart work harder than normal. Problems with the heart's electrical system, called arrhythmias, can make it hard for the heart to pump blood efficiently.

What Are The Lungs?

Your lungs are organs in your chest that allow your body to take in oxygen from the air. They also help remove carbon dioxide (a waste gas that can be toxic) from your body. The lungs' intake of oxygen and removal of carbon dioxide is called gas exchange. Gas exchange is part of breathing. Breathing is a vital function of life; it helps your body work properly. Other organs and tissues also help make breathing possible.

The Respiratory System

The respiratory system is a group of organs and tissues that help you breathe. The main parts of this system are the airways, the lungs and linked blood vessels, and the muscles that enable breathing.

Airways

The airways are pipes that carry oxygen-rich air to your lungs and carbon dioxide, a waste gas, out of your lungs. The airways include these components:

- Nose and linked air passages (called nasal cavities)
- Mouth
- Larynx, or voice box
- Trachea, or windpipe
- Tubes called bronchial tubes or bronchi, and their branches

Air first enters your body through your nose or mouth, which wets and warms the air. (Cold, dry air can irritate your lungs.) The air then travels through your voice box and down your windpipe. The windpipe splits into two bronchial tubes that enter your lungs.

A thin flap of tissue called the epiglottis covers your windpipe when you swallow. This prevents food or drink from entering the air passages that lead to your lungs.

Except for the mouth and some parts of the nose, all of the airways have special hairs called cilia that are coated with sticky mucus. The cilia trap germs and other foreign particles that enter your airways when you breathe in air.

These fine hairs then sweep the particles up to the nose or mouth. From there, they're swallowed, coughed, or sneezed out of the body. Nose hairs and mouth saliva also trap particles and germs.

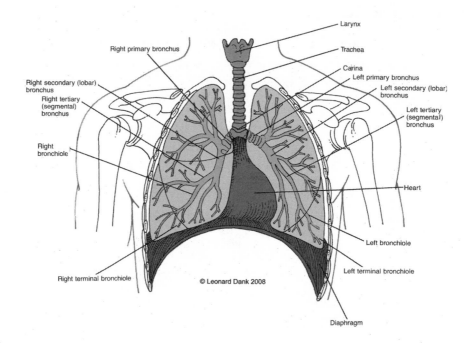

Figure 5.3. The Bronchial Tree. (Source: © 2008 Leonard Dank)

Lungs And Blood Vessels

Your lungs and linked blood vessels deliver oxygen to your body and remove carbon dioxide from your body. Your lungs lie on either side of your breastbone and fill the inside of your chest cavity. Your left lung is slightly smaller than your right lung to allow room for your heart.

Within the lungs, your bronchi branch into thousands of smaller, thinner tubes called bronchioles. These tubes end in bunches of tiny round air sacs called alveoli.

Each of these air sacs is covered in a mesh of tiny blood vessels called capillaries. The capillaries connect to a network of arteries and veins that move blood through your body.

The pulmonary artery and its branches deliver blood rich in carbon dioxide (and lacking in oxygen) to the capillaries that surround the air sacs. Inside the air sacs, carbon dioxide moves from the blood into the air. At the same time, oxygen moves from the air into the blood in the capillaries.

The oxygen-rich blood then travels to the heart through the pulmonary vein and its branches. The heart pumps the oxygen-rich blood out to the body.

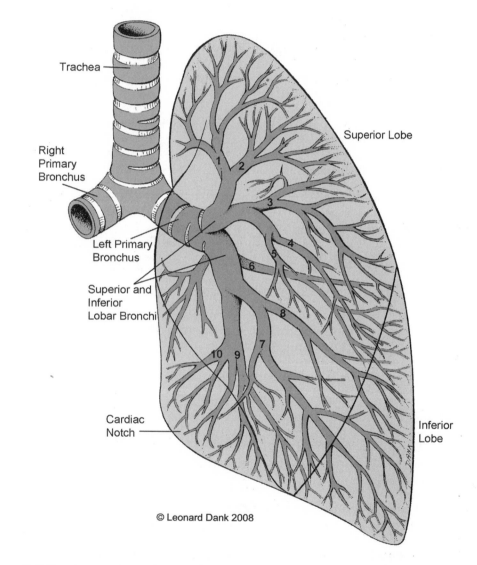

© Leonard Dank 2008

Figure 5.4. The Lungs, Bronchopulmonary Segments. (Source: © 2008 Leonard Dank)

The lungs are divided into five main sections called lobes. Some people need to have a diseased lung lobe removed. However, they can still breathe well using the rest of their lung lobes.

Muscles Used For Breathing

Muscles near the lungs help expand and contract (tighten) the lungs to allow breathing. These muscles include the diaphragm, intercostal muscles, abdominal muscles, and muscles in the neck and collarbone area.

The diaphragm is a dome-shaped muscle located below your lungs. It separates the chest cavity from the abdominal cavity. The diaphragm is the main muscle used for breathing.

The intercostal muscles are located between your ribs. They also play a major role in helping you breathe.

Beneath your diaphragm are abdominal muscles. They help you breathe out when you're breathing fast (for example, during physical activity).

Muscles in your neck and collarbone area help you breathe in when other muscles involved in breathing don't work well, or when lung disease impairs your breathing.

What Happens When You Breathe?

Breathing In (Inhalation)

When you breathe in, or inhale, your diaphragm contracts (tightens) and moves downward. This increases the space in your chest cavity, into which your lungs expand. The intercostal muscles between your ribs also help enlarge the chest cavity. They contract to pull your rib cage both upward and outward when you inhale.

As your lungs expand, air is sucked in through your nose or mouth. The air travels down your windpipe and into your lungs. After passing through your bronchial tubes, the air finally reaches and enters the alveoli (air sacs).

Through the very thin walls of the alveoli, oxygen from the air passes to the surrounding capillaries (blood vessels). A red blood cell protein called hemoglobin helps move oxygen from the air sacs to the blood.

At the same time, carbon dioxide moves from the capillaries into the air sacs. The gas has traveled in the bloodstream from the right side of the heart through the pulmonary artery.

Oxygen-rich blood from the lungs is carried through a network of capillaries to the pulmonary vein. This vein delivers the oxygen-rich blood to the left side of the heart. The left side of the heart pumps the blood to the rest of the body. There, the oxygen in the blood moves from blood vessels into surrounding tissues.

Breathing Out (Exhalation)

When you breathe out, or exhale, your diaphragm relaxes and moves upward into the chest cavity. The intercostal muscles between the ribs also relax to reduce the space in the chest cavity.

As the space in the chest cavity gets smaller, air rich in carbon dioxide is forced out of your lungs and windpipe, and then out of your nose or mouth.

Breathing out requires no effort from your body unless you have a lung disease or are doing physical activity. When you're physically active, your abdominal muscles contract and push your diaphragm against your lungs even more than usual. This rapidly pushes out the air in your lungs.

What Controls Your Breathing?

A respiratory control center at the base of your brain controls your breathing. This center sends ongoing signals down your spine and to the nerves of the muscles involved in breathing.

These signals ensure your breathing muscles contract (tighten) and relax regularly. This allows your breathing to happen automatically, without you being aware of it.

To a limited degree, you can change your breathing rate, such as by breathing faster or holding your breath. Your emotions also can change your breathing. For example, being scared or angry can affect your breathing pattern.

Your breathing will change depending on how active you are and the condition of the air around you. For example, you need to breathe more often when you do physical activity. In contrast, your body needs to restrict how much air you breathe if the air contains irritants or toxins.

To adjust your breathing to changing needs, your body has many sensors in your brain, blood vessels, muscles, and lungs.

Sensors in the brain and in two major blood vessels (the carotid artery and the aorta) detect carbon dioxide or oxygen levels in your blood and change your breathing rate as needed.

Sensors in the airways detect lung irritants. The sensors can trigger sneezing or coughing. In people who have asthma, the sensors may cause the muscles around the airways in the lungs to contract. This makes the airways smaller.

Sensors in the alveoli (air sacs) detect a buildup of fluid in the lung tissues. These sensors are thought to trigger rapid, shallow breathing.

Sensors in your joints and muscles detect movement of your arms or legs. These sensors may play a role in increasing your breathing rate when you're physically active.

Lung Diseases And Conditions

Many steps are involved in breathing. If injury, disease, or other factors affect any of the steps, you may have trouble breathing.

For example, the fine hairs (cilia) that line your upper airways may not trap all of the germs you breathe in. These germs can cause an infection in your bronchial tubes (bronchitis) or deep in your lungs (pneumonia). These infections cause a buildup of mucus and/or fluid that narrows the airways and limits airflow in and out of your lungs.

If you have asthma, breathing in certain substances that you're sensitive to can trigger your airways to narrow. This makes it hard for air to flow in and out of your lungs.

Over a long period, breathing in cigarette smoke or air pollutants can damage the airways and the air sacs. This can lead to a condition called COPD (chronic obstructive pulmonary disease). COPD prevents proper airflow in and out of your lungs and can hinder gas exchange in the air sacs.

An important step to breathing is the movement of your diaphragm and other muscles in your chest, neck, and abdomen. This movement lets you inhale and exhale. Nerves that run from your brain to these muscles control their movement. Damage to these nerves in your upper spinal cord can cause breathing to stop, unless a machine is used to help you breathe. (This machine is called a ventilator or a respirator.)

A steady flow of blood in the small blood vessels that surround your air sacs is vital for gas exchange. Long periods of inactivity or surgery can cause a blood clot called a pulmonary embolism (PE) to block a lung artery. A PE can reduce or block the flow of blood in the small blood vessels and hinder gas exchange.

Chapter 6

Teen Nutrition

What Teens Need

A healthy, balanced diet for children and teens (and adults, too), includes a mix of different foods. Here's what a healthy eating plan looks like.

Fruits

- How much each day: 2 cups (4 portions)
- Tip: Choose whole fruits (fresh, frozen, or canned) more often than fruit juice.

Vegetables

- How much each day: 2½ cups (5 portions)
- Tip: Aim for a variety of vegetables each week, including dark green vegetables (like spinach and broccoli), orange vegetables (like carrots), dry beans (such as lentils, white beans, and kidney beans), starchy vegetables (such as corn and sweet potatoes), and other vegetables.

Milk And Milk Products

- How much each day: 3 cups (3 portions) for children 9 years of age and older and adults (one portion = 1½ ounces of natural cheese or 2 ounces processed cheese)
- Tip: Milk and milk products include fat-free or low-fat milk, low-fat yogurt, and low-fat cheeses.

About This Chapter: Excerpted from *BodyWorks: A Toolkit for Healthy Teens and Strong Families*, Office on Women's Health (www.womenshealth.gov), 2006. Revised by David A. Cooke, MD, FACP, May 2012.

Whole Grains

- How much each day: 6 ounces total grains; whole grains: 3 ounces or more (at least half of total grains)

- Tip: Examples of whole grains include whole wheat, brown rice, oats/oatmeal, whole rye, corn, whole-grain barley, and popcorn. Remember: The whole grain should be first on the ingredients list. Wheat flour, enriched flour, and degerminated cornmeal are not whole grains.

Meat And Beans

- How much each day: 5½ ounces (2 portions)

- Tip: Try different types of foods. Examples include lean meats, poultry, and fish (grilled, baked, broiled), nuts, eggs, beans, peanut butter, and peas.

Fats, Salts, Sugars

- Tip: Read the Nutrition Facts labels to find foods low in saturated fats, trans fats, cholesterol, and sugars.

Serving Sizes

A *serving* is a unit of measure used to describe the amount of food recommended from each food group. You can check the servings on the Nutrition Facts labels found on packaged foods. A recommended serving for whole grains, for example, would be one slice of bread or one-half cup of bread or pasta.

The term *portion size* is also a common term, but it has a different meaning. Portion size refers to the amount of a specific food you choose to eat for a meal or snack.

Identifying Portion Sizes

- Fruit: 1 medium fruit is about the size of a baseball.

- Vegetables: ½ cup is about the size of a small computer mouse.

- Cheese (low-fat or fat-free): 1½ ounces is about the size of six dice.

- Pasta (cooked): ½ cup is about the size of a small computer mouse.

- Fish or lean meat: 2–3 ounces is about the size of a deck of cards.

Supersized Foods

You may be overeating without even knowing it. A recent study found that serving sizes of foods and beverages you often buy in restaurants and grocery stores have gotten a lot bigger. So much bigger, in fact, that you may be taking in far more calories than you realize. The following are just a few examples:

- The size of an average soft drink increased from 13 ounces to 20 ounces (144 calories to 193 calories).

- The average cheeseburger was once 5.8 ounces at 397 calories but is now 7.3 ounces at 533 calories.

- Salty snacks were once 1 ounce but are now about 1.6 ounces, resulting in an increase from 132 to 225 calories.

- A typical serving of French fries increased by a half ounce and 68 calories.

Using Nutrition Facts Labels

You can find important information about nutrition on the Nutrition Facts label.

Serving Size: Look at the serving size. In the case of the example shown in Figure 6.1, a serving is 1 cup.

Servings Per Container: In the example, there are two servings in the container. If you eat the entire container you have eaten two servings, and you double the calories and nutrients you have consumed.

Calories: The amount of calories and nutrients listed is the amount in one serving (not the amount in the container). Decide if this food is worth eating based on the number of calories and the amount of nutrients you are getting. More than 400 calories per serving is high for a single food item.

Fat, Cholesterol, Sodium: Limit your intake of total fat, saturated fat, trans fat, cholesterol, and sodium to help reduce the risk of heart disease.

Percent Daily Value (% DV): The %DV tells you if a serving of food is high or low in a nutrient. Keep nutrients like saturated fat, cholesterol, and sodium low. Aim for 100% DV of dietary fiber, vitamins A and C, calcium, and iron. Remember, 5% DV or less is low; 20% or more is high.

Grams Of Sugar: Read the ingredient list to make sure that sugars added to foods or drinks during processing or preparation are not one of the first few ingredients. Examples include brown sugar, corn sweetener, high fructose corn syrup, dextrose, fructose, fruit juice concentrates, maltose, dextrose, sucrose, honey, and maple syrup.

The Special Importance Of Nutrition For Teens

Adolescence is a time of major growth and development. That is why good nutrition is more important than ever. The following is a list of the major nutrients adolescents need to be healthy and strong.

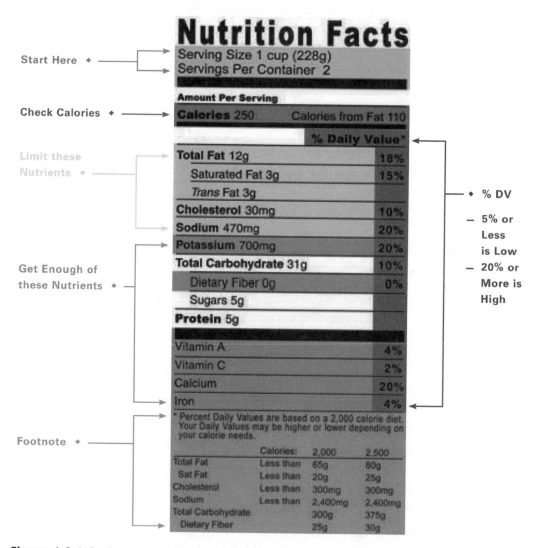

Figure 6.1. What you need to know about the Nutrition Facts label.

Vitamin A

- Benefits: Good vision, healthy skin and hair, helps you grow
- Some Food Sources: Fortified cereals (cereals that have vitamin A added to them), cantaloupe, green vegetables (like spinach), carrots, sweet potatoes, and pumpkin

Vitamin C

- Benefits: Healthy bones, gums, and teeth
- Some Food Sources: Strawberries, grapefruits, oranges, melons, mangos, tomatoes, broccoli, red sweet peppers, cauliflower, and sweet potatoes

Vitamin E

- Benefits: Protects body cells
- Some Food Sources: Nuts (such as almonds, hazelnuts, and peanuts) and vegetable oils

Calcium

- Benefits: Strong bones and teeth
- Some Food Sources: Low-fat or fat-free milk, yogurt, cheese, calcium-fortified cereals and juices, and calcium-fortified soymilk and tofu

Folate (also called folic acid)

- Benefits: Helps your body make red blood cells
- Some Food Sources: Cooked or dry beans, peas, peanuts, oranges, orange juice, dark-green leafy vegetables (like spinach), fortified cereals, and enriched grain products

Fiber

- Benefits: May help reduce risk for coronary heart disease and helps make you feel full and keep regular
- Some Food Sources: Beans, ready-to-eat bran cereals, sweet potatoes and baked potatoes with skin, and small fresh pears and apples with skin

Magnesium

- Benefits: Helps contract and relax muscles

- Some Food Sources: Ready-to-eat bran cereals, spinach, almonds, cashews, pine nuts, and halibut (a kind of fish)

Iron

- Benefits: Helps red blood cells carry oxygen to different parts of the body. This helps produce energy. Lack of iron in red blood cells (called anemia) can make you feel weak and tired.

- Some Food Sources: Beef, clams, oysters, shrimp, canned sardines, spinach

Potassium

- Benefits: Helps muscles work

- Some Food Sources: Baked white or sweet potatoes, cooked spinach, winter (orange) squash, bananas and plantains, many dried fruits, oranges and orange juice, cantaloupe, and honeydew melons

The Special Importance Of Calcium

Calcium is one of the most important nutrients for adolescents, especially girls. If they get enough calcium while they are young, they can strengthen their bones and reduce the risk of osteoporosis when they are older.

Good sources of calcium are low-fat or fat-free milk or other milk products like low-fat yogurt and cheese. The daily recommended amount for girls and boys nine years and older is 3 cups.

Foods With Calcium

Percent (%) daily value (DV) is listed on Nutrition Facts labels and tells you how much of the recommended amount of calcium a food has in one serving. Aim for foods and drinks with 20% or more DV for calcium. Foods with less than 5% DV for calcium provide only a small amount of the calcium needed each day.

- Plain yogurt, low-fat or fat-free; one serving = 1 cup; 45% Daily Value

- American cheese, low-fat or fat-free; one serving = 2 ounces; 35% Daily Value

- Ricotta cheese, part skim; one serving = ½ cup; 34% Daily Value

- Fruit yogurt, low-fat or fat-free; one serving = 1 cup; 31% Daily Value

- Milk, fat-free (skim) or low-fat (1%); one serving = 1 cup; 30% Daily Value

- Orange juice with added calcium; one serving = 1 cup; 30% Daily Value

- Cheddar cheese, low-fat; one serving = 1 ounce; 20% Daily Value

- White beans (boiled); one serving = 1 cup; 16% Daily Value

- Calcium-fortified cereal; one serving = 1 cup; 9% Daily Value

Calcium And Lactose Intolerance

For some people, drinking milk or eating dairy products leads to abdominal discomfort. This condition, known as lactose intolerance, happens when a person has trouble digesting lactose, the sugar found in milk and dairy foods. Lactose intolerance is not common among infants and young children but can occur in older children, teens, and adults. It is also more common among people of African-American, Hispanic, Asian, and American Indian and Alaska Native descent.

Tolerance to milk is individual. If a person cannot tolerate drinking a glass of milk, here are some other options:

- Drinking milk in small amounts and combining it with other foods such as cereal

- Eating other dairy products such as cheeses and yogurt, which cause fewer symptoms

- Using lactose-free milk products

- Using pills and drops that make it easier to digest milk and other dairy products

Some people are allergic to milk and dairy products and should not eat them. In this case, they can eat nondairy foods that are rich in calcium such as sardines and collards or calcium-fortified foods such as orange juice, soy drinks, and some cereals. Taking calcium supplements is also an option, although getting calcium from foods is recommended.

Breakfast Boost

Breakfast jumpstarts the brain and keeps children and teens (as well as adults) alert throughout the morning. After 8 to 12 hours without food at night, the American Heart Association says, "The body is essentially a cold furnace, waiting to be stoked." Children, who have a smaller physical system than adults, are especially sensitive to long periods without eating. Yet, many kids don't eat any breakfast at all.

Why Teens Should Eat Breakfast

Kids do better in school and are more alert when they eat breakfast, and kids who eat breakfast get the nutrients they need to grow and develop.

- Kids are more creative and perform better, with increased attention span and memory.

- Students have more energy by late morning, with less fatigue, irritability, and restlessness.

- Students take fewer trips to the school nurse's office complaining of headaches and stomach aches due to hunger.

- Kids who eat breakfast miss fewer days and are late less often.

- Adolescents who eat breakfast are more likely to be at a healthy weight.

- They are more likely to get adequate amounts of minerals, such as calcium and some vitamins, such as A, C, B12, and folate.

What To Eat

Most families are pretty rushed in the morning. Teens may not feel that they have time to eat a nutritious breakfast and that they have to eat on the run. But breakfast does not have to be French toast, home-made blueberry pancakes, or scrambled eggs. Kids on the go can have breakfast if they keep a few things handy to grab as they rush out the door: fresh fruit, low-fat or fat-free yogurt, hard-cooked eggs, or breakfast bars. Here are some other ideas for easy, nutritious breakfasts:

- Low-sugar whole-grain cereal with fruit and low-fat or fat-free milk or yogurt

- Whole-grain cereal with a cup of low-fat or fat-free yogurt

- Frozen waffles topped with peanut butter

- Instant oatmeal with low-fat or fat-free milk and dried fruit

- A whole-wheat pita stuffed with sliced hard-cooked eggs

- Breakfast burrito of scrambled eggs and veggies in a warm tortilla

Some kids may prefer less traditional breakfasts:

- Smoothie made in blender from banana, cup of orange or pineapple juice, ½ cup fat-free milk, and 3 ice cubes

- Yogurt smoothie made from 8 oz. container of low-fat vanilla or fruit yogurt, a banana or cup of berries, fresh or frozen

- Low-fat cheese and salsa rolled up in a soft flour tortilla

- Baked apples with low-fat or fat-free yogurt or cottage cheese and cinnamon

- Pita bread with low-fat cheese, cooked lean meat and vegetables heated in the microwave

- Melted low-fat or fat-free cheese on a slice of whole grain toast
- Peanut butter and jelly on a slice of whole wheat bread

Be cautious about breakfast foods high in fat, sugar, and/or sodium (salt), including bacon, ham, sausage, croissants, biscuits, donuts, cinnamon buns, hash browns, and most fast-food breakfast sandwiches.

Lunch Lift

Eating lunch at school poses nutritional challenges for students of all ages. Typical school cafeteria menus feature high-fat, high-calorie foods such as burgers, chicken nuggets, french fries, cookies, and cakes. Lunch lines are often long, and some students have as little as 20 minutes to eat before their next class. So many adolescents grab chips and a soda from the vending machine instead of enjoying a healthy meal.

A growing teenager needs a lunch that provides one-third of the day's nutritional needs. Teens can learn make healthy choices (if their cafeteria offers a wide variety of foods) or pack a lunch that provides them with protein, whole grains, fruits and vegetables, and low-fat or fat-free milk.

Brown Bag Makeover

Easy suggestions for a nutritional makeover of your brown bag lunch:

1. Choose 1% or fat-free milk.
2. Use cheese on sandwiches that is low-fat or fat-free.
3. Switch from bologna, ham, salami, pastrami and other high-fat luncheon meats to low-fat alternatives like turkey.
4. Include at least one serving of fruit in every lunch.
5. Add vegetables to your diet by using ones, like lettuce or slices of cucumber, tomato, and green pepper on sandwiches.
6. Use whole grain bread instead of white bread for sandwiches.
7. Limit cookies, snacks cakes, donuts, brownies, and other baked goods.
8. Pack baked chips, pretzels, bread sticks, or low-fat crackers instead of potato chips or corn chips that are fried.
9. Don't pack prepared lunch kits that are high in fat and sugar.
10. Pack water or a low-calorie flavored water, rather than fruit drinks that contain only 10 percent juice.

Liquid Candy

Soda has replaced milk and water as the beverage of choice for many children and adolescents. In fact, the number of adolescents who drink soda has increased by 65 percent in recent years.

Adolescents are missing out on important nutrients like calcium, by drinking more soda and less milk. Girls are especially for risk broken bones and osteoporosis later in life if they do not get adequate calcium intake.

Soda is also high in sugar and calories. Treat soda as an occasional treat, not a regular part of your diet. Limit the amount of soda you drink at home and at school. This includes diet soda, which should not take the place of healthier beverages. Replace the soda you drink with low-fat or fat-free milk, water, or a low-calorie flavored water.

Munch-A-Lunch Kit

Kids often ask for prepackaged lunch kits. A typical kit may include three soft flour tacos, seasoned ground beef, a cheese product, taco sauce, a chocolate bar, and a fruit drink. The kits save busy people the chore of packing a lunch.

However, people pay a high price for these kits. Not only are they expensive—about $2 to $4 per kit—but they are loaded with fat and sugar. Many contain up to 500 calories each, and most of these are empty calories, lacking vitamins and other nutrients that provide the energy kids need to get through the afternoon at school.

In addition, the prepackaged lunches are often high in salt. For some people, too much sodium can be a factor in high blood pressure. Also, the drinks included in the kit are either sugary sodas or fruit drinks that are only 10 percent fruit juice. A healthier alternative is low-fat or fat-free milk, a bottle of water, or low-calorie flavored water.

Here are ideas for some healthy options for bag lunches:

- Lean sandwich meats, such as roast turkey, chicken breast, lean ham, or roast beef
- Whole wheat bread or whole wheat crackers
- Individually packaged dairy products, such as low fat yogurt or string cheese
- Cut up vegetables and pieces of fruit
- Granola or cereal bars, graham crackers, or fig bars

These five easy lunches can carry you through the entire school week:

- Monday: Peanut butter and banana on whole wheat bread; carrot sticks with apple sauce cup, oatmeal raisin cookies

- Tuesday: Turkey and cream cheese on tortilla; baked potato chips; pear; red pepper slices

- Wednesday: Fruit yogurt; string cheese; whole wheat crackers or breadsticks; carrot sticks with low-fat dip

- Thursday: Chicken slices on pita with lettuce, tomato, cucumber and low-fat mayo; fruit cup; pretzels; fig bars

- Friday: Pasta salad with tomatoes and cucumbers and Italian dressing; hardboiled egg; apple

Fat Facts

Fat is an important nutrient, just like protein and carbohydrates. It helps the body function in many ways, including contributing to growth and development, serving as an important energy source, and maintaining healthy skin and hair. However, some fats are better than others. Unsaturated fats found in many vegetable oils do not raise blood cholesterol. They can be part of a healthy diet —as long as you don't eat too much since it is still high in calories. Unsaturated fats are found in olive, canola, safflower, sunflower, corn, and soybean oils as well as in fish and nuts.

Saturated fats cause "bad" cholesterol levels in your blood and increase your risk for heart disease. They are a major risk for heart disease so it is best to limit foods with too much saturated fat. These fats are found in animal products such as butter, cheese, whole milk, and fatty meats and also in coconut, palm, and palm kernel oils. Saturated fats can also be found in cakes, cookies, quick breads, donuts, and chips.

Trans fats also raise "bad" cholesterol levels in your blood and increase the risk of heart disease. There is no safe amount of trans fat. The best approach is to eat foods with as little trans fat as possible. Trans fat is often found in baked goods, snack foods, vegetable shortening, hard margarine, fried foods, and many processed foods.

How To Handle Fats

Read the ingredients and nutrition labels.

- Amounts of saturated fat and dietary cholesterol already are listed on nutrition panels. Remember, 5% of the daily value (%DV) or less is low and 20% or more is high.

- Read the ingredients and look for words such as shortening, partially hydrogenated vegetable oil, or hydrogenated vegetable oil. These are clues that the food contains trans fat.

Make good choices.

- Stick to olive, canola, soybean, corn, and sunflower oils.
- Choose soft margarines (liquid, tub, or spray) over solid shortenings, hard margarines, and animal fats, including butter.
- Eat more foods like nuts and fish.

Don't be afraid to ask questions when you eat out.

- Ask what oils and fats were used to prepare foods.
- Don't be shy—ask for replacements and substitutions.

Fast Foods

On average, teenagers eat at fast-food restaurants twice each week. As a result, they are probably taking in a lot of extra calories and fat. Just one supersized fast food meal of a sandwich, fries, and soda can have more calories, fat, and added sugar than people need in an entire day.

The best approach is to limit the amount of fast food you eat. And when you do eat at fast food restaurants, choose the healthier options.

Fast-Food Guide

- Order garden or grilled chicken salads with low-fat or fat-free dressings.
- Choose grilled over fried foods.
- Remove breading from fried chicken, which can cut half the fat.
- Choose chicken over beef. Grilled chicken is the best option.
- Buy the smallest sandwich available.
- Substitute mustard or ketchup for mayonnaise.
- Order water, orange juice, or low-fat or fat-free milk instead of soda.
- Skip the "value" and "supersize" meals.

Healthy Choices At Some Popular Fast-Food Restaurants

McDonald's

- Chicken McGrill sandwich without mayo: 340 calories, 7 grams of fat

- Grilled chicken caesar salad without dressing: 100 calories, 3 grams of fat

- Fruit 'n yogurt parfait (5.3 ounces) without granola: 130 calories, 2 grams of fat; with granola: 160 calories, 2 grams of fat

Burger King

- BK Veggie burger without mayonnaise: 330 calories, 7 grams of fat

- Fire-grilled shrimp garden salad with fat-free honey mustard dressing: 225 calories, 10 grams of fat

- Chicken Whopper Sandwich without reduced fat mayonnaise: 405 calories, 4 grams of fat

Wendy's

- Mandarin chicken salad: 170 calories, 2 grams of fat

- Plain baked potato: 270 calories, 0 grams of fat

- Small chili: 220 calories, 6 grams of fat

Kentucky Fried Chicken

- Tender roast sandwich without sauce: 270 calories, 6 grams of fat

- Corn on the cob: 150 calories, 2 grams of fat

- Baked beans: 190 calories, 3 grams of fat

What's It Mean?

Trans Fats: Trans fat is made when hydrogen is added to vegetable oil—a process called hydrogenation. This process increases the shelf life and flavor stability of foods containing these fats. The government requires food manufacturers to list the amount of trans fat on nutrition labels, just like saturated fat and dietary cholesterol.

Taco Bell

- Bean burrito: 370 calories, 10 grams of fat

- Chicken soft taco: 190 calories, 10 grams of fat

- Steak or chicken Gordito: 270 calories, 11 grams of fat

Other Tips For Eating Out

- Check the menu first. Are there choices that are low in sugar, fat, and sodium (salt)?

- Ask a server to explain a dish if you are not sure what it contains.

- Don't be embarrassed to ask for changes or substitutions to make a dish healthier.

- Watch out for hidden fats, such as full fat salad dressings and sauces.

- Take home half of what you are served—most restaurant meals are actually more than one serving.

- Avoid buffets—you may be tempted to eat too much.

- Eat out less often.

What $10 Can Buy

Healthy food, and snacks in particular, do not have to be expensive. (Check out the two shopping lists below.) You don't need a nutritional analysis to tell you that the second list is far more healthful and will stretch farther for snacks, packed lunches, or ingredients for salads.

Typical Snack Foods Cost

- 1 large bag (20oz.) potato chips $4.19
- 1 bag, chocolate chip cookies $3.79
- 2 liter bottle, cola $1.49
- 1 chocolate candy bar $0.65
- Total cost: $9.52*

Healthier Snack Foods Cost

- 6 bananas $1.00
- 2 large bunches of grapes $1.59
- 4 red apples $1.49
- 8 large carrots $1.00
- 4 oranges $1.20
- 1 cucumber $0.60
- ½ gallon orange juice $2.00
- 1 gallon spring water $0.69
- Total cost: $9.57*

*Costs are based on prices at a national chain grocery store in the metropolitan Washington, DC area.

Home-Cooking Short Cuts For People On The Run

- Learn how to cook. Ask your parents if you can help prepare meals. Learn new recipes and help shop for ingredients. Cookbooks for children, preteens, and older adolescents include *Honest Pretzels* by Molly Katzen, *There's a Chef in My Soup! Recipes for the Kid in Everyone* by Emeril Lagasse, and *The Teen's Vegetarian Cookbook* by Judy Krizmanic.

- Plan weekly. Take an hour to work with your parents and plan your meals for the week and then help with the shopping. Use a shopping list.

- Keep basic ingredients on hand. Stock up on dry beans, tuna, rice, pasta, spaghetti sauce, and other fixings for a quick meal. Buying extra frozen fruits and vegetables is also a good idea.

- Use a crock pot or slow cooker to save time. All you have to do is fill it up and turn it on. When you get home in the evening, dinner is ready.

- Try cooking big batches of food in advance. Block out a few hours during the weekend or during the week to make a big batch of chili, soup, casserole, or pasta. Refrigerate or freeze, depending on how soon you plan to eat the food. When you're ready, all you have to do is heat and serve.

- Use the microwave. Cooking with a microwave can be a safe, easy way to make a meal. There are plenty of recipes for microwave cooking.

Chapter 7

Weighty Issues

What Is A Healthy Weight?

Most doctors use special growth charts to determine if a child is underweight, overweight, or within a healthy weight range.

First, a child's body mass index (BMI) is calculated by dividing his or her weight in kilograms by height in meters squared. The BMI measurement is then compared to other children who are of the same age and gender. The comparisons are expressed as percentiles. For example, for a 12-year-old girl who is in the 50th percentile, 50 percent of girls her age weigh more and 50 percent weigh less.

The following cut-off points are used to evaluate a child's weight:

- Underweight: less than the 5th percentile
- At risk of overweight: 85th percentile and above
- Overweight: greater than or equal to the 95th percentile

However, BMI measurements are not always accurate in determining children's body fat percentages since body composition changes at different rates and different times as kids grow. For example, boys are usually leaner during growth spurts, while girls gain body fat during puberty.

Puberty And Weight

Girls are growing physically and emotionally during adolescence. Before age 11 or 12, girls may get taller and heavier and have more fat around their hips, waist, and breasts. Boys experience

About This Chapter: Excerpted from *BodyWorks: A Toolkit for Healthy Teens and Strong Families*, Office on Women's Health (www.womenshealth.gov), 2006. Reviewed by David A. Cooke, MD, FACP, May 2012.

their growth spurt from 10 to 16 years of age. They will get taller, gain weight, have broader shoulders, and develop muscles. During this time, pre-teens may become sensitive about their appearance, particularly as they begin comparing themselves to peers and images in the media. They need to be reassured that some of this weight gain is a normal part of puberty.

For these reasons, a pediatrician or family doctor is the best person to determine if a child is overweight. If overweight is an issue, the goal will be to reduce the rate of body weight gain while allowing for normal growth and development. It is also important that parents let children know that they are accepted, no matter how much they weigh.

Weight Across Cultures

Overweight affects children and youth from all races and ethnicities. However, some ethnic and racial groups have higher rates among adolescents ages 12 to 19: 17.4 percent of white (non-Hispanic), 21.8 percent of black (non-Hispanic), 16.3 percent of Mexican descent, 39 percent of American Indian children, 50 percent of children from Guam are overweight.

Weight And Emotions

Eating is often about more than being hungry. It is a way to celebrate a happy event, follow cultural traditions, or socialize with friends. For some people, however, eating is a way to deal with difficult feelings such as stress, depression, and anxiety. This is called emotional eating, and it can lead to overeating, or even eating disorders.

Like adults, children and adolescents may eat for emotional reasons. One study, for example, found that 11-year-old school children who were stressed tended to eat more unhealthy foods and eat fewer nutritious meals and snacks.

Researchers are now also finding links between serious emotional problems and overweight:

- Depressed adolescents may actually be at greater risk of becoming obese.

- Children who develop serious behavioral problems may be five times more likely to become overweight two years later.

- Overweight girls are more likely to feel bad about their bodies. These feelings place them at a greater risk of having low self-esteem, depression, and problems with anxiety.

- Teasing about body weight is associated with feeling badly about one's appearance, low self-esteem, depression, and even thinking about and attempting suicide.

Talk to your parents about your feelings and how they may be connected to eating habits. Consult a pediatrician or family doctor if you think you may be suffering from more serious emotional problems. A doctor can help you determine if you need to talk to a mental health professional.

Smoking And Weight Control

Research shows that people under age 30 are more likely to smoke if they are trying to lose weight, even though many want to stop smoking.

Teen girls may be especially open to the risks of smoking to control their weight. Cigarettes are often marketed as "slims" or "thins" to play into the social pressures on young women to control their weight, manage stress, and look grown up. One study found that girls who had dieted up to one time each week were twice as likely to become smokers, and girls who dieted more often had four times the odds of becoming smokers.

Adolescent girls need to be warned that using tobacco is not a good way to lose weight. There are healthier ways to control weight.

The Diet Trap

Many adolescent girls are unhappy with their bodies and try to lose weight by using unhealthy dieting practices such as skipping meals, fasting, smoking, severely restricting calories, or eliminating whole classes of foods such as starches and sugars. Some girls are using even more extreme methods, such as making themselves vomit and using diet pills and laxatives.

The best approach is to adopt healthy eating practices and regular physical activity. Diets do not provide the right kind of nutrition girls need to grow.

Also, diets may cause some girls to gain more weight and develop lifelong unhealthy eating habits. One study, for example, found that children who diet actually gain more weight in the long term than children who do not diet. This is because dieting may cause a cycle in which children eat very little and then overeat or binge eat (eating large amounts of food in a short period of time, usually alone, without being able to stop when full).

Girls who feel dissatisfied with their bodies and use unhealthy dieting methods are also at increased risk for eating disorders, obesity, poor nutrition, growth impairments, and emotional problems such as depression.

What To Do?

How can you begin adopting habits that lead to a healthy weight? The following are some general tips to help you get started:

- Talk to your parents about healthy eating habits for your whole family.

- Avoid unhealthy eating habits such as skipping meals to lose weight, complaining about your body, or using food as a reward or to make yourself feel better.

- Learn to control your eating. Stop eating when full. Some practices such as being forced to eat certain foods, being required to "clean your plate," and being forbidden particular foods may actually lead to overeating. Discuss these concerns with your parents if necessary.

- Include in your diet a variety of healthy foods at meals and snack times, including fruits, vegetables, whole grains, and other foods that are low in sugar, sodium (salt), and saturated fat.

- Eat meals with your family. Meals are an important social outlet.

- Participate in physical activities with your family. Visit parks, beaches, and other places where you can be physically active. Take walks, hikes, or bike rides as a family.

- Limit time spent watching television. Television encourages you to be inactive and exposes you to many food advertisements. Don't keep a television in your bedroom.

Chapter 8

Mental Wellness

Your mental health is very important. You will not have a healthy body if you don't also take care of your mind. People depend on you. It's important for you to take care of yourself so that you can do the important things in life—whether it's working, learning, taking care of your family, volunteering, enjoying the outdoors, or whatever is important to you.

Good mental health helps you enjoy life and cope with problems. It offers a feeling of well-being and inner strength. Just as you take care of your body by eating right and exercising, you can do things to protect your mental health. In fact, eating right and exercising can help maintain good mental health. You don't automatically have good mental health just because you don't have mental health illness. You have to work to keep your mind healthy.

Nutrition And Mental Health

Visit www.ChooseMyPlate.gov to help find personalized eating plans and other interactive tools to help you make good food choices.

The food you eat can have a direct effect on your energy level, physical health, and mood. A "healthy diet" is one that has enough of each essential nutrient, contains many foods from all of the basic food groups, provides the right amount of calories to maintain a healthy weight, and does not have too much fat, sugar, salt, or alcohol.

By choosing foods that can give you steady energy, you can help your body stay healthy. This may also help your mind feel good. The same diet doesn't work for every person. In order to find the best foods that are right for you, talk to your health care professional.

About This Chapter: From "Mental Health," Office on Women's Health (www.womenshealth.gov), March 29, 2010.

Some vitamins and minerals may help with the symptoms of depression. Experts are looking into how a lack of some nutrients—including folate, vitamin B12, calcium, iron, selenium, zinc, and omega-3—may contribute to depression in new mothers. Ask your doctor or another health care professional for more information.

Exercise And Mental Health

Regular physical activity is important to the physical and mental health of almost everyone, including older adults. Being physically active can help you continue to do the things you enjoy and stay independent as you age. Regular physical activity over long periods of time can produce long-term health benefits. That's why health experts say that everyone should be active every day to maintain their health.

If you are diagnosed with depression or anxiety, your doctor may tell you to exercise in addition to taking any medications or receiving counseling. This is because exercise has been shown to help with the symptoms of depression and anxiety. Your body makes certain chemicals, called endorphins, before and after you work out. They relieve stress and improve your mood. Exercise can also slow or stop weight gain, which is a common side effect of some medications used to treat mental health disorders.

Sleep And Mental Health

Your mind and body will feel better if you sleep well. Your body needs time every day to rest and heal. If you often have trouble sleeping—either falling asleep, or waking during the night and being unable to get back to sleep—one or several of the following ideas might be helpful to you:

- Go to bed at the same time every night and get up at the same time every morning. Avoid sleeping in (sleeping much later than your usual time for getting up). It will make you feel worse.

- Establish a bedtime ritual by doing the same things every night for an hour or two before bedtime so your body knows when it is time to go to sleep.

- Avoid caffeine, nicotine, and alcohol.

- Eat on a regular schedule and avoid a heavy meal prior to going to bed. Don't skip any meals.

- Eat plenty of dairy foods and dark green leafy vegetables.

- Exercise daily, but avoid strenuous or invigorating activity before going to bed.

- Play soothing music on a tape or CD that shuts off automatically after you are in bed.

- Try a turkey sandwich and a glass of milk before bedtime to make you feel drowsy.

- Try having a small snack before you go to bed, something like a piece of fruit and a piece of cheese, so you don't wake up hungry in the middle of the night. Have a similar small snack if you awaken in the middle of the night.

- Take a warm bath or shower before going to bed.

- Place a drop of lavender oil on your pillow.

- Drink a cup of herbal chamomile tea before going to bed.

You need to see your doctor if any of the following conditions describe you:

- You often have difficulty sleeping and the solutions listed above are not working for you.

- You awaken during the night gasping for breath.

- You snore loudly.

- You wake up feeling like you haven't been asleep.

- You fall asleep often during the day.

Stress And Mental Health

Stress can happen for many reasons. Stress can be brought about by a traumatic accident, death, or emergency situation. Stress can also be a side effect of a serious illness or disease.

There is also stress associated with daily life, the workplace, and family responsibilities. It's hard to stay calm and relaxed in our hectic lives. With all we have going on in our lives, it seems almost impossible to find ways to de-stress. But it's important to find those ways. Your health depends on it.

These are some common symptoms:

- Headache

- Sleep disorders

- Difficulty concentrating

- Short-temper

- Upset stomach

- Job dissatisfaction

- Low morale

- Depression

- Anxiety

Remember to always make time for you. It's important to care for yourself. Think of this as an order from your doctor, so you don't feel guilty. No matter how busy you are, you can try to set aside at least 15 minutes each day in your schedule to do something for yourself, like taking a bubble bath, going for a walk, or calling a friend.

Chapter 9

Sleep Is Important For Fitness

How Much Sleep Do I Need?

Most teens need about 8½ to more than 9 hours of sleep each night. The right amount of sleep is essential for anyone who wants to do well on a test or play sports without tripping over their feet. Unfortunately, though, many teens don't get enough sleep.

Why Aren't Teens Getting Enough Sleep?

Until recently, teens were often given a bad rap for staying up late, oversleeping for school, and falling asleep in class. But recent studies show that adolescent sleep patterns actually differ from those of adults or kids.

These studies show that during the teen years, the body's circadian rhythm (sort of like an internal biological clock) is temporarily reset, telling a person to fall asleep later and wake up later. This change in the circadian rhythm seems to be due to the fact that the brain hormone melatonin is produced later at night for teens than it is for kids and adults. This can make it harder for teens to fall asleep early.

These changes in the body's circadian rhythm coincide with a time when we're busier than ever. For most teens, the pressure to do well in school is more intense than when they were kids, and it's harder to get by without studying hard. And teens also have other time demands—everything from sports and other extracurricular activities to fitting in a part-time job to save money for college.

About This Chapter: "How Much Sleep Do I Need?," May 2009, reprinted with permission from www.kidshealth.org. This information was provided by KidsHealth®, one of the largest resources online for medically reviewed health information written for parents, kids, and teens. For more articles like this, visit www.KidsHealth.org or www.TeensHealth.org. Copyright © 1995-2012 The Nemours Foundation. All rights reserved.

Early start times in some schools may also play a role in this sleep deficit. Teens who fall asleep after midnight may still have to get up early for school, meaning that they may only squeeze in 6 or 7 hours of sleep a night. A couple hours of missed sleep a night may not seem like a big deal, but can create a noticeable sleep deficit over time.

Can sleep boost creativity?

A recent study found that getting enough sleep helps people solve problems more creatively.

Why Is Sleep Important?

This sleep deficit impacts everything from a person's ability to pay attention in class to his or her mood. According to the National Sleep Foundation's 2006 Sleep in America poll, more than one quarter of high school students fall asleep in class, and experts have been able to tie lost sleep to poorer grades. Lack of sleep also damages teens' ability to do their best in athletics.

Slowed responses and concentration from lack of sleep don't just affect school or sports performance, though. More than half of teens surveyed reported that they have driven a car drowsy over the past year and 15% of students in the 10th to 12th grades drive drowsy at least once a week. The National Highway Safety Traffic Administration estimates that more than 100,000 accidents, 40,000 injuries, and 1,500 people are killed in the U.S. every year in crashes caused by drivers who are simply tired. Young people under the age of 25 are far more likely to be involved in drowsy driving crashes.

Lack of sleep has also been linked to emotional troubles, such as feelings of sadness and depression. Sleep helps keep us physically healthy, too, by slowing our body's systems enough to re-energize us after everyday activities.

How Do I Know If I'm Getting Enough?

Even if you think you're getting enough sleep, you may not be. Here are some of the signs that you may need more sleep:

- Difficulty waking up in the morning
- Inability to concentrate
- Falling asleep during classes
- Feelings of moodiness and even depression

How Can I Get More Sleep?

Recently, some researchers, parents, and teachers have suggested that middle- and high-school classes begin later in the morning to accommodate teens' need for more sleep. Some schools have already implemented later start times. You and your friends, parents, and teachers can lobby for later start times at your school, but in the meantime you'll have to make your own adjustments.

Here are some things that may help you to sleep better:

- **Set a regular bedtime.** Going to bed at the same time each night signals to your body that it's time to sleep. Waking up at the same time every day can also help establish sleep patterns. So try to stick as closely as you can to your sleep schedule even on weekends. Don't go to sleep more than an hour later or wake up more than two to three hours later than you do during the week.

- **Exercise regularly.** Try not to exercise right before bed, though, as it can rev you up and make it harder to fall asleep. Finish exercising at least three hours before bedtime. Many sleep experts believe that exercising in late afternoon may actually help a person sleep.

- **Avoid stimulants.** Don't drink beverages with caffeine, such as soda and coffee, after 4 p.m. Nicotine is also a stimulant, so quitting smoking may help you sleep better. And drinking alcohol in the evening can also cause a person to be restless and wake up during the night.

- **Relax your mind.** Avoid violent, scary, or action movies or television shows right before bed—anything that might set your mind and heart racing. Reading books with involved or active plots may also keep you from falling or staying asleep.

- **Unwind by keeping the lights low.** Light signals the brain that it's time to wake up. Staying away from bright lights (including computer screens!), as well as meditating or listening to soothing music, can help your body relax. Try to avoid TV, computer and telephone at least one hour before you go to bed.

- **Don't nap too much.** Naps of more than 30 minutes during the day may keep you from falling asleep later.

- **Avoid all-nighters.** Don't wait until the night before a big test to study. Cutting back on sleep the night before a test may mean you perform worse than you would if you'd studied less but got more sleep.

- **Create the right sleeping environment.** Studies show that people sleep best in a dark room that is slightly on the cool side. Close your blinds or curtains (and make sure they're heavy enough to block out light) and turn down the thermostat in your room (pile on extra blankets or wear PJs if you're cold). Lots of noise can be a sleep turnoff, too.

- **Wake up with bright light.** Bright light in the morning signals to your body that it's time to get going. If it's dark in your room, it can help to turn on a light as soon as your alarm goes off.

If you're drowsy, it's hard to look and feel your best. Schedule "sleep" as an item on your agenda to help you stay creative and healthy.

Part Two
Making And Maintaining A Fitness Plan

Chapter 10

Tips For Getting Started On A Path To Fitness

Getting Started And Staying Active

If you think getting fit is difficult, you are not alone. Many people find it hard to get started, for many different reasons. Do any of these reasons sound like you?

- I can't exercise because I don't have any equipment

- I don't have time to exercise

- I don't know how to exercise

- My parents/guardian aren't active

- Exercise sounds so boring to me

- Equipment or health clubs cost too much

If you can relate to any of these statements, it is important that you read on for tips on leading an active lifestyle. You don't have to be an athlete or be involved in an organized sport to be fit. You just have to sit less and move more! It is also important to get other members of your family moving, too.

Make A Fitness Plan

There are lots of other things that might get in the way of regular exercise. You might think your schedule is full or you are not sure how to get started. For each situation, there is a solution.

About This Chapter: From "Fitness," Office on Women's Health (www.girlshealth.gov), October 2009.

No More Excuses

Make fitness work for you. Check out these exercise challenges and solutions:

I am too busy.

Try exercising after school, or pick a time that works best for you each day. It's up to you to make the time and effort.

Exercise bores me.

Try out different activities. Sick of jogging? Try rollerblading. Not interested in lifting weights? Try Pilates You could also schedule different activities for different days of the week to keep things interesting. For example, you could swim on Saturdays and do yoga on Tuesdays. Here's a list of fun activities:

- Kickboxing
- Skateboarding
- Surfing
- Salsa dancing
- Scuba diving
- Yoga
- Rock climbing
- Snowboarding
- Mountain biking
- Sandboarding
- Kayaking
- Pilates
- T'ai chi

You will need permission from your parents/guardian to invest time and money (many require safety equipment) for most of these sports. Also, these activities carry risks for serious injury and it is important to learn the proper techniques before trying them out on your own. Make sure to learn from certified teachers to stay safe.

It's hard to stick with it.

Try exercising with a friend or a family member to give one another support. If someone else is counting on you to workout or play catch, you'll be less likely to skip exercising.

I don't have equipment or access to a health club.

Choose activities that don't require special equipment, such as jogging or walking. Find resources within your community that are either low-cost or free, such as park and recreation programs. Can you use your school's gym or swimming pool after school or on weekends? You could also take your dog (or borrow a neighbor's pup!) for a long walk or an easy jog. Try jumping rope. There are lots of ways to exercise that don't require a gym membership—be creative!

I don't know how.

Start with activities that you don't have to learn new skills for, such as walking, climbing stairs, or jogging. Exercise with friends who are either beginners like you, or who are more experienced and can teach you what they know. Take a class to learn new things, such as a Pilates class at your community center or health club.

Once you get past these challenges, decide when you are going to exercise and which activities you would like to do.

Fitness As A Lifestyle

Once you get past these challenges, decide when you are going to exercise and which activities you would like to do. When you think about a new physical activity, ask yourself these questions:

- Will you enjoy it?
- Is it safe?
- Is it available to you?
- Do you have the time to do it?
- Do you have friends who do it, too?

If you answered "no" to these questions, find another activity. It is better to find something that fits into your schedule, that you will enjoy, and that you can do safely. The important thing is that you get moving and there are lots of ways to get started! Walk when you talk on the phone, use the stairs instead of an elevator, and walk or bike to school.

Don't worry if you don't have athletic equipment. You don't need anything special to exercise. You can use canned foods as weights, go for power walks or run around your neighborhood or the school track, or use your own body weight to strength train by doing push-ups, sit-ups, tricep dips, and lunges. There are many different exercises to work all parts of your body.

Working Different Muscle Groups

Different kinds of exercises work different muscle groups. You should try to work all of your muscles each week. Some exercises work many muscles, so this is not as hard as you might think!

Below is a list of exercises and the kinds of muscles used for each exercise, if you do the exercise correctly (Source: American Council on Exercise):

- Push-ups: Chest, shoulders, arms, abdominals

- Sit-ups: Abdominals

- Jumping Jacks: Calves (lower leg), inner/outer thigh, butt

- Running: Calves, front/back thigh, abdominals

- Jumping rope: Calves, thighs, abdominals, shoulders, arms

- Swimming: Nearly all major muscles

- Dancing: Nearly all major muscles (depending on type of dance)

- Walking: Arms, calves, front/back thigh, abdominals

- Squats: Calves, front/back thigh, butt

- Inline Skating: Inner/outer thigh, butt

- Hula Hoop: Lower back, abdominals

Chapter 11

Fitness Self-Assessment

How Fit Are You?

Keeping active can improve your health and wellbeing and lower your risk of developing major chronic diseases.

The Department of Health [UK] recommends that adults should do 150 minutes of physical activity a week. Those aged 18 and under should be doing an hour each day.

Are you doing enough?

Use this assessment to find out.

Questions

1. How old are you?

a) 18 and under (0 points). If you are under 18 you should be active for at least one hour a day

b) 19 to 30 (0 points). Adults should do at least 150 minutes moderate or 75 minutes vigorous physical activity a week.

c) 31 to 45 (0 points). Adults should do at least 150 minutes moderate or 75 minutes vigorous physical activity a week.

d) 46 to 64 (0 points). Adults should do at least 150 minutes moderate or 75 minutes vigorous physical activity a week.

About This Chapter: "Fitness Self-Assessment," reprinted with permission from NHS Choices, www.nhs.uk, © 2011. All rights reserved.

e) 65 plus (0 points). Over 65s should take particular care to keep moving and retain their mobility through daily activity—at least 30 minutes, five days a week.

Physical Activity For The Under 5s

For those under five, being active is important for growth and development.

For babies it's important to make sure they can move as much as possible, for example letting them lie them on their stomach so they can kick their legs and stretch their arms.

For children who can walk, they should be active for at least three hours every day. The good news is they get a lot of this by just playing at the playground or park, climbing and jumping, running, and chasing.

Growth And Development

Regular health exams and tests can help find problems before they start. They also can help find problems early, when chances for treatment and cure are better. By getting the right health services, screenings, and treatments, teens can take steps that help their chances for living a longer, healthier life. Family history, lifestyle choices (what they eat, how active they are), and other important factors influence what and how often teens need health services and screenings.

Insufficient sleep is associated with a number of chronic diseases and conditions, such as diabetes, cardiovascular diseases, obesity, and depression. Students who are working or studying long hours may experience episodes of sleep deprivation. This can cause daytime sleepiness, sluggishness, and difficulty concentrating or making decisions. Teens and young adults who do not get enough sleep are at risk for problems, such as automobile crashes, poor grades and school performance, depressed moods, and problems with friends, fellow students, and adult relationships.

Quick Tips

- Avoid stimulants like caffeine and nicotine. The stimulating effects of caffeine in coffee, colas, teas, and chocolate can take as long as eight hours to wear off fully.
- Have a good sleeping environment. Get rid of anything that might distract you from sleep, such as noises or bright lights.
- Stick to a sleep schedule. Go to bed and wake up at the same time each day, even on the weekends.
- See your health provider if you continue to have trouble sleeping.
- Avoid pulling an all-nighter to study.

Source: "Physical Health: Growth and Development," U.S. Department of Health and Human Services (www.hhs.gov), 2011.

For Adults Only (that is, respondents answer b, c ,d, or e to question 1)

2. The Department of Health recommends adults are moderately active for 150 minutes or vigorously active for 75 minutes each week. In an average week, how close are you to achieving this?

a) You achieve this every week (3 points). By meeting the recommended levels of physical activity, the risk of heart disease, stroke, and type 2 diabetes is reduced by up to 50%.

b) You're almost there, but not quite (2 points). Upping your physical activity levels to 150 minutes a week will lower your risk of heart disease, stroke, and type 2 diabetes—by up to 50%.

c) You do around half of what's recommended (1 point). Upping your physical activity levels to 150 minutes a week will lower your risk of heart disease, stroke, and type 2 diabetes—by up to 50%.

d) You're a long way off doing what's recommended (0 points). It's very important that you start being more active to reduce your risk of heart disease, stroke, and type 2 diabetes.

What Moderate And Vigorous Mean

- **Moderate:** Physical activity that increases your heart rate, makes you warm and slightly out of breath but allows you to maintain a conversation.

- **Vigorous:** Physical activity that increases your heart rate, causes you to breathe rapidly, and makes a conversation difficult.

Adults should do a minimum of 150 minutes moderate or 75 minutes vigorous physical activity a week. This activity should last for at least 10 minutes, could be a combination of both, and can be spread out over the week.

For 18 And Under

3. Those aged between 5 and 18 should be active for 60 minutes every day. On an average day, how close are you to achieving this?

a) You achieve this every day (3 points). Being active when you're young helps to build strong muscles and healthy bones.

b) You're almost there but not quite (2 points). You need to up your levels to an hour a day. Being active when you're young helps to build strong muscles and healthy bones.

c) You do around half of what's recommended (1 point). You need to up your levels to an hour a day. Being active when you're young helps to build strong muscles and healthy bones.

d) You're a long way off (0 points). It's very important that you start being more active. Being active when you're young helps to build strong muscles and healthy bones, can help improve self-confidence, and will help maintain a healthy weight.

For Adults Only

4. How many days a week do you do activities that strengthen your muscles?

a) At least two days (2 points). You're already working on strengthening your muscles which is great for your health.

b) One day (1 point). You're already working on your muscle strength which is great for your health. By increasing it to two days a week you'll gain maximum health benefits.

c) Hardly ever (0 point). You need to work on your muscle strength. Try doing exercises that use your body weight for resistance.

Fitness Training Tips: What are muscle strengthening activities?

Besides aerobic activity, you need to do things to strengthen your muscles at least two days a week. These activities should work all the major muscle groups of your body (legs, hips, back, chest, abdomen, shoulders, and arms).

Examples include lifting weights, doing exercises that use your body weight for resistance (for example, sit-ups, push-ups), heavy gardening or manual work, yoga, or tai chi.

To gain health benefits, muscle-strengthening activities need to be done to the point where it's hard for you to do another repetition without help.

For 18 And Under

4. How many days a week do you do activities that strengthen your muscles?

a) At least three days (2 points). You're already working on strengthening your muscles which is great for your health.

b) One or two days (1 point). You're already working on your muscle strength which is great for your health. By increasing it to three days a week you'll gain maximum health benefits.

c) Hardly ever (0 point). You need to work on your muscle strength. Try doing exercises that use your body weight for resistance.

Fitness Training Tips: What are muscle strengthening activities?

Besides aerobic activity, you need to do things to strengthen your muscles and bones at least three days a week. These activities should work all the major muscle groups of your body (legs, hips, back, chest, abdomen, shoulders, and arms).

This could include resistance exercises using body weight or resistance bands, rope or tree climbing, and sports such as gymnastics, basketball, volleyball, and tennis.

Younger children might also try games such as tug of war, swinging on playground equipment/bars and hopping, skipping and jumping.

5. If you're not doing enough physical activity, which of the following best describes why? (You can pick more than one)

a) "I don't have time" (0 point). Consider building activities into your daily routine, like walking more or cycling to work.

b) "I'm too tired" (0 point). Exercise can boost energy levels and even improve your sleep. Try to do a little each day.

c) "I don't have the willpower" (0 point). Setting a goal can really help strengthen your willpower and achieving it will have great mental as well as physical health benefits.

d) "I don't like to exercise" (0 point). Try out lots of different activities to find something you can enjoy on a regular basis.

e) "It's hard work" (0 point). As well having physical health benefits, keeping active can boost mental wellbeing so try to do a little rather than avoiding it.

f) "None of these" (0 point).

6. How would you describe the way you feel after climbing a flight of stairs?

a) Great (4 points).

b) Ok (3 points).

c) Breathless (2 points). Avoid taking the lift or escalator every time and start using the stairs. It's an easy way to build activity into your day.

d) Exhausted (1 points). Try to make small changes in your day to increase your activity levels. Over time you'll be able to climb stairs without feeling exhausted.

e) Can't do it (0 points). Not being able to climb stairs may suggest you need to see your family doctor for a health check.

7. How many of the following could you do easily? (You can pick more than one.)

a) 10 sit-ups (2 points)

b) 5 push-ups (2 points)

c) Touch your toes (1 point)

d) 20 star jumps (2 points)

e) None of these (0 points)

Results

12–16 points: Based on your responses today, you are close to meeting or exceeding the recommended levels of physical activity. This is great for your health. Keep up the good work.

7-12 points: Based on your responses today, you're physically active but not quite meeting recommended levels.

0–6 points: Based on your responses today you're not very active and struggling with motivation. Start small and build up. You'll soon gain in confidence and feel better.

Chapter 12

Fitness Guidelines For Children And Adolescents

Active Children And Adolescents

Regular physical activity in children and adolescents promotes health and fitness. Compared to those who are inactive, physically active youth have higher levels of cardiorespiratory fitness and stronger muscles. They also typically have lower body fatness. Their bones are stronger, and they may have reduced symptoms of anxiety and depression.

Youth who are regularly active also have a better chance of a healthy adulthood. Children and adolescents don't usually develop chronic diseases, such as heart disease, hypertension, type 2 diabetes, or osteoporosis. However, risk factors for these diseases can begin to develop early in life. Regular physical activity makes it less likely that these risk factors will develop and more likely that children will remain healthy as adults.

Youth can achieve substantial health benefits by doing moderate- and vigorous-intensity physical activity for periods of time that add up to 60 minutes (one hour) or more each day. This activity should include aerobic activity as well as age-appropriate muscle- and bone-strengthening activities. Although current science is not complete, it appears that, as with adults, the total amount of physical activity is more important for achieving health benefits than is any one component (frequency, intensity, or duration) or specific mix of activities (aerobic, muscle-strengthening, bone-strengthening). Even so, bone-strengthening activities remain especially important for children and young adolescents because the greatest gains in

About This Chapter: Excerpted from "Chapter 3: Active Children and Adolescent," *2008 Physical Activity Guidelines for Americans*, U.S. Department of Health and Human Services (www.health.gov/paguidelines), 2008. Text under the heading "Getting Started" is excerpted and adapted from *BodyWorks: A Toolkit for Healthy Teens and Strong Families*, Office on Women's Health, U.S. Department of Health and Human Services, 2006. Reviewed by David A. Cooke, MD, FACP, May 2012.

bone mass occur during the years just before and during puberty. In addition, the majority of peak bone mass is obtained by the end of adolescence.

Key Guidelines For Children And Adolescents

Children and adolescents should do 60 minutes (one hour) or more of physical activity daily.

- *Aerobic:* Most of the 60 or more minutes a day should be either moderate-or vigorous-intensity aerobic physical activity, and should include vigorous-intensity physical activity at least three days a week.

- *Muscle-strengthening:* As part of their 60 or more minutes of daily physical activity, children and adolescents should include muscle-strengthening physical activity on at least three days of the week.

- *Bone-strengthening:* As part of their 60 or more minutes of daily physical activity, children and adolescents should include bone-strengthening physical activity on at least three days of the week.

It is important to participate in physical activities that are age appropriate, that are enjoyable, and that offer variety.

Types Of Activity For Young People

Each type of physical activity has important health benefits.

- *Aerobic* activities are those in which young people rhythmically move their large muscles. Running, hopping, skipping, jumping rope, swimming, dancing, and bicycling are all examples of aerobic activities. Aerobic activities increase cardiorespiratory fitness. Children often do activities in short bursts, which may not technically be aerobic activities. However, this chapter will also use the term aerobic to refer to these brief activities.

- *Muscle-strengthening* activities make muscles do more work than usual during activities of daily life. Muscle-strengthening activities can be unstructured and part of play, such as playing on playground equipment, climbing trees, and playing tug-of-war. Or these activities can be structured, such as lifting weights or working with resistance bands.

- *Bone-strengthening* activities produce a force on the bones that promotes bone growth and strength. This force is commonly produced by impact with the ground. Running, jumping rope, basketball, tennis, and hopscotch are all examples of bone-strengthening activities. As these examples illustrate, bone-strengthening activities can also be aerobic and muscle-strengthening.

Why aren't teens active?

Kids are most often physically active through free play, but nowadays they have less opportunity. In some cases, children have no safe means of getting to and from youth sport and other recreational programs. In many cases, kids are not physically active because they are sitting in front of televisions and computers during their free time. In fact, one study found that children and teens spend several hours every day watching TV, playing video games, and using the internet and other forms of media.

Even when kids are involved in physical education classes (P.E.) in school or other organized sport activities, they may not be getting enough vigorous exercise. In softball or volleyball, for example, players don't have to be moving around very much.

Source: Excerpted from *BodyWorks: A Toolkit for Healthy Teens and Strong Families*, Office on Women's Health, U.S. Department of Health and Human Services, 2006. Reviewed by David A. Cooke, MD, FACP, May 2012.

How Age Influences Physical Activity

Children and adolescents should meet physical activity guidelines by doing activity that is appropriate for their age. Their natural patterns of movement differ from those of adults. For example, children are naturally active in an intermittent way, particularly when they do unstructured active play. During recess and in their free play and games, children use basic aerobic and bone-strengthening activities, such as running, hopping, skipping, and jumping, to develop movement patterns and skills. They alternate brief periods of moderate- and vigorous-intensity activity with brief periods of rest. Any episode of moderate- or vigorous-intensity physical activity, however brief, counts.

Children also commonly increase muscle strength through unstructured activities that involve lifting or moving their body weight or working against resistance. Children don't usually do—or need—formal muscle-strengthening programs, such as lifting weights.

As children grow into adolescents, their patterns of physical activity change. They are able to play organized games and sports and are able to sustain longer periods of activity. But they still commonly do intermittent activity, and no period of moderate- or vigorous-intensity activity is too short to count.

Adolescents may meet physical activity guidelines by doing free play, structured programs, or both. Structured exercise programs can include aerobic activities, such as playing a sport, and muscle-strengthening activities, such as lifting weights, working with resistance bands, or using body weight for resistance (such as push-ups, pull-ups, and sit-ups). Muscle-strengthening activities count if they involve a moderate to high level of effort and work the major muscle groups of the body: legs, hips, back, abdomen, chest, shoulders, and arms.

Levels Of Intensity For Aerobic Activity

Children and adolescents can meet physical activity guidelines by doing a combination of moderate- and vigorous-intensity aerobic physical activities or by doing only vigorous-intensity aerobic physical activities.

Youth should not do only moderate-intensity activity. It's important to include vigorous-intensity activities because they cause more improvement in cardiorespiratory fitness.

The intensity of aerobic physical activity can be defined on either an absolute or a relative scale. Absolute intensity is based on the rate of energy expenditure during the activity, without taking into account a person's cardiorespiratory fitness. Relative intensity uses a person's level of cardiorespiratory fitness to assess level of effort.

Relative intensity describes a person's level of effort relative to his or her fitness. As a rule of thumb, on a scale of 0 to 10, where sitting is 0 and the highest level of effort possible is 10, moderate-intensity activity is a 5 or 6. Young people doing moderate-intensity activity will notice that their hearts are beating faster than normal and they are breathing harder than normal. Vigorous-intensity activity is at a level of 7 or 8. Youth doing vigorous-intensity activity will feel their heart beating much faster than normal and they will breathe much harder than normal.

Examples Physical Activities For Adolescents

Some activities, such as bicycling, can be moderate or vigorous intensity, depending upon level of effort.

What Happened To P.E.?

The school P.E. class is an important way for teens to be physically active. Unfortunately, P.E. is no longer part of the schedule at many middle and high schools around the country. Experts recommend that teens participate in P.E. class every day, yet only 29 percent of students in grades 9–12 actually do so. And even when P.E. classes are available, most students do not spend enough time being active.

Source: Excerpted from *BodyWorks: A Toolkit for Healthy Teens and Strong Families*, Office on Women's Health, U.S. Department of Health and Human Services, 2006. Reviewed by David A. Cooke, MD, FACP, May 2012.

Moderate-Intensity Aerobic

- Active recreation, such as canoeing, hiking, skateboarding, rollerblading
- Brisk walking
- Bicycle riding (stationary or road bike)
- Housework and yard work, such as sweeping or pushing a lawn mower
- Games that require catching and throwing, such as baseball and softball

Vigorous-Intensity Aerobic

- Active games involving running and chasing, such as flag football
- Bicycle riding
- Jumping rope
- Martial arts, such as karate
- Running
- Sports such as soccer, ice or field hockey, basketball, swimming, tennis
- Vigorous dancing
- Cross-country skiing

Muscle-Strengthening

- Games such as tug-of-war
- Push-ups and pull-ups
- Resistance exercises with exercise bands, weight machines, hand-held weights
- Climbing wall
- Sit-ups (curl-ups or crunches)

Bone-Strengthening

- Hopping, skipping, jumping
- Jumping rope
- Running
- Sports such as gymnastics, basketball, volleyball, tennis

Physical Activity And Healthy Weight

Regular physical activity in children and adolescents promotes a healthy body weight and body composition.

Exercise training in overweight or obese youth can improve body composition by reducing overall levels of fatness as well as abdominal fatness. Research studies report that fatness can be reduced by regular physical activity of moderate to vigorous intensity three to five times a week, for 30 to 60 minutes.

Physical Fitness Guidelines For American Youth

American youth vary in their physical activity participation. Some don't participate at all, others participate in enough activity to meet physical fitness guidelines, and some exceed guidelines.

One practical strategy to promote activity in youth is to replace inactivity with activity whenever possible. For example, where appropriate and safe, young people should walk or bicycle to school instead of riding in a car. Rather than just watching sporting events on television, young people should participate in age-appropriate sports or games.

Reduce TV Time And Get Moving

A good way to get moving is to decrease TV time. The American Academy of Pediatrics suggests no more than an hour or two each day of good quality TV programming, video, and computer games combined.

Many families don't allow TV on school nights and limit hours during weekends. Other parents restrict TV until homework is finished and do not permit watching TV during meals. Keeping the TV out of your bedroom can also help by eliminating the temptation associated with unlimited access

Tape your favorite shows to view later. You can cut TV viewing time by planning to watch specific shows, rather than just zoning out on whatever is on. You can also fast forward through the commercials.

Replace after-school TV watching with other activities. Find other ways to spend your free time, especially activities that involve a physical activity such as walking. There are many good after-school programs in most communities that involve physical activity, from individual and team sports to dance, Double Dutch, and martial arts. Check with local schools, churches, and community groups.

Source: Excerpted and adapted from *BodyWorks: A Toolkit for Healthy Teens and Strong Families*, Office on Women's Health, U.S. Department of Health and Human Services, 2006. Reviewed by David A. Cooke, MD, FACP, May 2012.

- Children and adolescents who do not meet the guidelines should slowly increase their activity in small steps and in ways that they enjoy. A gradual increase in the number of days and the time spent being active will help reduce the risk of injury.

- Children and adolescents who meet the guidelines should continue being active on a daily basis and, if appropriate, become even more active. Evidence suggests that even more than 60 minutes of activity every day may provide additional health benefits.

- Children and adolescents who exceed the guidelines should maintain their activity level and vary the kinds of activities they do to reduce the risk of overtraining or injury.

Children and adolescents with disabilities are more likely to be inactive than those without disabilities. Youth with disabilities should work with their health-care provider to understand the types and amounts of physical activity appropriate for them. When possible, children and adolescents with disabilities should meet the physical activity guidelines. When young people are not able to participate in appropriate physical activities to meet the guidelines, they should be as active as possible and avoid being inactive.

Getting Started

Research shows that young people are more likely to be active if their parents or siblings are active and if their parents support their participation in physical activities. Talk to your family about ways you can all become more active together by planning leisure activities such as walking or bicycling. Even birthday parties and vacations can involve some physical activity. And, don't forget your friends. Get fit with friends by planning a physical activity together like bike riding each week.

How Much Activity?

Physical activity can be part of play, games, sports, or recreation—in short it should be part of every teen's daily life.

Adolescents should be physically active for 60 minutes every day, or most every day. Setting aside 60 consecutive minutes each day is one way to get in enough physical activity. Teens can also break it up into a few 10- or 15-minute sessions of moderate-to-intensive activity.

Vigorous-intensity physical activity (jogging or other aerobic exercise) causes a person to sweat and breathe hard and generally provides more benefits than moderate-intensity physical activity. However, moderate-intensity physical activity is also helpful. Moderate-intensity physical activity is exercising while you can talk, but not so lightly that you can sing. Walking two miles, shooting baskets, or biking five miles in 30 minutes would all be considered moderate-intensity physical activities.

Resistance exercise (such as weight training, using weight machines and resistance band workouts) increases muscular strength and endurance and maintains or increases muscle mass, when performed two or more days a week. Weight-bearing exercises include any activity in which your feet and legs carry your own weight. Examples include running, jumping rope, dancing, climbing stairs, skating, racquet sports, and team sports, like soccer and basketball.

Ideas For Moderate-To-Vigorous Activities

The following list is arranged so that it begins with less vigorous activities and more time and ends with more vigorous activities and less time:

- Playing volleyball for 45 minutes
- Playing touch football for 30–45 minutes
- Wheeling self in wheelchair for 30–40 minutes
- Walking 1¾ miles in 35 minutes (20 min/mile)
- Basketball (shooting baskets) for 30 minutes
- Bicycling 5 miles in 30 minutes
- Dancing fast (social) for 30 minutes
- Walking 2 miles in 30 minutes (15 min/mile)
- Water aerobics for 30 minutes
- Swimming laps for 20 minutes
- Wheelchair basketball for 20 minutes
- Basketball (playing a game) for 15–20 minutes
- Bicycling 4 miles in 15 minutes
- Jumping rope for 15 minutes
- Running 1½ miles in 15 minutes (10 min/mile)
- Stairwalking for 15 minutes

Doing chores around the house may not be fun, but they can help teens to be more physically active. Here are some examples:

- Washing and waxing a car for 45–60 minutes
- Washing windows or floors for 45–60 minutes
- Gardening for 30–45 minutes
- Raking leaves for 30 minutes
- Shoveling snow for 15 minutes

Finding The Best Exercise

What is the best exercise? The one that you are actually going to do!

Walking

Getting in your exercise for the day can be as simple as walking. Experts recommend that people walk 10,000 steps to get in enough physical activity for the day. Most people who do not exercise regularly walk between 4,000 and 6,000 steps per day. Taking 10,000 steps means you are walking about two extra miles.

Here are some tips to help you get in extra walking time:

- Pacing while talking on the phone
- Taking a walk after dinner
- Parking further from the entrance to a store
- Getting off the bus one or two stops early and walking the rest of the way home

Yoga

Yoga can help increase flexibility, relieve stress, and increase self-esteem. It also helps teens to learn about themselves and their bodies. Yoga is especially good for girls and boys who don't like organized sports or shy away from competitive sports.

Resistance Training

Resistance or strength training is a great way for teens to strengthen their muscles and get in a moderate-intensity physical activity. Strength training involves using your muscles against some form of resistance, such as barbells, dumb bells, exercise machines, or even your own body weight. Milk jugs filled with water or sand will also do. Teens will get best results by training two to three times each week, resting one day in between workouts to give muscles a chance to recover.

Safety is important when strength training. Before getting started, teens should talk to a school gym instructor, coach, or health club counselor to make sure the training program is safe and appropriate. A friend or spotter should be nearby at all times when *free weights*, such as dumbbells or barbells, are used.

Chapter 13

A Formula For Fitness

The Formula

Overload principle sounds like something you might do at an all-you-can-eat pizza party or what might happen when an unpopular teacher hands out homework. Actually, the overload principle is part of the formula for fitness. If you don't use it, you won't get faster, stronger, or more flexible.

What's operation overload?

The overload principle says that to improve your fitness level, you have to work a little harder than you are used to every time you exercise. This can help you build your cardiorespiratory fitness, muscle strength and endurance, and flexibility. The idea is to challenge your body to jump farther, lift a little more weight, do one more push-up, or do one more hamstring stretch than you did last time. Of course, you don't want to push too hard and end up hurting yourself. Slow and steady progress is the goal here.

What if I don't overload every time?

The overload principle helps you improve your fitness level. You can maintain your current fitness level without overloading, but you probably won't get any faster, stronger, or more flexible.

About This Chapter: This chapter begins with "Formula For Fitness," reprinted with permission from www.iEmily. com. © 2008 iEmily.com. All rights reserved. It also includes "Test Your Fitness Flair," reprinted with permission from www.iEmily.com. © 2008 iEmily.com. All rights reserved.

What if it's too hard?

Improving your fitness level isn't easy. And using the overload principle means you will sweat a little more, breathe a little faster, and push yourself a little harder every time you exercise. The good news is that you'll notice that your fitness level is improving little by little all the time.

Think EFIT

You can be your own personal trainer! Just keep the EFIT formula in mind when putting together your exercise program. EFIT stands for exercise, frequency, intensity, and time.

Exercise

The exercises you choose should help you accomplish your fitness goals. If you want stronger arms, spend more time doing bicep curls, tricep dips, and push-ups rather than running. On the other hand, running is a good way to improve your cardiorespiratory fitness if that is your goal.

Frequency

Do some form of exercise three to five times a week. Devote the other days to rest, and maybe a little stretching. You deserve it! Even if you want to exercise more often, it's important that you don't do strength training more than three times a week or two days in a row. Your muscles need time to recover.

Intensity

Intensity is the measure of how hard your body is working. It isn't always easy to tell how hard you are working, but it's important to figure it out if you want to get the most out of your workout. Using a heart rate monitor is a good way to measure how hard you're working. Some exercise equipment, like treadmills and elliptical trainers, have a built in monitor or you can buy a portable model at a sporting goods store. You can monitor your own energy level: On a scale of 1 to 10, think of 0 as your lowest level of effort (vegging) and 10 as your highest (gasping for breath). Aim for an intensity of 7 or 8 on this scale to improve your fitness level.

Maybe the easiest way to monitor your energy level is to take the talk test. While you are exercising, say a short sentence out loud, like "Are we almost done?" If you can speak briefly without gasping or running out of breath, you're getting the most out of your workout. If you can talk for as long as you want, pick up the pace. Try it out with a workout buddy if you feel goofy talking to yourself.

Time

Exercise nonstop for at least 20 to 30 minutes at a challenging pace. If you have a heart rate monitor, make sure you stay in your target heart rate zone. This is especially important for improving your cardiorespiratory fitness. If you stop exercising to say "hi" to friends, go to the bathroom, or slack off, reset that timer and start over again.

Test Your Fitness Flair

Not sure if you're fit? Try our fun quiz that tests your physical fitness.

Cardiorespiratory Health

Run up a flight of stairs (at least 16 steps) without stopping. Then see how you feel.

a. I can talk comfortably and could run up another flight.

b. I'm too winded to talk.

c. I could use an ambulance.

Muscle Strength And Endurance

Do as many push-ups in a row as you can. Be sure to keep your hands under your shoulders and your toes on the ground.

a. I can do 10 push-ups and keep going.

b. I can do 5 push-ups.

c. I think I'll just lie here on the floor.

Flexibility

Stand up straight, then reach for the floor. Try to touch your toes without bending your knees.

a. I can touch my toes.

b. I can touch my knees.

c. I can hardly bend over without getting dizzy.

Overall Fitness

How do you feel after completing this test?

a. What test? I feel great!

b. I'm a little bit sore and tired.

c. I'm ready for a vacation.

If your answers were mostly a's, you're an animal! Go to the head of the class!

If your answers were mostly b's, you're a good sport! Get ready to shape up!

If your answers were mostly c's, you're a fitnessphobe! Prepare for the new you!

Change Takes Time

Making big changes in your life is not easy. It takes about three months to change a behavior and about six months to make a new behavior part of your everyday routine.

It's important that you begin by taking a few small steps.

- Think about your reasons for making healthy lifestyle changes. Keep these reasons in mind as you begin to make these changes.
- Build on what you already do. Think about the healthy activities you already enjoy, and start from there.
- Figure out what may get in the way of making these changes so you are prepared to deal with them. Examples include lack of support from other family members and busy schedules.
- Decide on two or three small changes. Add one or two more goals after a few weeks. Remember to write your goals down and refer back to them regularly.
- Keep a daily activity journal. Journals help to keep you on track and check your progress.
- Know that you can do it!

Remember, change happens gradually. Don't be discouraged by slips—they are a normal part of changing behavior. Just get back on track.

Source: Excerpted and adapted from *BodyWorks: A Toolkit for Healthy Teens and Strong Families*, Office on Women's Health, U.S. Department of Health and Human Services, 2006. Reviewed by David A. Cooke, MD, FACP, May 2012.

Chapter 14

When Is The Right Time To Work Out?

Question

When is the best time of the day to work out? I exercise first thing in the morning, without eating anything beforehand. I just drink water before, during, and after my workout and then eat breakfast about a half hour after I get back from the gym. Am I compromising my workout in any way by not "fueling up" beforehand?

—Early Bird Exerciser

Answer

The best time to exercise is the time that's right for you. Morning workouts really get some people going, release endorphins, and enhance mood. If you enjoy starting your day with a workout, or find that it's the only time you can fit it into your schedule, stick with it. Others find afternoon or evening workouts productive and stress-relieving. When we wake up, our body temperature and blood sugar levels are low, so our muscles aren't as "loose" as later in the day. In a perfect world, our muscles are warmer and fueled by a few meals (hopefully) later, well after we awake.

There isn't really a "simple" answer to your second query. It will be helpful, though, to ask yourself the following questions: How hard do you work out (intensity)? How long are your sessions (duration)? What are your exercise activities? How soon after you awake do you begin exercising? Your answers are important in determining what may enhance your performance.

For some people, exercising with no fuel (food) beforehand may cause lightheadedness, dizziness, and early fatigue. Research shows that eating before exercise, as opposed to exercising on an empty stomach, improves athletic performance. If you have three hours until your workout, have a normal breakfast. However, if you're going straight to a workout after waking up, here are a few suggestions:

- If your exercise session is less than an hour, just snack on any foods that are easy to digest, such as bread, crackers, or a banana.

- If your session is one hour or longer, get up a little earlier and have something small to eat—perhaps around 250–300 calories—such as toast and fruit or a small bowl of cereal and skim milk.

- Drinking some water before and during exercise is important for hydration.

If you eat before exercising, make sure you allow your body some time to digest and absorb the food. During digestion, our bodies send blood to the stomach to help out with this process. When we exercise, our muscles need the blood flow, so our stomach becomes a second class citizen and digestion is slowed. If too much food is in the stomach while we're exercising, we may be uncomfortable.

Also take into account the type of food you eat and the activities you do. Some people tolerate liquids more easily because they leave the stomach more quickly than solid food. Some exercisers, such as runners, for example, would prefer not to have the internal "sloshing" around that liquids may cause.

General guidelines for eating before exercising are:

- Three or four hours before exercising, a large meal is fine (600 calories or more).

- Two or three hours beforehand, a smaller meal is suitable (400–500 calories).

- One or two hours before, a liquid meal is appropriate (300–400 calories).

- With less than one hour, a small snack will do (200–300 calories).

In addition, people tolerate foods differently, and the composition of the food matters. Fats stay in the stomach longest, followed by protein and high fiber carbohydrate, then low fiber complex carbohydrates, and finally simple sugars, which are absorbed fastest.

Sugary foods, such as sodas and candy, are absorbed quickly by the body and produce a sugar high within an hour of a workout. Along with a quick "sugar high" comes a quick "sugar low." People who eat sugar 15–30 minutes before exercising may experience a "low," with lightheadedness and fatigue, during their workout. If you feel that you absolutely must have juice or some sugary snack before exercising, have it only five or ten minutes before you begin. This way, there isn't enough time for your body to secrete insulin, a hormone which lowers blood sugar, causing fatiguing symptoms. Since everyone reacts differently, try various strategies to determine what helps you the most. No matter what, drink water before, during, and after exercise. And, have breakfast afterwards, especially if you haven't had anything to eat earlier, since this will replace glycogen stores and will keep you going all morning long.

Columbia University Copyright Information

Chapter 15

Health Clubs And Fitness Friends

Make A Fitness Friend

Wouldn't it be great to have your own personal trainer to encourage you when you don't feel like exercising or to get you to do just one more abdominal crunch? Wouldn't you like to have someone to keep you company while you work out and motivate you to be your best? Well, why not? When you and a friend become Fitness Friends, exercise can be twice as fun and rewarding. And Fitness Friends watch out for each other. This can keep both of you safe from injury, especially when one of you is doing something challenging like lifting a heavier weight or climbing a steep hill.

What is a Fitness Friend?

A Fitness Friend is someone you make an exercise "date" with on a regular basis. Maybe you meet every Saturday morning for a long walk. Or you take a yoga class and then practice at home together once or twice a week. A Fitness Friend can be a girl or a guy, or even someone you don't know very well, but would like to. You and your Fitness Friend don't even have to have the same fitness goals. You just need to make a commitment to exercising together and to being in shape.

How can a Fitness Friend help me?

Your Fitness Friend is there to motivate you. And you're there to motivate him or her. That means if he or she feels like skipping your afternoon run, you can make sure you both get some exercise. If your Fitness Friend is too tired to run, you might suggest a walk instead. Or make it a strength training day. You're both more likely to stick with your fitness program when you've made a "date" to workout. And you may find that by exercising with a Fitness Friend, you have the energy to do that exercise video, even though you didn't think you could drag yourself off the couch an hour earlier.

Can a Fitness Friend push me to work harder?

Definitely! A Fitness Friend can help you run faster, jump farther, or do one more bicep curl than you might have by yourself. You'll push yourself harder because you have a Fitness Friend to challenge and encourage you to do your best. On your own, you might quit running halfway around the track. But when you're with a friend, you'll probably dig a little deeper and push yourself to finish that last lap. Or you might not think that you can do one more abdominal crunch, but with your Fitness Friend cheering you on, you make it! The great thing about being Fitness Friends is that you bring out the best in each other.

How can I find a Fitness Friend?

A Fitness Friend can be someone you know from school, your neighborhood, or a gym or club that you belong to. He or she can be another teen or an adult you trust. You might even find a Fitness Friend in your own family! If you don't know who to ask, put an item in your school's paper or tell a coach that you're looking for someone to work out with. If you go to a public gym like a YMCA, you can post a note seeking a Fitness Friend. Or ask someone you see exercising if she or he would be interested in working out with you.

Joining A Health Club: Is It For You?

Joining a health club can be a fun fitness option if you're serious about exercising several days a week. Clubs offer a variety of exercise classes, cardio exercise equipment, and strength training options. Some even have pools, saunas, and showers. But health clubs aren't for everybody. A family membership can be expensive. And you may find the health club is crowded at the time of day you like to work out. Some clubs place restrictions on the hours when teens can use the facility as well. Before your family signs up, you might want to think about whether a health club can help you meet your fitness goals.

What are the advantages of health clubs?

Private health clubs generally have a wide variety of services and fairly new equipment. But your family will pay more for those benefits than you will to join a public gym or school program. Joining a health club is no guarantee that you will get fit, but there are some advantages.

- A good health club always has a trainer on the floor to answer your questions about proper weight lifting form and to teach you how to use the equipment.

- Because health clubs have a variety of options, you will be less likely to get bored doing the same exercise all the time.

- You will meet people who are interested in the same thing you are—fitness! Who knows, you might even make a Fitness Friend.

What are the disadvantages of health clubs?

Joining a health club isn't the only way to get in shape. In fact, there are several disadvantages to belonging to one.

- If you prefer exercising alone or feel self-conscious about working out in front of other people, a health club may not be right for you.

- If you have to get a ride to the health club or if it's a hassle to get there, you're more likely to miss a workout.

- If you don't like the fitness staff or the other people who work out there, you're probably not going to go.

- If you love being outdoors, exercising inside a club might not be your thing.

How do you join a health club?

If you want to join a health club because your best friend goes there or you like its ads, you may regret it. Remember, the only good health club is the health club you like to use! Before you ask your family to put money down, ask yourself these questions:

- Is the club at a convenient location? Will I still go if I have to walk or get a ride there?

- Is it open during the times I want to use it? Some big city gyms are open 24 hours a day, seven days a week, while others close early on weekends or have limited hours.

- Will I have to pay for extras like towels or a locker? These can add up quickly!

- Does it offer the kinds of classes that I want? Check the class schedule to make sure the class you want is offered at a time that's good for you.

- Are the facilities clean, and is the equipment well maintained? You can't use broken equipment. And moldy showers are a sure sign that the club isn't concerned about your health.

Chapter 16

Selecting And Using
A Fitness Facility

The health/fitness facility should provide a variety of equipment and programs to meet your personal fitness goals and interests. First, be sure to establish your exercise/fitness goals before talking to personnel to see if they provide the programs and equipment you seek.

Selecting A Facility

According to the International Health, Racquet and Sportsclub Association (IHRSA), there are more than 17,000 health clubs in the U.S. with a membership representing more than 33 million individuals. These facilities can offer an attractive, safe and effective venue for exercise and health promotion. The quality of the facilities, staffing and programs vary greatly; therefore, you will want to thoroughly evaluate the facility before making your decision. The facility should conform to all relevant laws, regulations, and published standards, including U.S. federal laws (ADA and OSHA), local government laws and regulations and local building codes and ordinances.

A quality facility provides a safe environment for exercise. It will allow you to use state-of-the-art exercise equipment and participate in any number of activity programs. Group exercise programs will give you opportunities to meet new people and exercise in a social environment.

About This Chapter: Information in this chapter is from "Selecting and Effectively Using A Health/Fitness Facility," reprinted with permission of the American College of Sports Medicine. Copyright © 2011 American College of Sports Medicine. This brochure was created and updated by Hank Williford, Ed.D., FACSM, and Michelle Olson, Ph.D., FACSM, and is a product of ACSM's Consumer Information Committee. Visit ACSM online at www.acsm.org.

Before Joining

Visit several facilities prior to making your investment. Some facilities offer a trial membership for a day or a week. Before joining, take a tour and ask questions.

Observe the classes and programs. Take into consideration whether the facility is located in an area that is convenient for you. Also, consider the following:

- Does the facility offer the type of exercise or program in which you are interested?
- Do qualified exercise instructors develop the programs?
- Will staff members modify the programs to meet your needs?
- Does the facility offer programs to address medical conditions?
- Does the facility offer programs for the age group in which you are interested?
- Does the facility offer fitness assessments and a personalized exercise program or prescription?

Safety

The staff of the facility should be able to respond to any reasonable emergency situation that threatens the safety of its members. Staff should also provide you with any information regarding potential risks associated with using the facility. Check for these safety features:

- Does the facility have a posted emergency response evacuation plan?
- Is staff qualified to execute the emergency response evacuation plan?
- Does the facility have automated external defibrillators (AEDs) onsite?
- Is the facility clean and well-maintained?
- Is the facility free from physical or environmental hazards?
- Is the facility appropriately lit?
- Does the facility have adequate heating, cooling and ventilation?
- Does the facility have adequate parking?

Pre-Activity Screening

Every adult member should be offered a pre-activity screening. Check to see if the facility provides for or adheres to the following:

- Does the facility offer a pre-activity screening, such as the PAR-Q (Physical Activity Readiness Questionnaire), to assess whether members have medical conditions or risk factors that should be addressed by a physician?

- Aside from an initial general health and wellness screening, does the facility have a health and fitness screening method appropriate for the type of exercise you will undertake?

- Does the facility offer fitness assessments?

Special Needs

If you have special needs, it is important to see if the staff of the facility can meet your needs regarding modification of equipment, facilities and programs.

A Complete Physical Activity Program

A well-rounded physical activity program includes aerobic exercise and strength training exercise, but not necessarily in the same session. This blend helps maintain or improve cardiorespiratory and muscular fitness and overall health and function. Regular physical activity will provide more health benefits than sporadic, high intensity workouts, so choose exercises you are likely to enjoy and that you can incorporate into your schedule.

The American College of Sports Medicine (ACSM)'s physical activity recommendations for healthy adults, updated in 2011, recommend at least 30 minutes of moderate-intensity physical activity (working hard enough to break a sweat, but still able to carry on a conversation) five days per week, or 20 minutes of more vigorous activity three days per week. Combinations of moderate- and vigorous-intensity activity can be performed to meet this recommendation.

Examples of typical aerobic exercises are:

- Walking
- Running
- Stair climbing
- Cycling
- Rowing
- Cross country skiing
- Swimming.

In addition, strength training should be performed a minimum of two days each week, with 8–12 repetitions of 8–10 different exercises that target all major muscle groups. This type of training can be accomplished using body weight, resistance bands, free weights, medicine balls or weight machines.

Personnel And Certification

The facility should have a professional staff that has the appropriate education and training related to their duties. Professional qualifications should include a college degree in a health-related field such as exercise science, physical education or kinesiology. Additionally, staff members should hold a certification from a nationally recognized organization such as the American College of Sports Medicine. Any certification should be based upon job-related performance criteria which have been validated by scientific research in the field and analyzed for reliability. Many certification programs do not comply with industry standards. It is important to inquire about how the certification examination was developed and administered and what the prerequisites were for participating in the certification program. Check to make sure the entire staff has credentials and education from credible institutions.

Checklist For Personnel

- Do staff members have appropriate education, certification and training recognized by the industry and the public as representing a high level of competence and credibility?

- Is there sufficient staff on site?

- Are staff members easy to recognize?

- Are the staff members friendly and helpful?

- Do staff members receive ongoing professional training?

- Do staff members provide each new member with an orientation to the equipment and/or facility?

- Are the staff members trained in cardiopulmonary resuscitation (CPR), in the use of automated external defibrillators (AEDs) and in first aid?

- Are the staff members knowledgeable about your health conditions?

- Can staff help me set realistic exercise goals?

Youth Services

If you are interested in a facility with youth programs, they should be appropriately supervised at all times. In certain parts of the country, background screening, specific training and licensure is required. Check to make sure that the facility meets your needs regarding childcare and youth programs.

Staying Active Pays Off!

Those who are physically active tend to live longer, healthier lives. Research shows that moderate physical activity—such as 30 minutes a day of brisk walking—significantly contributes to longevity. Even a person with risk factors like high blood pressure, diabetes, or even a smoking habit can gain real benefits from incorporating regular physical activity into their daily life.

As many dieters have found, exercise can help you stay on a diet and lose weight. What's more, regular exercise can help lower blood pressure, control blood sugar, improve cholesterol levels and build stronger, denser bones.

The First Step

Before you begin an exercise program, take a fitness test, or substantially increase your level of activity, make sure to answer the following questions. This physical activity readiness questionnaire (PAR-Q) will help determine if you're ready to begin an exercise routine or program.

- Has your doctor ever said that you have a heart condition or that you should participate in physical activity only as recommended by a doctor?
- Do you feel pain in your chest during physical activity?
- In the past month, have you had chest pain when you were not doing physical activity?
- Do you lose your balance from dizziness? Do you ever lose consciousness?
- Do you have a bone or joint problem that could be made worse by a change in your physical activity?
- Is your doctor currently prescribing drugs for your blood pressure or a heart condition?
- Do you know of any reason you should not participate in physical activity?

If you answered yes to one or more questions, if you are over 40 years of age and have recently been inactive, or if you are concerned about your health, consult a physician before taking a fitness test or substantially increasing your physical activity. If you answered no to each question, then it's likely that you can safely begin exercising.

Prior To Exercise

Prior to beginning any exercise program, including the activities depicted in this brochure, individuals should seek medical evaluation and clearance to engage in activity. Not all exercise programs are suitable for everyone, and some programs may result in injury. Activities should be carried out at a pace that is comfortable for the user. Users should discontinue participation in any exercise activity that causes pain or discomfort. In such event, medical consultation should be immediately obtained.

Business Practices

Before signing a contract, consider the following:

- Does the staff pressure you into purchasing a membership?

- Does the membership fee fit into your budget?

- Is there a trial membership program?

- Is there a grace period in which you can cancel your membership and receive a refund?

- Are there different membership options and are all the fees for services posted?

- Does the facility provide you with a written set of rules and policies, which govern the responsibilities of members as well as the facility?

- Does the facility have a procedure to inform members of any changes in charges, services or policies?

- Make sure you read and understand everything before signing a contract. Do not rely on verbal responses.

Ask a lot of questions so that you will have accurate information when you are making a decision.

Making an informed decision can help you avoid choosing a facility that does not fit your needs. Selecting a facility with professional and qualified staff, state-of-the-art equipment and a variety of programs is a sound investment of your money and in your health.

Chapter 17

Exercise Caution Before Spending Money On Fitness Products

Health Spas, Your Rights

Joining a health spa, fitness center, gym, or sports club can be a great way to improve your physical condition.

Nearly 33 million people are members of some 17,000 health clubs in the U.S. today, according to the International Health, Racquet & Sportsclub Association. And, although many consumers who join health clubs are pleased with their choices, others are not. They've complained to the Federal Trade Commission (FTC) about high-pressure sales tactics, misrepresentations of facilities and services, broken cancellation and refund clauses, and lost membership fees as a result of spas going out of business.

To avoid these kinds of problems, it's best to look closely at the spa's fees, contractual requirements and facilities before you join. Here are some suggestions to help you make the right choice.

Inspect The Spa

Visit the spa during the hours you would normally use it to see if it's overcrowded. Notice whether the facilities are clean and well-maintained, and note the condition of the equipment.

Ask about these items:

- Trial periods. Is there some time when you can sample the services and equipment for free?

About This Chapter: This chapter includes "Health Spas: Exercise Your Rights," May 2001, and "How's That Work-Out Working Out? Tips on Buying Fitness Gear," September 2011, both produced by the Federal Trade Commission (www.ftc.gov). Reviewed by David A. Cooke, MD, FACP, May 2012.

- Number of members. Many spas set no membership limits. While the spa may not be crowded when you visit, it may be packed during peak hours or after a membership drive.

- Hours of operation. Some spas restrict men's use to certain days and women's to others. Some may limit lower-cost memberships to certain hours.

- Instructors and trainers. Some spas hire trainers and instructors who have special qualifications. If you're looking for professionals to help you, ask about staff qualifications and longevity.

Review The Contracts

Some spas ask you to join—and pay—the first time you visit and offer incentives like special rates to entice you to sign on the spot.

Resist. Wait a few days before deciding. Take the contract home and read it carefully. Before you sign, ask yourself these questions:

- Is everything that the salesperson promised written in the contract? If a problem arises after you join, the contract probably will govern the dispute. And if something is not written in the contract, it's going to be difficult to prove your case.

- Is there a "cooling-off" period? Some spas give customers several days to reconsider after they've signed the contract.

- Could you get a refund for the unused portion of your membership if you had to cancel, say, because of a move or an injury? What if you simply stopped using the spa? Will the spa refund your money? Knowing the spa's cancellation policies is especially important if you choose a long-term membership.

- Can you join for a short time only? It may be to your advantage to join on a trial basis, say, for a few months, even if it costs a little more each month. If you're not enjoying the membership or using it as much as you had planned, you won't be committed to years of payments.

- Can you afford the payments? Consider the finance charges and annual percentage rates when you calculate the total cost of your membership. Break down the cost to weekly and even daily figures to get a better idea of what it really will cost to use the facility.

Research The Spa's History

Finally, before you join a health club, contact your local consumer protection office, state Attorney General or Better Business Bureau to find out whether they have received any complaints about the business, or whether there are state laws regulating health club memberships. If problems arise after you join, these offices also may be able to help you resolve your complaints.

Tips on Buying Fitness Gear

The benefits of exercise are well-documented. Unfortunately, that's not always the case with advertising claims for work-out gear and exercise equipment. Ready to put your best foot forward in evaluating promises you see in ads? The Federal Trade Commission, the nation's consumer protection agency, offers these tips to separate fitness facts from physical fiction.

Some advertisers say—without evidence—that their shoes, clothing, equipment, or other exercise add-ons offer a quick, easy way to shape up and lose weight. The truth is, there's no such thing as a no-work, no-sweat way to a fit, healthy body. What really gets the job done is the exercise, not how you're geared up while working out.

Looking for fitness advice that hits the spot? Avoid promises of spot reduction. Losing weight in one problem area requires regular exercise that works the whole body. Promises to effortlessly burn a spare tire or melt fat from hips and thighs—without a regular work-out routine—should cause you to raise an eyebrow.

Be skeptical of before-and-after photos from "satisfied" customers. Their experiences may not reflect the results users get.

As for those celebrity endorsements? They're no proof that the product will work as claimed, either. And what about the chiseled models in the ads? Is that six-pack the result of the product they're peddling—or months in the gym and years of healthy habits?

Shopping for work-out equipment? After you've evaluated the advertised claims—but before you buy—consider how the product fits your fitness goals. Basements, closets, and rec rooms are stocked with pricey purchases that just didn't suit the buyer's lifestyle. The only gear worth getting is something that will help you make a consistent commitment to conditioning. Before buying, give different kinds of equipment a test drive at a local gym, recreation center, or retailer.

Do the math. Some companies advertise "three easy payments of..." or "try it free for a month." But if they're not up-front about the price, what else are they hiding? The advertised price may not include sales tax, shipping, and delivery charges. Ask about refund policies, factoring in restocking fees or how much it might cost to send something back.

Consider the source. That "gotta have it" fitness product may be available at a better price from a local retailer. Or perhaps you can pocket a few bucks by comparing prices online. The benefit of working out is the "work." If a company claims it's just their product—and not your effort—that provides the benefit, keep walking. It's a sign their puffed-up ad claims could use some toning down.

For More Information

The Federal Trade Commission (FTC) works to prevent fraudulent, deceptive and unfair business practices in the marketplace and to provide information to help consumers spot, stop, and avoid them.

To file a complaint or get free information on consumer issues, visit ftc.gov or call toll-free, 877-FTC-HELP (877-382-4357); TTY: 866-653-4261. Watch a video, "How to File a Complaint," at ftc.gov/video to learn more.

Chapter 18

A Physically Active Lifestyle

What Is Physical Activity?

Physical activity is any body movement that works your muscles and requires more energy than resting. Walking, running, dancing, swimming, yoga, and gardening are a few examples of physical activity.

According to the Department of Health and Human Services' *2008 Physical Activity Guidelines for Americans*, physical activity generally refers to movement that enhances health.

Exercise is a type of physical activity that's planned and structured. Lifting weights, taking an aerobics class, and playing on a sports team are examples of exercise.

Physical activity is good for many parts of your body. This chapter focuses on the benefits of physical activity for your heart and lungs. The chapter also provides tips for getting started and staying active, and it discusses physical activity as part of a heart healthy lifestyle.

Outlook

Being physically active is one of the best ways to keep your heart and lungs healthy. Following a healthy diet and not smoking are other important ways to keep your heart and lungs healthy.

Many Americans are not active enough. The good news, though, is that even modest amounts of physical activity are good for your health. The more active you are, the more you will benefit.

About This Chapter: Information in this chapter is reprinted from "What Is Physical Activity?" National Heart Lung and Blood Institute (www.nhlbi.nih.gov), September 2011.

Types Of Physical Activity

The four main types of physical activity are aerobic, muscle-strengthening, bone-strengthening, and stretching. Aerobic activity benefits your heart and lungs the most.

Aerobic Activity

Aerobic activity moves your large muscles, such as those in your arms and legs. Running, swimming, walking, biking, dancing, and doing jumping jacks are examples of aerobic activity. Aerobic activity also is called endurance activity.

Aerobic activity makes your heart beat faster than usual. You also breathe harder during this type of activity. Over time, regular aerobic activity makes your heart and lungs stronger and able to work better.

Other Types Of Physical Activity

The other types of physical activity—muscle-strengthening, bone strengthening, and stretching—benefit your body in other ways.

Muscle-strengthening activities improve the strength, power, and endurance of your muscles. Doing push-ups and sit-ups, lifting weights, climbing stairs, and digging in the garden are examples of muscle-strengthening activities.

With bone-strengthening activities, your feet, legs, or arms support your body's weight, and your muscles push against your bones. This helps make your bones strong. Running, walking, jumping rope, and lifting weights are examples of bone-strengthening activities.

Muscle-strengthening and bone-strengthening activities also can be aerobic. Whether they are depends on whether they make your heart and lungs work harder than usual. For example, running is an aerobic activity and a bone-strengthening activity.

Stretching helps improve your flexibility and your ability to fully move your joints. Touching your toes, doing side stretches, and doing yoga exercises are examples of stretching.

Levels Of Intensity In Aerobic Activity

You can do aerobic activity with light, moderate, or vigorous intensity. Moderate- and vigorous-intensity aerobic activity is better for your heart than light-intensity activity. However, even light-intensity activity is better than no activity at all.

The level of intensity depends on how hard you have to work to do the activity. People who are less fit usually have to work harder to do an activity than people who are more fit. Thus, what is light-intensity activity for one person may be moderate-intensity for another.

Light- And Moderate-Intensity Activities

Light-intensity activities are common daily tasks that don't require much effort. Moderate-intensity activities make your heart, lungs, and muscles work harder than usual.

On a scale of 0 to 10, moderate-intensity activity is a 5 or 6. It causes noticeable increases in breathing and heart rate. A person doing moderate-intensity activity can talk but not sing.

Vigorous-Intensity Activities

Vigorous-intensity activities make your heart, lungs, and muscles work hard. On a scale of 0 to 10, vigorous-intensity activity is a 7 or 8. A person doing vigorous-intensity activity can't say more than a few words without stopping for a breath.

Examples Of Aerobic Activities

Below are examples of aerobic activities. Depending on your level of fitness, they can be light, moderate, or vigorous in intensity:

- Gardening, such as digging or hoeing that causes your heart rate to go up
- Walking, hiking, jogging, and running
- Water aerobics or swimming laps
- Biking, skateboarding, rollerblading, and jumping rope
- Ballroom dancing and aerobic dancing
- Tennis, soccer, hockey, and basketball

Benefits Of Physical Activity

Physical activity has many health benefits. These benefits apply to people of all ages and races and both sexes. For example, physical activity helps you maintain a healthy weight and makes it easier to do daily tasks, such as climbing stairs and shopping.

Physically active adults are at lower risk for depression and declines in cognitive function as they get older. (Cognitive function includes thinking, learning, and judgment skills.) Physically active children and teens may have fewer symptoms of depression than their peers.

Physical activity also lowers your risk for many diseases, such as coronary heart disease (CHD), diabetes, and cancer. Many studies have shown the clear benefits of physical activity for your heart and lungs.

Physical Activity Strengthens Your Heart And Improves Lung Function

When done regularly, moderate- and vigorous-intensity physical activity strengthens your heart muscle. This improves your heart's ability to pump blood to your lungs and throughout your body. As a result, more blood flows to your muscles, and oxygen levels in your blood rise.

Capillaries, your body's tiny blood vessels, also widen. This allows them to deliver more oxygen to your body and carry away waste products.

Physical Activity Reduces Coronary Heart Disease Risk Factors

When done regularly, moderate- and vigorous-intensity aerobic activity can lower your risk for coronary heart disease (CHD). CHD is a condition in which a waxy substance called plaque builds up inside your coronary arteries. These arteries supply your heart muscle with oxygen-rich blood.

Plaque narrows the arteries and reduces blood flow to your heart muscle. Eventually, an area of plaque can rupture (break open). This causes a blood clot to form on the surface of the plaque.

If the clot becomes large enough, it can mostly or completely block blood flow through a coronary artery. Blocked blood flow to the heart muscle causes a heart attack.

Certain traits, conditions, or habits may raise your risk for CHD. Physical activity can help control some of these risk factors because it has these effects:

- Can lower blood pressure and triglyceride levels. Triglycerides are a type of fat in the blood.

- Can raise HDL cholesterol levels. HDL sometimes is called "good" cholesterol.

- Helps your body manage blood sugar and insulin levels, which lowers your risk for type 2 diabetes.

- Reduces levels of C-reactive protein (CRP) in your body. This protein is a sign of inflammation. High levels of CRP may suggest an increased risk for CHD.

- Helps reduce overweight and obesity when combined with a reduced-calorie diet. Physical activity also helps you maintain a healthy weight over time once you have lost weight.

- May help you quit smoking. Smoking is a major risk factor for CHD.

Inactive people are nearly twice as likely to develop CHD as people who are physically active. Studies suggest that inactivity is a major risk factor for CHD, just like high blood pressure, high blood cholesterol, and smoking.

Physical Activity Reduces Heart Attack Risk

For people who have CHD, aerobic activity done regularly helps the heart work better. It also may reduce the risk of a second heart attack in people who already have had heart attacks. Vigorous aerobic activity may not be safe for people who have CHD. Ask your doctor what types of activity are safe for you.

Risks Of Physical Activity

In general, the benefits of regular physical activity far outweigh risks to the heart and lungs.

Rarely, heart problems occur as a result of physical activity. Examples of these problems include arrhythmias, sudden cardiac arrest, and heart attack. These events generally happen to people who already have heart conditions.

The risk of heart problems due to physical activity is higher for youth and young adults who have congenital heart problems. The term "congenital" means the heart problem has been present since birth.

Congenital heart problems include hypertrophic cardiomyopathy, congenital heart defects, and myocarditis. People who have these conditions should ask their doctors what types of physical activity are safe for them.

For middle-aged and older adults, the risk of heart problems due to physical activity is related to coronary heart disease (CHD). People who have CHD are more likely to have a heart attack when they're exercising vigorously than when they're not.

The risk of heart problems due to physical activity is related to your fitness level and the intensity of the activity you're doing. For example, someone who isn't physically fit is at higher risk for a heart attack during vigorous activity than a person who is physically fit.

If you have a heart problem or chronic (ongoing) disease—such as heart disease, diabetes, or high blood pressure—ask your doctor what types of physical activity are safe for you. You also should talk with your doctor about safe physical activities if you have symptoms such as chest pain or dizziness. Discuss ways that you can slowly and safely build physical activity into your daily routine.

Recommendations For Physical Activity

The U.S. Department of Health and Human Services (HHS) has released physical activity guidelines for all Americans aged 6 and older. The *2008 Physical Activity Guidelines for*

Americans explain that regular physical activity improves health. They encourage people to be as active as possible.

The guidelines recommend the types and amounts of physical activity that children, adults, older adults, and other groups should do. The guidelines also provide tips for how to fit physical activity into your daily life. The information below is based on the HHS guidelines.

Guidelines For Children And Youth

- Children and youth should do 60 minutes or more of physical activity every day. Activities should vary and be a good fit for their age and physical development. Children are naturally active, especially when they're involved in unstructured play (like recess). Any type of activity counts toward the advised 60 minutes or more.

- Most physical activity should be moderate-intensity aerobic activity. Examples include walking, running, skipping, playing on the playground, playing basketball, and biking.

- Vigorous-intensity aerobic activity should be included at least three days a week. Examples include running, doing jumping jacks, and fast swimming.

- Muscle-strengthening activities should be included at least three days a week. Examples include playing on playground equipment, playing tug-of-war, and doing push-ups and pull-ups.

- Bone-strengthening activities should be included at least three days a week. Examples include hopping, skipping, doing jumping jacks, playing volleyball, and working with resistance bands.

Children and youth who have disabilities should work with their doctors to find out what types and amounts of physical activity are safe for them. When possible, these children should meet the recommendations in the guidelines.

Some experts also advise that children and youth reduce screen time because it limits time for physical activity. They recommend that children aged 2 and older should spend no more than two hours a day watching television or using a computer (except for school work).

Getting Started And Staying Active

Physical activity is an important part of a heart healthy lifestyle. To get started and stay active, make physical activity part of your daily routine, keep track of your progress, be active and safe, and talk with your doctor if you have a chronic (ongoing) health condition.

Make Physical Activity Part Of Your Daily Routine

You don't have to be a marathon runner to benefit from physical activity. Do activities that you enjoy, and make them part of your daily routine.

If you haven't been active for a while, start slowly and build up your level of activity. Many people like to start with walking and slowly increase their time and distance. You also can take other steps, such as those described below, to make physical activity part of your routine.

Personalize The Benefits

People value different things. Some people may highly value the health benefits from physical activity. Others want to be active because they enjoy recreational activities or they want to look better or sleep better.

Some people want to be active because it helps them lose weight or it gives them a chance to spend time with friends. Figure out which benefits of physical activity you value, and focus on those.

Be Active With Friends And Family

Friends and family can help you stay active. For example, go hiking with a friend, take dancing lessons, or play ball with your friends. The possibilities are endless.

Make Everyday Activities More Active

You can make your daily routine more active. For example, take the stairs instead of the elevator. Rake the leaves in your yard instead of using a leaf blower.

Reward Yourself With Time For Physical Activity

Sometimes going for a bike ride or a long walk relieves stress after a long day. Think of physical activity as a special time to refresh your body and mind.

Keep Track Of Your Progress

Consider keeping a log of your activity. A log can help you track your progress. Many people like to wear pedometers (small devices that counts steps) to track how much they walk every day. These tools can help you set goals and stay motivated.

Be Active And Safe

Physical activity is safe for almost everyone. You can take steps to make sure it's safe for you. For example:

- Be active on a regular basis to raise your fitness level.

- Do activities that fit your health goals and fitness level. Start slowly and build up your activity level over time. As your fitness improves, you will be able to increase the length and intensity of your activity.

- Spread out your activity over the week and vary the types of activity you do.

- Use the proper gear and equipment to protect yourself. For example, use bike helmets, elbow and knee pads, and goggles.

- Be active in safe environments. Pick well-lit and well-maintained places that are clearly separated from car traffic.

- Follow safety rules and policies, such as always wearing a helmet when biking.

- Make sensible choices about when, where, and how to be active. Consider weather conditions (such as how hot or cold it is), and change your plans as needed.

Talk With Your Doctor If Needed

Healthy people who don't have heart problems may not need to check with their doctors before starting moderate-intensity physical activities. If you have a heart problem or chronic disease—such as heart disease, diabetes, or high blood pressure—ask your doctor what types of physical activity are safe for you. You also should ask your doctor about safe physical activities if you have symptoms such as chest pain or dizziness.

Physical Activity As Part Of A Heart Healthy Lifestyle

Physical activity is one part of a heart healthy lifestyle. A healthy lifestyle also involves maintaining a healthy weight, following a healthy diet, and not smoking.

Maintain A Healthy Weight

Being overweight or obese increases your risk for heart disease, even if you have no other risk factors. Overweight or obesity also raises your risk for other diseases that play a role in heart disease, such as diabetes and high blood pressure.

Your weight is the result of a balance between energy IN and energy OUT. Energy IN is the energy, or calories, you take in from food. Energy OUT is the energy you use for things like breathing, digestion, and physical activity.

- If you have the same amount of energy IN and energy OUT over time, your weight stays the same

- If you have more energy IN than energy OUT over time, you will gain weight

- If you have more energy OUT than energy IN over time, you will lose weight

To maintain a healthy weight, your energy IN and energy OUT should balance each other. They don't have to be the same every day; it's the balance over time that matters.

Balancing energy IN and energy OUT with diet or physical activity alone is possible. However, research shows that being physically active and following a healthy diet is a better way to reach and stay at a healthy weight.

People who want to lose more than 5 percent of their body weight need to do a lot of physical activity unless they also reduce their calorie intake. The same is true for people who are trying to keep off a lot of weight that they have lost.

Many people need to do more than 300 minutes (5 hours) of moderate-intensity activity a week to meet their weight-control goals.

Follow A Healthy Diet

Following a healthy diet can help you maintain good health. A healthy diet includes a variety of vegetables and fruits. These foods can be fresh, canned, frozen, or dried. A good rule is to try to fill half of your plate with vegetables and fruits.

A healthy diet also includes whole grains, fat-free or low-fat dairy products, and protein foods, such as lean meats, poultry without skin, seafood, processed soy products, nuts, seeds, beans, and peas.

Choose and prepare foods with little sodium (salt). Too much salt can raise your risk for high blood pressure. Studies show that following the Dietary Approaches to Stop Hypertension (DASH) eating plan can lower blood pressure.

Try to avoid foods and drinks that are high in added sugars. For example, drink water instead of sugary drinks, like soda.

Also, try to limit the amount of solid fats and refined grains that you eat. Solid fats are saturated fat and trans fatty acids. Refined grains come from processing whole grains, which results in a loss of nutrients (such as dietary fiber).

If you drink alcohol, do so in moderation. Too much alcohol can raise your blood pressure and triglyceride level. (Triglycerides are a type of fat found in the blood.) Alcohol also adds extra calories, which can cause weight gain.

Don't Smoke

People who smoke are up to six times more likely to have a heart attack than people who don't smoke. The risk of having a heart attack increases with the number of cigarettes smoked each day. Smoking also raises your risk for stroke and lung diseases, such as COPD (chronic obstructive pulmonary disease) and lung cancer.

Quitting smoking can greatly reduce your risk for heart and lung diseases. Ask your doctor about programs and products that can help you quit. Also, try to avoid secondhand smoke.

If you have trouble quitting smoking on your own, consider joining a support group. Many hospitals, workplaces, and community groups offer classes to help people quit smoking.

10 Ideas To Stay Active

We know you've got a lot of homework, but take it from us, you can fit activity into your life. Here are some easy ways to get started.

- Take your dog for a walk.
- Start up a playground kickball game.
- Join a sports team.
- Go to the park with a friend.
- Help your parents with yard work.
- Play tag with kids in your neighborhood.
- Ride your bike to school.
- Walk to the store.
- See how many jumping jacks you can do.
- Race a friend to the end of the block.

Source: "Get Motivated: 10 Ideas To Stay Active," reprinted with permission from www.presidentschallege.org. © 2012 The President's Challenge.

Part Three
Exercise Fundamentals

Chapter 19

Kinds of Exercise

You need to exercise for about 60 minutes every day. Setting aside 60 minutes all at once each day is one way to get in enough exercise. If you wait until the end of the day to squeeze it in, you probably won't exercise enough or at all. If you're not active for 60 minutes straight, it's okay to exercise for 10 or 20 minutes at a time throughout the day.

Different Exercises

No matter what your shape—apple, pear, ruler, or hourglass—there's an exercise for you!

- Pick exercises you like to do and choose a few different options so you don't get bored.

- Aim to exercise most days of the week. If you're not very active right now, start slowly and work your way up to being active every day.

Children and adolescents should do 60 minutes (1 hour) or more of physical activity daily. You should combine the different kinds of exercise below to total 60 minutes each day. For example, you could do 35 minutes of swimming, 10 minutes of push-ups, and 15 minutes of jumping rope to reach 60 minutes.

Even if you have a disability, you should also exercise at least 60 minutes each day. Talk to your doctor about what exercises are right for you. Read more about staying active with a disability.

There are many levels and kinds of exercise that can keep your body healthy. Learn more about different kinds of exercise and how they work!

About This Chapter: Information in this chapter is reprinted from "Fitness Basics," Office on Women's Health (www.girlshealth.gov), October 9, 2010.

Table 19.1. Guidelines For Different Exercises

Exercise Type	How often?	What is it?	Why do it?
Aerobic exercise	Most of your 60 minutes of daily exercise, at least 3 days a week.	Aerobic activities are those in which young people regularly move their muscles. Running, hopping, skipping, jumping rope, swimming, dancing, and biking are all examples of aerobic activity.	It makes your heart and lungs strong.
Muscle-strengthening exercise (3 or more days each week)	As part of your 60 minutes of exercise each day, at least 3 days a week.	Muscle-strengthening activities make muscles do more work than usual. This is called "overload" and it makes your muscles stronger. Climbing trees, yoga, rock climbing, lifting weights, or working with resistance bands are all muscle-strengthening exercises	It increases your strength and builds muscle.
Bone-strengthening exercise (3 or more days each week)	As part of your 60 minutes of exercise each day, at least 3 days a week.	Bone-strengthening activities push on your bones and help them grow and be strong. This push usually comes from impact with the ground. Running, jumping rope, basketball, tennis, and hopscotch are all bone-strengthening exercises. (These exercises can also be aerobic and muscle-strengthening.)	It will make your bones stronger. Your bones get strongest in the years just before and during puberty.

Levels Of Exercise

There are three levels of physical activity.

- **Light:** Not sweating; not breathing hard (slow walking, dancing)

- **Moderate:** Breaking a sweat; can talk but can't sing (walking fast, dancing)

- **Vigorous:** Sweating, breathing hard, can't talk or sing (running, swimming laps)

No matter what level at which you are exercising, the activity can be one of three types: aerobic exercise, muscle-strengthening exercise, or bone-strengthening exercise.

It's important to remember that as you exercise more and more, activities that were once vigorous may become moderate. Don't be afraid to challenge yourself! After several weeks or months of training, try jogging for longer distances or at a faster rate.

Table 19.2. Examples of moderate- and vigorous-intensity aerobic physical activities and muscle- and bone-strengthening activities for children and adolescents

Type of Physical Activity	Age Group Children	Age Group Adults
Moderate–intensity aerobic	• Active recreation, such as hiking, skateboarding, roller-blading • Bicycle riding • Brisk walking	• Active recreation, such as canoeing, hiking, skateboarding, rollerblading • Brisk walking • Bicycle riding (stationary or road bike) • Housework and yard work, such as sweeping or pushing a lawn mower • Games that require catching and throwing, such as baseball and softball
Vigorous–intensity aerobic	• Active games involving running and chasing, such as tag • Bicycle riding • Jumping rope • Martial arts, such as karate • Running • Sports such as soccer, ice or field hockey, basketball, swimming, tennis • Cross-country skiing	• Active games involving running and chasing, such as flag football • Bicycle riding • Jumping rope • Martial arts, such as karate • Running • Sports such as soccer, ice or field hockey, basketball, swimming, tennis • Vigorous dancing • Cross-country skiing
Muscle-strengthening	• Games such as tug-of-war • Modified push-ups (with knees on the floor) • Resistance exercises using body weight or resistance bands • Rope or tree climbing • Sit-ups (curl-ups or crunches) • Swinging on playground equipment/bars	• Games such as tug-of-war • Push-ups and pull-ups • Resistance exercises with exercise bands, weight machines, hand-held weights • Climbing wall • Sit-ups (curl-ups or crunches)
Bone-strengthening	• Games such as hopscotch • Hopping, skipping, jumping • Jumping rope • Running • Sports such as gymnastics, basketball, volleyball, tennis	• Hopping, skipping, jumping • Jumping rope • Running • Sports such as gymnastics, basketball, volleyball, tennis

Note: Some activities, such as bicycling, can be moderate or vigorous intensity, depending upon level of effort

Source: *2008 Physical Activity Guidelines for Americans*, Chapter 3.

What Kind Of Exercise Does Your Body Need?

Exercise should increase your heart rate and move the muscles in your body. Examples include swimming, dancing, skating, playing soccer, or riding a bike.

Exercise should include something from each of these four basic fitness areas:

Cardio-respiratory endurance is the same thing as aerobic endurance. It means using your heart and lungs nonstop. When you exercise, your heart beats faster, sending more needed oxygen throughout your body. If you are not fit, your heart and lungs have to work harder during exercise. Long runs and swims are examples of activities that can help your heart and lungs work better over a long period of time.

Muscular strength is the ability to move a muscle against a resistance. To become stronger, you need to push or pull against resistance, such as your own weight (like in push-ups), using free weights (note: talk to an instructor before using weights), or even pushing the vacuum cleaner. Regular exercise keeps all of your muscles strong and makes it easier to do daily physical tasks.

Muscular endurance is the ability of a muscle, or a group of muscles, to keep pushing against resistance for a long period. Push-ups are often used to test endurance of arm and shoulder muscles. Aerobic exercise also helps to improve your muscular endurance. Activities such as running increase your heart rate and make your heart muscle stronger.

Flexibility exercises stretch your muscles and make them long. Reaching for your toes is a good measure of flexibility of the lower back and backs of the upper legs. When you are flexible, you are able to bend and reach with ease. Being flexible can help prevent injuries like pulled muscles. This is why warming up and stretching are so important. If you force your body to move in a way that you aren't used to, you risk tearing muscles, as well as ligaments and tendons (other parts of your musculoskeletal system). Yoga increases muscle-strength and flexibility.

Chapter 20

Cardiovascular (Cardio) Exercise

With a large percentage of Americans overweight, it's clear that many of us are not following the latest exercise guidelines that prescribe an hour of exercise a day. In fact, there was no doubt a collective groan when people realized they would now have to find an hour each day to do something they can't seem to find five minutes for. How important are these guidelines and what can you do to make them fit into your life?

The Simple Facts About Cardio

Before we talk about how much cardio you should do, you should at least know why it's so important. Cardiovascular exercise simply means that you're involved in an activity that raises your heart rate to a level where you're working, but can still talk (aka, in your Target Heart Rate Zone). Here's why cardio is so important:

- It's one way to burn calories and help you lose weight.

- It makes your heart strong so that it doesn't have to work as hard to pump blood.

- It increases your lung capacity.

- It helps reduce risk of heart attack, high cholesterol, high blood pressure, and diabetes.

- It makes you feel good.

- It helps you sleep better.

- It helps reduce stress.

About This Chapter: "Cardio 101—The Facts About Cardio," © 2012 About.com. Used with permission of About, Inc. which can be found online at www.About.com. All rights reserved.

- I could go on all day, but you get the point.

Bottom line: You need cardio if you want to get your weight under control and get your stress to a tolerable level.

Choosing Your Cardio

Your first step is to choose what kind of activities you'd like to do. The trick is to think about what's accessible to you, what fits your personality, and what you'd feel comfortable fitting into your life. If you like to go outdoors, running, cycling, hiking or walking are all good choices. If you like the gym, you'll have access to stationary bikes, elliptical trainers, treadmills, rowing machines, Stairmasters, and more.

For the home exerciser, there are a number of excellent exercise videos to try and you don't need much equipment to get a great home cardio workout.

Just about any activity will work, as long as it involves a movement that gets your heart rate into your Target Heart Rate Zone. Remember:

- There is no "best" cardio exercise. Anything that you enjoy and that gets your heart rate up fits the bill
- It's not what you do, but how hard you work. Any exercise can be challenging if you make it that way
- Do something you enjoy. If you hate gym workouts, don't force yourself onto a treadmill. If you like socializing, consider sports, group fitness, working out with a friend, or a walking club.
- Choose something you can see yourself doing at least three days a week.
- Be flexible, and don't be afraid to branch out once you get comfortable with exercise.

How Long Should You Exercise?

After you choose what to do, the most important element of your workout will now be how long you do it. You should work on duration before you work on anything else—it's more important to work on continuous exercise than to worry about how fast you're going or how hard you're working. If you're a beginner, start with 10–20 minutes and add more time to each workout until you're up to 30 minutes.

The official guidelines say to work out for 30–60 minutes most days of the week, but don't feel like you have to start at that level if you're not ready. Feel free to:

- Split your workouts into smaller workouts throughout the day.

- Take a few minutes here and there for some stair-climbing or speed walking.

- Do all those things you know you should be doing: take the stairs, walk more, stop driving around looking for that front row parking space, etc.

- Make the time. People who work out don't have more time than people who don't. They've just practiced making exercise a priority. Scheduling your workouts and treating them like any other appointment you wouldn't miss may help you stick to your program.

- Pay someone to make you exercise. Finding a good personal trainer can make a difference when it comes to motivation and reaching your goals.

- Do something...anything. If you think five minutes isn't enough time to work out, you couldn't be more wrong. Whether it's five minutes, 10 minutes or 60 minutes, every single minute counts.

Keep in mind that doing too much cardio is a no-no as well and can actually backfire. There is a point of diminishing returns, so keep it reasonable (3–6 days a week, depending on your fitness level), vary your intensity, and don't forget to take rest days when needed.

How Often Should You Exercise?

The frequency of your workouts will depend on your fitness level and your schedule. Beginners should start with about three nonconsecutive days of cardio and work their way up to more frequent sessions. The general guidelines are:

- To maintain current fitness level: 2–4 days a week (at least 20 minutes)

- To lose weight: Four or more days a week (at least 30 minutes)

- To train for a triathlon: A whole lot.

What happens if you can't follow the guidelines? If you're still working on building the endurance and conditioning, it may take a few weeks to work your way up to more frequent exercises. If it's a busy schedule that stands in your way or other obstacles, do your best to work out as many days as you can try to squeeze something in, even if it's just a five or ten-minute brisk walk, on the other days.

Keep in mind that if you can't follow the guidelines because of your busy schedule, you may have trouble reaching your weight loss goals. If you can't do the work required to reach your goals, you may have to change your lifestyle or, if that isn't working, change your goal to fit where you are in your exercise or weight loss experience.

How Hard Do You Need To Work?

Once you've gotten used to exercise (and are up to 30 minutes of continuous movement) you can start working on your intensity. How hard you work is a crucial factor in your workout because:

- How hard you work is directly related to how many calories you burn.

- Raising intensity is the best way to burn more calories when you're short on time..

- It's an easy part of your workout to change—all you do is work harder.

- It's easy to monitor with a heart rate monitor or perceived exertion scale.

So how hard should you work? That depends on several factors including your fitness level and your goals. There are three different levels of intensity you can focus on during your workouts, and you can even incorporate all of these levels into the same workout:

- **High Intensity Cardio:** This falls between about 75–85% of your maximum heart rate (MHR) if you're using heart rate zones, or a 7 to 8 on this perceived exertion scale. What this translates to is exercise at a level that feels challenging and leaves you too breathless to talk much. If you're a beginner, you may want to work up to this level or try interval training so that you work harder for shorter periods of time.

- **Moderate Intensity Cardio:** This level falls between about 60–70% of your MHR (a level 4 to 6 on this perceived exertion scale). The American College of Sports Medicine (ACSM) often recommends this level of intensity in its exercise guidelines. This is the level you typically want to shoot for during your workouts.

- **Low Intensity Cardio:** This type of exercise is considered to be below about 50–55% of your MHR, or about a level 3 to 5 on this perceived exertion scale. This is a good level to work at during your warm ups or when you're squeezing in other activities, like walking, throughout the day.

Keep in mind that your target heart rate calculation isn't 100% accurate so you might want to use a combination of perceived exertion and your heart rate to find a range that works for you.

Chapter 21

Start Running

Tips For Beginning Runners

Take stock of your current health and fitness level.

If you have been sedentary, have or suspect health problems such as heart disease, diabetes, high blood pressure, high cholesterol, joint problems, etc., (or for adults who are over 40), it is recommended that you have a physical with your doctor before starting a vigorous exercise program. If you know you have no major health problems, starting a light to moderate intensity exercise program such as brisk walking usually does not require a physical, but check with your doctor for his or her opinion in your specific case. Remember that the health risks of a sedentary lifestyle are much greater than the risks of exercise. A renowned exercise physiologist, Per Olaf Astrand, quipped that if one plans a sedentary lifestyle, one should have a physical to see if the heart can stand it!

Be safe.

Don't run/walk in high crime areas. When running after dark, be sure to wear reflective clothing, carry a small flashlight, and assume drivers don't see you. Well-lighted neighborhoods are a good choice. Women should run with a partner, or a dog if possible, and consider carrying pepper spray. Runners and walkers should never use headphones outdoors, as it makes it impossible to hear traffic or an approaching attacker. Always carry ID.

About This Chapter: "Starting a Running Program," by Matt Rogers, MS, CSCS, U.S. Department of Homeland Security (www.cbp.gov), February 26, 2009.

Start slowly and build up gradually.

Most people should start with a brisk walking program and progress to a mix of alternating walking and jogging. Eventually you should be able to run the entire distance you desire at a comfortable pace. At that point you can increase weekly mileage about 10% every third week, depending on your goals. For health and fitness there is generally no need to run more than about 15 miles per week, along with some strength and flexibility training. Those wishing to progress to competitive running should seek out experienced runners or coaches for advice. Check the Road Runners Club of America website for a running club in your area (http://www.rrca.org).

Using the right type of shoes helps prevent injuries.

Shin splints and runner's knee are preventable with proper conditioning AND the right running shoe type. There are three basic types for different running mechanics:

- **Motion Control:** Generally best choice for flat feet and "floppy ankles" (over pronation or rolling too far to the inside after foot touches down). Shoes should be straight lasted and often will have a full board last inside plus a harder rubber or plastic area on the inner (arch support) side of heel to control excess movement.

- **Stability:** Generally best for normal arches, will have a semi-curved last and a moderate amount of motion control.

- **Cushioned:** Generally best for high arches and "clunk foot"; these feet are usually very rigid and under pronate, that is, feet do not roll to the inside far enough after foot touches down and therefore make poor shock absorbers. Shoes should have a curved or semi-curved last, extra cushioning, a full slip last (no board inside), and be very flexible.

Another choice, for off road running are trail running shoes. These are made low to the ground and more stable to help prevent ankle sprains, have good traction, and help prevent foot bruises from roots, rocks, etc.

Don't use any type running shoes for other sports, as they are not made for lateral movements, making ankle sprains more likely. They also last longer and maintain cushioning better if only used for running. Use only good quality court shoes or cross-trainers for other conditioning activities. Wrestling shoes are recommended for defensive tactics training on matted floors.

Do the "wet test" to see what type of foot you have.

Wet feet and step onto some paper on a hard surface. (Even better is to run a short distance barefoot on sand.) A "blob" footprint with little arch indicates flat feet. Two "islands" with a lot of space between the heel and ball indicates high arches. A normal arch will look like the classic cartoon footprint.

Make sure the shoe fits!

The best shoe for you is one that fits your foot type and running mechanics and also is the right length and width. Try on running shoes with the socks you plan to run in and toward the end of the day when feet are larger. You should have about one thumb's width of room between your longest toe and the end of the shoe. Shoes should be wide enough that foot does not feel pinched on the sides, but not a sloppy fit or one that slips at the heel. Jog a bit in the store to see how the shoes feel and fit. Most running specialty stores will have the expertise and take the time to fit you properly in several models and watch you run in them before you choose. Don't count on the employees of a general sporting goods or discount footwear store understanding any of the above running shoe information.

Dress for the weather.

In cold weather wear several lightweight layers, hat, and gloves to trap body heat. You can unzip or remove layers if you get too warm. In hot weather wear as little as the law allows, and don't forget the sunscreen. Drink plenty of fluids throughout the day to avoid dehydration and plan ahead so you can get fluids during longer runs.

Run with good form.

Shoulders should be relaxed with elbows bent to about 90 degrees as arms swing smoothly forward and back with no twisting of the torso. Arms should not cross the center of body and hands should pass just above the hip pocket on each forward and backward motion. The upper body should be nearly upright, with a very slight forward lean. Don't run on the toes or hit hard with the heel, but rather land as softly as possible with foot nearly flat. The foot should be flexed upward slightly just before foot lands. Breathe naturally through both the nose and mouth. If you're gasping for air—slow down!

Most running injuries are avoidable!

Following the tips on proper footwear, form, and starting slowly will greatly reduce your chances of common beginners' complaints such as shin splints and knee pain. Basic strength and flexibility exercises can prevent and correct muscle imbalances responsible for most running injuries. If you do have a running injury, find the cause rather than just treating the symptoms.

Ignore the myths.

The bulk of scientific evidence shows that running, even in ultra-marathon runners, does not cause osteoarthritis in the hips or knees if these joints were healthy to begin with. In fact, weight-bearing exercise such as running probably prevents arthritis, since the incidence in long-time runners is about half that of non-runners, including swimmers.

Chapter 22

Calisthenics

Calisthenics are a type of repetitive, rhythmic exercise. Calisthenics are an integral part of a well-rounded physical fitness program because they develop both muscular and aerobic endurance. They are used to warm up and limber the body for sports activities or weight-resistant training and also for cooling down afterward. Calisthenics are low-resistance, high-repetition training.

Individuals can test their level of fitness with push-ups, toe touches, knee-bends, or sit-ups. Beginners will find that more than just a few repetitions require a combination of strength and muscular endurance. Certain calisthenics are helpful in training for particular sports. For example, pushups develop the upper body endurance needed for rowing. Special equipment is not necessary and the exercises allow for concentration on particular areas of the body.

Stair climbing and jumping rope are not considered to be calisthenics but may supplement a calisthenics routine. Computerized stationary climbers such as the StairMaster® are excellent for aerobic training and provide a good workout for the legs. Hand rails are used for maintaining balance (users are cautioned not to grip the hand rails tightly). The Versa Climber is a ladder-like stationary climbing device that works the upper and lower body while training the cardiovascular system. Many athletes jump rope as part of their warm-up and cool-down routines. Jumping rope develops strength, coordination, and endurance.

About This Chapter: Excerpted and Adapted from "Physical Fitness: A Guide for Individuals with Lower Limb Loss," U.S. Department of Veterans Affairs, 1993. Reviewed by David A. Cooke, MD, FACP, May 2012.

Jump Rope

Jump rope is just a fun game that girls play in their backyards or on the playground, right? No way!

Jump rope works the upper and lower legs, heart and lungs, and upper arms. In addition to being a great aerobic workout, jumpers of all ages can compete nationally in categories such as speed, freestyle, and double dutch—which is where two ropes are turned like an egg-beater by two turners, while one or two people jump within the moving ropes.

Ropes

Not all ropes are actually made of rope. Ropes come in cloth (regular rope), speed (skinny cord), beaded (plastic beads that clack when they hit the ground), and even electric.

Play It Safe

Avoid spills—set the right length for your rope. To find out what that is, stand on the center of the cord and pull the handles up so they fit right under your arms. When you jump over the rope, the rope should just brush the floor under your feet. If it doesn't touch the floor, it's too short. If it hits the floor in front of your feet, it's too long.

Source: Excerpted from "Jump Rope Activity Card," Body And Mind (BAM!), Centers for Disease Control and Prevention (www.bam.gov); accessed May 19, 2012.

Jumping Jacks

Purpose

- Warm-up and/or cool-down exercise for the entire body.

Procedure

- Begin by standing with feet together and hands at sides.

- Simultaneously bring your hands together directly above your head, jump, and split both legs wider than shoulder-width

- Without stopping, jump both legs back together and bring arms down to the sides of the body.

- Gradually work up to at least 20 repetitions.

Neck Rolls

Purpose

- Stretches and exercises the neck muscles.

Procedure (Clockwise Rotation)

This exercise may be done while standing or seated.

- Bend the neck until the chin touches the chest.
- Roll the head to the right until the right ear touches the right shoulder.
- Roll the head back, bringing the chin up as far as possible.
- Roll the head to the left until the left ear touches the left shoulder.
- Repeat first four steps.
- Rest (20–30 seconds); then perform the exercise in two counter-clockwise rotations.
- Fifteen to 20 repetitions are recommended for each rotation sequence.

Free-Hand Neck Resistance

Purpose

- Develops strength in the neck muscles. This exercise is often used as a warm-up for weightlifting exercise.

Procedure: Front

- Interlock fingers and place both hands with the backs of the hands against the forehead.
- Push the hands and head against each other.
- Start with the head back and push forward.

Procedure: Back

- Interlock fingers and place both hands with the palm side on the back of the head.
- Again push the hands against the head.
- Start with the head forward and push backward.

Procedure: Sides

- Place the right palm against the right side of the head.

- Start with the head on the left shoulder and push it against the hand as the hand resists.

- Continue until the head is resting on the right shoulder.

- Do the same with the left hand on the left side of the head.

- Repeat the entire sequence (front to back to sides) 15 to 20 times.

Arm Circles

This exercise may be performed while either standing or sitting.

Purpose

- Exercises the shoulders, arms, and the upper back.

Procedure

- Stand with the feet shoulder-width apart and arms full length at each side. Bring both arms to shoulder height and move them in a small circular motion.

- Begin by circling forward for 15 to 20 repetitions, then circle the arms backward for 15 to 20 repetitions.

- Bring both arms down to the sides of the body and relax for about 10 seconds before beginning a second set of the exercise.

- Vary the size of the circles from small to large and increase the speed. This will assist in limbering the shoulders and upper back.

Alternating Toe Touches With Bar

Purpose

- Warm-up and cool-down exercise for muscles of the upper body, shoulders, arms, abdominal muscles, and the hamstrings. The bar helps to keep the shoulders straight while performing this exercise.

Procedure

- Place a bar (about 36 inches in length) on the shoulders and hold it on both ends by wrapping arms around.
- Bend from the waist, keeping the torso approximately parallel to the floor. (Try not to bend the knees.)
- Twist the body in a smooth motion so that the left hand touches the right foot. The right arm will be extended in the air.
- Raise to an upright position and repeat for the other side.
- Fifteen to 20 repetitions are recommended.
- Suggested sequence: Toe touch left hand to right foot. Upright. Toe touch right hand to left foot. Upright. Repeat the sequence 15 to 20 times.

Caution: Stretch gradually, do not bounce. Bouncing may stretch the muscles too far and possibly cause injury.

Trunk Twists

Purpose

- Helps develop muscle tone on the waistline and upper body, including increased flexibility of the neck.

Procedure

- Keep the feet planted on the floor and spaced a bit wider than the shoulders.
- Raise both arms to chest height, keeping the elbows slightly bent.
- Twist side to side from the waist. Try to rotate far enough so that each shoulder reaches at least the midline of the body.
- Twist on both sides 15 to 20 times.

Variation

- Place a bar (about 36 inches in length) on the shoulders and hold it at both ends.
- Keeping both feet on the floor with knees straight but relaxed keep hips still and twist from the waist to each side.

Caution: Stretch gradually, do not bounce. Bouncing may stretch the muscles too far and possibly cause injury.

Abductor/Adductor Leg Raise

Purpose

- Works the muscles of the inner thigh and outer thigh.

Procedure 1: Abductors

- Lie on one side with one arm holding the head up and the other resting at the waist (beginners may use this arm as additional support by placing the palm of the hand on the floor).
- Keeping both legs straight, raise the top leg about 12 to 15 inches from the floor.
- Hold at the high position for a few seconds before lowering the leg.
- Raise the leg up only high enough to maintain tension on the abductors.
- Fifteen to 20 repetitions are recommended.

Procedure 2: Adductors

- Lift the bottom leg in front of the other leg. (You will not be able to raise it as high as you were able to raise the top leg.)
- Hold the high position for a few seconds before lowering the leg.
- Fifteen to 20 repetitions are recommended.

Prone Leg Extension

Purpose

- Develops the hamstring and gluteal muscles.

Procedure

- Lie on the floor in a prone position.
- Alternate raising one leg at a time by extending from the hip. Keep both legs as straight as possible.

- Bring each leg up as high as possible in order to gain the full benefit from the exercise before lowering the leg.

- Work each leg separately doing 15 to 20 repetitions per set, then switch legs. No rest is necessary between sets.

Variation

- Hold the fully raised position for a few seconds, contracting the muscles of the hamstring and gluteus. Then lower the leg slowly to the floor.

Caution: Low back hypertension against resistance can cause undue stress to the spine. Observe caution; do not strain this area.

Standing One-Legged Toe Raise

Purpose

- Develops strength and definition in the gastrocnemius/soleus muscles.

Procedure

- Stand with your feet close together. Hold onto a support with one or both hands.

- Raise up on your toes on one side. Hold the position at the top for a few seconds before lowering the heel.

- Perform this exercise in a slow, controlled motion.

- For full calf development use three positions: Point toes straight ahead to work calf muscle in general. Point toes inward to work outer calf specifically. Point toes outward to work inner calf specifically.

- Fifteen to 20 repetitions on each side are recommended.

Variation

- For a greater range of motion, stand on a raised step with your heel off the edge so that it may be lowered further. The standing toe raise may also be done while using barbells.

Chapter 23

Strength Training

Strength training is a vital part of a balanced exercise routine that includes aerobic activity and flexibility exercises.

Regular aerobic exercise, such as running or using a stationary bike, makes your muscles use oxygen more efficiently and strengthens your heart and lungs. When you strength train with weights, you're using your muscles to work against the extra pounds (this concept is called resistance). This strengthens and increases the amount of muscle mass in your body by making your muscles work harder than they're used to.

Most people who work out with weights typically use two different kinds: *free weights* (including barbells, dumbbells, and hand weights) and *weight machines*. Free weights usually work a group of muscles at the same time; weight machines typically are designed to help you isolate and work on a specific muscle.

Most gyms or weight rooms set up their machines in a *circuit*, or group, of exercises that you perform to strengthen different groups of muscles.

People can also use resistance bands and even their own body weight (as in pushups, sit-ups, or body weight squats) for strength training.

Many people tend to lump all types of weightlifting together, but there's a big difference between strength training, powerlifting, and competitive bodybuilding!

About This Chapter: "Strength Training," May 2009, reprinted with permission from www.kidshealth.org. This information was provided by KidsHealth®, one of the largest resources online for medically reviewed health information written for parents, kids, and teens. For more articles like this, visit www.KidsHealth.org or www.TeensHealth.org. Copyright © 1995-2012 The Nemours Foundation. All rights reserved.

Strength training uses resistance methods like free weights, weight machines, resistance bands, or a person's own weight to build muscles and strength. Olympic lifting, or powerlifting, which people often think of when they think of weightlifting, concentrates on how much weight a person can lift at one time. Competitive bodybuilding involves evaluating muscle definition and symmetry, as well as size.

Powerlifting, competitive weightlifting, and bodybuilding are not recommended for teens who are still maturing. That's because these types of activity can cause serious injuries to growing bones, muscles, and joints.

Getting Started

If you've started puberty, your body will have begun making the hormones necessary to help build muscle in response to weight training. If you haven't started puberty, though, you'll still be able to get stronger—you just won't see your muscles getting bigger.

Before you start strength training, you should be checked out by your doctor to make sure it's safe for you to lift weights.

Any time you start a new sport or activity, start out slowly so that your body gets used to the increase in activity. Even if you think you're not exerting yourself very much, if you've never lifted weights before, your muscles may be sore when you wake up the next day. And, because of something called delayed onset muscle soreness, the pain may be at its worst two or three days after you first exercise.

Before you begin any type of strength training routine, get some guidance and expert advice. Your coach or trainer can give you advice on how many times a week you should lift and what kinds of warm-up and cool-down activities you should do before and after lifting to avoid soreness or injury. Many trainers who work at schools, gyms, and in weight rooms are knowledgeable about strength training, but it's best to get advice from someone who is a certified fitness expert and experienced working with teens.

When lifting weights—either free weights or on a machine—make sure that there's always someone nearby to supervise, or *spot*, you. This person, called a spotter, encourages you and also can act as your coach, telling you if you're not doing a particular exercise correctly.

Having a spotter nearby is particularly important when using free weights. Even someone in great shape sometimes just can't make that last rep. It's no big deal if you're doing bicep curls; all you'll have to do is drop the weight onto the floor. But if you're in the middle of a bench press—a chest exercise where you're lying on a bench and pushing a loaded barbell away from your chest—it's easy to become trapped under a heavy weight. A spotter can keep you from dropping the barbell onto your chest.

Many schools offer weight or circuit training as units in their gym classes. Check to see if you can sign up. Don't be afraid to ask for pointers and tips about how much weight to start with and how to develop a routine.

What Are Some Dangers of Strength Training?

You may love the challenge of lifting, especially if you and your friends do it together. You'll definitely see results over a few months in your ability to progressively lift more weight. But there are a few things to look out for.

Because your bones, joints, and tendons are still growing and developing, it's easy to overdo it and strain or even permanently damage them. When you're in the middle of a strength-training session and something doesn't feel right to you, you feel pain, or if you hear or feel a "pop" when you're in the middle of a workout, stop what you're doing and have a doctor check it out before you resume training. It's possible you may need to modify your training or even stop lifting weights for a while to allow the injury to heal.

Another danger surrounding strength training is the use of anabolic steroids or other performance-enhancing drugs and preparations that supposedly help muscles develop. Steroid use is widespread in many sports—including football, swimming, biking, track and field, and baseball. But because many of their long-term effects on the body are still unknown (and because they are linked to health problems like cancer, heart disease, and sterility), resist the urge to try them. The benefit is definitely not worth the risk!

Benefits of Strength Training

- Increases endurance and strength for sports and fitness activities
- Improves focus and concentration, which may result in better grades
- Reduces body fat and increases muscle mass
- Helps burn more calories even when not exercising
- May reduce the risk of short-term injuries by protecting tendons, bones, and joints
- Helps prevent long-term medical problems such as high cholesterol or osteoporosis (weakening of the bones) when you get older

What Is a Healthy Routine?

If you take a few minutes to watch the guys and girls lift weights at your school, you'll see there are lots of different ways to train with weights. Try a few good basic routines that you can modify as you start to train harder later on.

If you're just starting out in the weight room, most fitness experts recommend you begin by training three sessions a week, ranging from 20 minutes to one hour (including warm-up and cool-down periods), allowing at least a day off between sessions. It's best to work only two or three muscle groups during each session. For example, you can work your leg muscles one day, your chest, shoulders, and triceps at the next session, and your back and biceps on the last.

Before you head for the weight bench, warm up your muscles by spending 5–10 minutes pedaling on a stationary bicycle or by taking a brisk walk around the gym. After finishing your workout, cool down by stretching all the major muscle groups to avoid injuries and keep your muscles flexible.

You can use many different exercises for each body part, but the basics—like bench presses, lat pull-downs, and squats—are great to start with. Learn proper technique first, without any added weight. Perform three sets of 8–10 repetitions (or reps) of each exercise, starting out with a light weight to warm up and increasing the weight slightly with the second and third sets. (Add more weight only after you can successfully perform 8–15 repetitions in good form.) Perform two to three different exercises for each body part to make sure you work each muscle in the group effectively.

Here are some basic rules to follow in strength training:

1. Start with body weight exercises for a few weeks (such as sit-ups, pushups, and pull-ups) before using weights.

2. Work out with weights about three times a week. Avoid weight training on back-to-back days.

3. Warm up for 5–10 minutes before each session.

4. Spend no more than 40 minutes in the weight room to avoid fatigue or boredom.

5. Work more reps; avoid maximum lifts. (A coach or teacher can give you specifics based upon your needs.)

6. Ensure you're using proper technique through supervision. Improper technique may result in injuries, particularly in the shoulder and back.

7. Cool down for 5–10 minutes after each session, stretching the muscles you worked out.

Cool Down

After finishing your workout, cool down by stretching all the major muscle groups to avoid injuries and to enhance and maintain flexibility.

Don't rely on strength training as your only form of exercise. You still need to get your heart and lungs working harder by doing some kind of additional aerobic exercise for a minimum of 20–30 minutes per session. Doctors recommend an hour a day of moderate to vigorous activity—so on days when you're not lifting weights, you may want to get more aerobic activity.

Strength training is a great way to improve strength, endurance, and muscle tone. But remember to start slowly, use proper form, avoid heavy weights, and increase workouts gradually to prevent injury. Just a few short sessions a week will really pay off—besides better muscle tone and definition, you may find that you have more energy and focus in both sports and school.

Chapter 24

Stretching

Why Is Stretching Important?

Stretching is important to help lengthen and loosen your muscles. People used to think that stretching was the first thing you should do before exercising. Now we know that you should warm up for 5–10 minutes by doing some light exercises and then you should stretch. The reason for this is that stretching cold muscles can directly contribute to pulled and torn muscles.

Here are some different kinds of stretches you can do after you've warmed up with light exercise (if you'd like to see pictures of the stretches, go online and visit http://www.girlshealth.gov/fitness/exercise/stretching.cfm):

Cross Shoulder Stretch

Stand up straight, with knees slightly bent. Place feet hip distance apart. Make sure toes are pointing forward. Keep shoulders even as you complete this stretch. Bend right arm at elbow joint, extend arm across chest. Place left hand on the right elbow to gently support the arm during this stretch. Feel the stretch in your right arm and shoulder. Inhale (breathe in) through your nose, and exhale (breathe out) through your mouth, as you complete this stretch. Hold stretch for a count of 8. Repeat this stretch on opposite side, using right hand to stretch left arm and shoulder.

Triceps Stretch

Stand up straight, with knees slightly bent. Place feet hip distance apart. Make sure toes are pointing forward. Keep shoulders even as you complete this stretch. Bend right arm at elbow joint, lift arm next to your head. Position right fingers so they touch the shoulder blade area.

About This Chapter: From "Stretching Exercises," Office on Women's Health (http://girlshealth.gov), October 9, 2009.

Place left arm across top of head, and place left hand on the right elbow to gently support the arm during this stretch. Feel the stretch in your right triceps. Inhale (breathe in) through your nose, and exhale (breathe out) through your mouth, as you complete this stretch. Hold stretch for a count of 8. Repeat this stretch on the opposite side, using right hand to stretch left triceps.

Chest Stretch

Stand up straight, with knees slightly bent. Place feet hip distance apart. Make sure toes are pointing forward. Keep shoulders even as you complete this stretch. Place arms behind your back. Clasp your hands together, extending your arms behind your back and hold this position. Feel the stretch in your chest. Inhale (breathe in) through your nose, and exhale (breathe out) through your mouth, as you complete this stretch. Hold stretch for a count of 8.

Quadriceps Stretch

Stand facing a wall, about 1 foot away from it. Keep yourself up by putting your right hand against the wall. Raise your left leg behind you and grab your foot with your left hand. Pull your heel slightly up toward your bottom, stretching the muscles in the front of your left thigh for 20 seconds. Keep your thighs close together to keep your knee aligned and stretch effective. Repeat the stretch with your right leg.

Hamstring Stretch

Lie down with your back flat on the floor, with both of your knees bent. Place your feet flat on the floor, about 6 inches apart. Bend your right knee up to your chest and hold onto your right thigh with both hands placed behind your knee. Slowly straighten your right leg, feeling slight stretching in the back of your leg. Hold the stretch for 20 seconds, and then repeat the stretch with your left leg.

Groin Stretch

Squat down and put both hands on the floor in front of you. Stretch your left leg straight out behind you. Keep your right foot flat on the floor and lean forward with your chest into your right knee, then move your weight back to your left leg, keeping it as straight as you can. Do not move your right knee farther than your right ankle. Hold the stretch for 20 seconds, and then repeat the stretch with your right leg behind you.

Calf Stretch

Stand facing a wall, about 2 feet away from it. Keeping your heels flat and your back straight, lean forward and press your hands and forehead to the wall. Make sure your knee does not move forward of your ankle. Do this slowly. You should feel stretching in the muscles in the back of your lower legs, above your heels. If you need a bigger stretch, move your back farther away from the wall. Hold this position for 20 seconds and then relax. Repeat.

After you exercise, you need to cool down for about 5 to 10 minutes by doing some of the stretches you did to warm up.

Chapter 25

Pilates And Yoga

Pilates

Pilates is a body conditioning routine that seeks to build flexibility, strength, endurance, and coordination without adding muscle bulk.

For decades, it's been the exercise of choice for dancers and gymnasts (and now Hollywood actors), but it was originally used to rehabilitate bedridden or immobile patients during World War I.

What Is Pilates?

Pilates (pronounced: puh-lah-teez) improves mental and physical well-being, increases flexibility, and strengthens muscles through controlled movements done as mat exercises or with equipment to tone and strengthen the body.

In addition, Pilates increases circulation and helps to sculpt the body and strengthen the body's "core" or "powerhouse" (torso). People who do Pilates regularly feel they have better posture, are less prone to injury, and experience better overall health.

Joseph H. Pilates, the founder of the Pilates exercise method, was born in Germany. As a child he was frail, living with asthma in addition to other childhood conditions. To build his body and grow stronger, he took up several different sports, eventually becoming an accomplished athlete. As a nurse in Great Britain during World War I, he designed exercise methods and equipment for immobilized patients and soldiers.

About This Chapter: "Pilates," October 2010, and "Yoga," January 2012, reprinted with permission from www .kidshealth.org. This information was provided by KidsHealth®, one of the largest resources online for medically reviewed health information written for parents, kids, and teens. For more articles like this, visit www.KidsHealth .org or www.TeensHealth.org. Copyright © 1995-2012 The Nemours Foundation. All rights reserved.

In addition to his equipment, Pilates developed a series of mat exercises that focus on the torso. He based these on various exercise methods from around the world, among them the mind-body formats of yoga and Chinese martial arts.

Joseph Pilates believed that our physical and mental health are intertwined. He designed his exercise program around principles that support this philosophy, including concentration, precision, control, breathing, and flowing movements.

There are two ways to exercise in Pilates:

1. Today, most people focus on the mat exercises, which require only a floor mat and training. These exercises are designed so that your body uses its own weight as resistance.

2. The other method uses a variety of machines to tone and strengthen the body, again using the principle of resistance.

Getting Started

The great thing about Pilates is that just about everyone—from couch potatoes to fitness buffs—can do it. Because Pilates has gained lots of attention recently, lots of classes are available.

The Hundred: For Beginners

Pose #1: Lie on your back, knees bent toward your chest. Breathe in deeply; as you breathe out, concentrate on feeling your chest and stomach sink toward the floor

Tip: Imagine a large weight pushing our torso onto the mat, and keep that posture for the full exercise.

Pose #2: Move your arms to the sides, palms toward the floor. Lift your head from the shoulders (not the neck) until the tips of your shoulder blades are pressing into your mat and you are looking at your belly button. Straighten your legs upward.

Knee Tip: You can keep your knees bent to begin with if this feels more comfortable.

Shoulder Tip: Don't strain your neck. If your neck hurts rest your head back on the mat.

Pose #3: Elongate your arms, as if reaching for the far side of the room, and pump your straightened arms up and down to the count of five, inhaling for five and exhaling for fie. The goal is 100 strokes, but start with fewer. Keep your belly flat and your back flat on the floor.

Tip: Focus on keeping your shoulders open. Don't lift them so they curl inward.

Pose #4: Cool down. Relax your head and pull your knees back to your chest.

Source: "Pilates," October 2010. Copyright © 1995-2012 The Nemours Foundation.

Many fitness centers and YMCAs offer Pilates classes, mostly in mat work. Some Pilates instructors also offer private classes that can be purchased class by class or in blocks of classes; these may combine mat work with machine work. If your health club makes Pilates machines available to members, make sure there's a qualified Pilates instructor on duty to teach and supervise you during the exercises.

The fact that Pilates is hot and classes are springing up everywhere does have a downside, though: inadequate instruction. As with any form of exercise, it is possible to injure yourself if you have a health condition or don't know exactly how to do the moves. Some gyms send their personal trainers to weekend-long courses and then claim they're qualified to teach Pilates (they're not!), and this can lead to injury.

So look for an instructor who is certified by a group that has a rigorous training program. These instructors have completed several hundred hours of training just in Pilates and know the different ways to modify the exercises so new students don't get hurt.

The Pilates mat program follows a set sequence, with exercises following on from one another in a natural progression, just as Joseph Pilates designed them. Beginners start with basic exercises and build up to include additional exercises and more advanced positioning.

Keep these tips in mind so that you can get the most out of your Pilates workout.

- **Stay focused.** Pilates is designed to combine your breathing rhythm with your body movements. Qualified instructors teach ways to keep your breathing working in conjunction with the exercises. You will also be taught to concentrate on your muscles and what you are doing. The goal of Pilates is to unite your mind and body, which relieves stress and anxiety.

- **Be comfortable.** Wear comfortable clothes (as you would for yoga—shorts or tights and a T-shirt or tank top are good choices), and keep in mind that Pilates is usually done without shoes. If you start feeling uncomfortable, strained, or experience pain, you should stop.

- **Let it flow.** When you perform your exercises, avoid quick, jerky movements. Every movement should be slow, but still strong and flexible. Joseph Pilates worked with dancers and designed his movements to flow like a dance.

- **Don't leave out the heart.** The nice thing about Pilates is you don't have to break a sweat if you don't want to—but you can also work the exercises quickly (bearing in mind fluidity, of course!) to get your heart rate going. Or, because Pilates is primarily about strength and flexibility, pair your Pilates workout with a form of aerobic exercise like swimming or brisk walking.

Most fans of Pilates say they stick with the program because it's diverse and interesting. Joseph Pilates designed his program for variety—people do fewer repetitions of a number of exercises rather than lots of repetitions of only a few. He also intended his exercises to be something people could do on their own once they've had proper instruction, cutting down the need to remain dependent on a trainer.

Before you begin any type of exercise program, it's a good idea to talk to your doctor, especially if you have a health problem.

Yoga

Are you looking for a workout program that's easy to learn, requires little or no equipment, and soothes your soul while toning your body? If strengthening your cardiovascular system, toning and stretching your muscles, and improving your mental fitness are on your to-do list, keep reading to learn more about the basics of yoga.

What Is Yoga?

It seems like a hot new trend, but yoga actually began more than 3,000 years ago in India. The word yoga is Sanskrit (one of the ancient languages of the East). It means to "yoke," or unite, the mind, body, and spirit.

Although yoga includes physical exercise, it is also a lifestyle practice for which exercise is just one component. Training your mind, body, and breath, as well as connecting with your spirituality, are the main goals of the yoga lifestyle.

The physical part of the yoga lifestyle is called hatha yoga. Hatha yoga focuses on *asanas*, or poses. A person who practices yoga goes through a series of specific poses while controlling his or her breathing. Some types of yoga also involve meditation and chanting.

There are many different types of hatha yoga, including:

- **Ashtanga Yoga:** Ashtanga yoga is a vigorous, fast-paced form of yoga that helps to build flexibility, strength, concentration, and stamina. When doing Ashtanga yoga, a person moves quickly through a set of predetermined poses while remaining focused on deep breathing.

- **Bikram Yoga:** Bikram yoga is also known as "hot yoga." It is practiced in rooms that may be heated to more than 100° F (37.8° C) and focuses on stamina and purification.

- **Gentle Yoga:** Gentle yoga focuses on slow stretches, flexibility, and deep breathing.

- **Kundalini Yoga:** Kundalini yoga uses different poses, breathing techniques, chanting, and meditation to awaken life energy.

- **Iyengar Yoga:** This type of yoga focuses on precise alignment of the poses. Participants use "props" like blankets, straps, mats, blocks, and chairs.

- **Restorative Yoga:** This practice allows the body to fully relax by holding simple postures passively for extended periods of time.

- **Vinyasa/Power Yoga:** Similar to Ashtanga yoga, these are also very active forms of yoga that improve strength, flexibility, and stamina. This type of yoga is popular in the United States.

Yoga has tons of benefits. It can improve flexibility, strength, balance, and stamina. In addition, many people who practice yoga say that it reduces anxiety and stress, improves mental clarity, and even helps them sleep better.

To reap the benefits of yoga, it's best to practice regularly. If you're new to yoga, start by learning some basic poses and build from there. Many people find that regular practice helps decrease stress and increase well-being.

Source: "Yoga," January 2012, Copyright © 1995-2012 The Nemours Foundation.

Getting Started

Many gyms, community centers, and YMCAs offer yoga classes. Your neighborhood may also have a specialized yoga studio. Some yoga instructors offer private or semi-private classes for students who want more personalized training.

Before taking a class, check whether the instructor is registered with the Yoga Alliance, a certification that requires at least 200 hours of training in yoga techniques and teaching. You may also want to sit in and observe the class that interests you.

You could also try using a yoga DVD. Websites, DVDs, and books can't compare to learning yoga poses from a teacher, but they can help you find out more. They can be especially helpful if you have already taken yoga classes and want to practice at home.

Dress comfortably for your first yoga session in clothing that allows you to move your body fully. Stretchy shorts or pants and a T-shirt or tank top are best. Yoga is practiced barefoot, so you don't have to worry about special shoes.

If you're doing your yoga workout on a carpeted floor, you probably don't need any equipment, although many people like to use a yoga mat or "sticky" mat. This special type of mat provides cushioning and grip while you do your poses. You can buy yoga mats in sporting goods stores or often at the yoga class location.

What can you expect at a yoga class or when you watch a yoga video? To begin the class, the instructor may lead you through a series of poses like Sun Salutations to warm up your arms, legs, and spine. After that, you'll concentrate on specific poses that work different areas of your body. Most yoga sessions end with some type of relaxation exercise.

Before you begin any type of exercise program, it's a good idea to talk to your doctor, especially if you have a health problem. Be sure to let your instructor know about any orthopedic problems or special needs you may have before the class begins. A good instructor will be able to provide modified poses for students who are just beginning or who have special needs.

Staying on Track

Your schedule's already packed—so how are you supposed to fit in time for yoga? Here are a few tips:

- **Break it down.** If you can't do a half hour of yoga in one sitting, try doing it in chunks. How about 15 minutes after you get up and 15 minutes before bed? Or try three 10-minute workouts to break up a long study session.

- **Do what works for you.** Some people have more success working out in the morning before the day's activities sidetrack them; others find that an after-school workout is the perfect way to unwind. Experiment with working out at different times of the day and find the time that fits your schedule and energy level best.

- **Find a workout buddy.** Doing your yoga routines with a friend is a great way to stay motivated. You'll be less likely to miss your workout if you have an appointment with a friend. You and your buddy can compare tips on healthy eating and exercise habits, evaluate each other's poses for form, and keep each other on track.

- **Consistency is key.** If you want to reap the benefits that yoga provides, you'll have to do it consistently. A once-a-month yoga workout may relieve some stress, but for benefits like increased flexibility and stamina, you should aim to practice yoga three or four times a week.

- **Set some goals.** The same routine every week may become monotonous, so set some goals to help you stay focused. Perhaps you'd like to incorporate power yoga into your routine so you get a better cardiovascular workout. Maybe you've always gone to yoga class and your goal is to start practicing on your own at home. Whatever you choose as your goal, make sure you reward yourself when you accomplish it.

The great thing about yoga is it can be as vigorous or as gentle as you want it to be. That makes it a good choice for anybody.

Chapter 26

Measuring Exercise Intensity

What Exactly Does Moderate Intensity Mean?

Question: I've seen a gazillion articles lately about exercising for "30 minutes at moderate intensity," but they always describe moderate intensity as walking at 4 miles an hour. I can't walk at 4 miles an hour because of mechanics; my legs seem to be just the length to have to switch from walking to jogging at about 4 miles an hour, so I can't do the walk to be able to figure out what "moderate intensity" feels like. Can you give any other measure for what is "moderate" and what is "intense"—percentage of maximum heart rate or METS or anything like that? —Confused

Answer: The American College of Sports Medicine (ACSM) defines exercise intensity by percentage of maximum heart rate, rate of perceived exertion, and METS (metabolic equivalents) in their Position Stand, Recommended Quantity and Quality of Exercise for Development and Maintenance of Cardiorespiratory and Muscular Fitness and Flexibility in Healthy Adults. Moderate activity has been defined as 55–69 percent of maximum heart rate (MHR). ACSM defines "hard" exercise at 70–89 percent MHR, and "very hard" at 90 percent and above, with 100 percent being maximal exertion. Check out minimum and maximum heart rate for aerobic exercise in the Go Ask Alice! archive to learn the calculations and more (http://goaskalice.columbia.edu/minimum-and-maximum-heart-rate-aerobic-exercise).

About This Chapter: This chapter begins with "What Exactly Does Moderate Intensity Mean?" reprinted with permission from *Go Ask Alice!* Columbia University's Health Q&A Internet Resource, at www.goaskalice .columbia.edu. Copyright © 2012 by The Trustees of Columbia University. (See full copyright information at the end of this document.) The chapter continues with excerpts from "General Physical Activities Defined by Level of Intensity," Centers for Disease Control and Prevention (www.cdc.gov), 1999. Reviewed by David A. Cooke, MD, FACP, May 2012.

You can also use the "Rate of Perceived Exertion" (RPE), a subjective rating that a person can use to rate his or her exercise intensity. If someone doesn't have any other way to rate workout intensity (i.e., has no watch to use to count heartbeats, or doesn't know how fast s/he is walking or running), RPE is a low-tech method of determining this calculation. For example, a person can consider walking at a leisurely pace a 6, and perhaps a mad dash to catch a bus or a flyaway $100 bill a 19; so, rating activity in-between is a way to rate one's exercise intensity. The ACSM Position Stand uses the original scale from 6–19 to identify the perceived level of difficulty of physical activity, as follows:

6–8:	Very, very light
9–10:	Very light
11–12:	Fairly light
13–14:	Somewhat hard
15–16:	Hard
17–18:	Very hard
19:	Very, very hard

Moderate intensity, using this scale of a person's self-perception of his or her own exercise difficulty, is 12–13; hard exercise is 14–16; and very hard activity is at 17–19.

The last measure—METS—has nothing to do with baseball players from New York; instead, it refers to metabolic equivalents. One MET is equivalent to your resting metabolic rate; 2 METS is any activity that requires two times your metabolic rate, etc. This measure is determined by the amount of oxygen consumed, which indicates the level of intensity a person is working. At 1 MET, an average man would be consuming 250 milliliters (ml) of oxygen per minute; an average woman would be consuming 200 ml of oxygen per minute. For those of you who wish to be even more exact, one MET is equal to 3.5 ml of oxygen per kilogram (kg) of body weight per minute (1 kg = 2.2 pounds). Since we are not going around measuring how much oxygen a person's body is consuming, assigning a MET equivalent can give us an idea as to how intense an activity is. At 1 MET (resting metabolic rate), a 55 kg female would use about 60 calories per hour, and a 65 kg male would use about 70 calories per hour. Two METS would be double that intensity, or consuming twice the amount of oxygen than at 1 MET. In other words, 2 METS means that one is working at twice his or her resting metabolic rate (which is relatively easy or achievable), 3 METS is 3 times someone's resting metabolic rate, and so on.

The ACSM rates moderate intensity using METS as decreasing with age. For men, moderate intensity by age is shown in Table 26.1.

Table 26.1. Moderate Intensity by Age, For Men.

Age (years)	# METS (moderate)	#METS (hard)	# METS (very hard)
20–39	4.8–7.1	7.2–10.1	>10.2
40–64	4.0–5.9	6.0–8.4	>8.5
65–70	3.2–4.7	4.8–6.7	>6.8
80 and over	2.0–2.9	3.0–4.25	>4.25

For women, mean values are 1–2 METS lower than for men.

Some examples of how METS are associated with activity are shown in Table 26.2.

Table 26.2. Examples of METS Associated with Activity

METS	Activity
1	Resting quietly, watching TV, reading
1.5	Eating, writing, desk work, driving, showering
2	Light moving, strolling, light housework
3	Level walking (2.5 mph), cycling (5.5 mph), bowling, golfing using a cart, heavy housework
4	Walking (3 mph), cycling (8 mph), raking leaves, doubles tennis
5	Walking (4 mph), cycling (10 mph), ice or roller skating, digging in the garden
6	Walking (5 mph), cycling (11 mph), singles tennis, splitting wood, shoveling snow
7	Jogging (5 mph), cycling (12 mph), basketball
8	Running (5.5 mph), cycling (13 mph), vigorous basketball
9	Competitive handball or racquetball
10	Running (6 mph)

The Centers for Disease Control and Prevention (CDC) standards for moderate activity are more succinct, defining moderate intensity as an activity allowing for sustained, rhythmic movements that are carried out at these rates:

- An RPE of 11–14, or

- 3–6 METS, or

- 3.5–7.0 calories expended per minute (The number of calories per minute depends on a person's estimated body weight, fitness level, and intensity. Many charts are on the internet that calculate energy expenditure for various activities, including the Fitness Partner calculator (http://www.primusweb.com/fitnesspartner/calculat.htm). An abundance of software, as well as exercise books, are also available for people who want to track this measure.)

Examples of such activity as defined by the CDC include mowing the lawn, dancing, swimming, or biking on a level surface.

Hope these explanations motivate you into moderate activity, so you can reap all its benefits.

Columbia University Copyright Information

General Physical Activities Defined By Level of Intensity

The following is in accordance with CDC and ACSM guidelines. Activity levels are given for an average person, defined here as 70 kilograms or 154 pounds. The activity intensity levels portrayed are most applicable to men aged 30 to 50 years and women aged 20 to 40 years. For younger individuals, the classification of activity intensity might be lower. Intensity is a subjective classification.

The data were available only for adults. Therefore, when children's games are listed, the estimate intensity level is for adults participating in children's activities.

Source: U.S. Department of Health and Human Services, Public Health Service, Centers for Disease Control and Prevention, National Center for Chronic Disease Prevention and Health Promotion, Division of Nutrition and Physical Activity. Promoting physical activity: a guide for community action. Champaign, IL: Human Kinetics, 1999. (Adapted from Ainsworth BE, Haskell WL, Leon AS, et al. Compendium of physical activities: classification of energy costs of human physical activities. *Medicine and Science in Sports and Exercise* 1993;25(1):71-80. Adapted with technical assistance from Dr. Barbara Ainsworth.)

Moderate Activity: 3.0 To 6.0 METs (3.5 to 7 kcal/min)

- Walking at a moderate or brisk pace of 3 to 4.5 mph on a level surface inside or outside, such as walking to class, work, or the store; walking for pleasure; or walking the dog.

- Walking downstairs or down a hill

- Racewalking—less than 5 mph

- Using crutches

- Hiking

- Roller skating or in-line skating at a leisurely pace

- Bicycling 5–9 mph, level terrain, or with few hills

- Stationary bicycling—using moderate effort

- Aerobic dancing—high impact

- Water aerobics

- Calisthenics—light

- Yoga

- Gymnastics

- General home exercises, light or moderate effort, getting up and down from the floor

- Jumping on a trampoline

- Using a stair climber machine at a light-to-moderate pace

- Using a rowing machine—with moderate effort

- Weight training and bodybuilding using free weights, Nautilus- or Universal-type weights

- Boxing—punching bag

- Dancing (ballroom, line, square, folk, and modern dancing like disco, and ballet)

- Table tennis—competitive

- Tennis—doubles

- Golf, wheeling or carrying clubs

- Softball—fast pitch or slow pitch

- Basketball—shooting baskets

- Volleyball—competitive
- Playing Frisbee
- Juggling
- Curling
- Cricket—batting and bowling
- Badminton
- Archery (nonhunting)
- Fencing
- Downhill skiing—with light effort
- Ice skating at a leisurely pace (9 mph or less)
- Snowmobiling
- Ice sailing
- Swimming—recreational
- Treading water—slowly, moderate effort
- Diving—springboard or platform
- Aquatic aerobics
- Waterskiing
- Snorkeling
- Surfing, board or body
- Canoeing or rowing a boat at less than 4 mph
- Rafting—whitewater
- Sailing—recreational or competition
- Paddle boating
- Kayaking—on a lake, calm water
- Washing or waxing a powerboat or the hull of a sailboat
- Fishing while walking along a riverbank or while wading in a stream—wearing waders

- Hunting deer, large or small game
- Pheasant and grouse hunting
- Hunting with a bow and arrow or crossbow—walking
- Horseback riding—general
- Saddling or grooming a horse
- Playing on school playground equipment, moving about, swinging, or climbing
- Playing hopscotch, 4-square, dodgeball, T-ball, or tetherball
- Skateboarding
- Roller-skating or in-line skating—leisurely pace
- Playing instruments while actively moving; playing in a marching band; playing guitar or drums in a rock band
- Twirling a baton in a marching band
- Singing while actively moving about—as on stage or in church
- Gardening and yard work: raking the lawn, bagging grass or leaves, digging, hoeing, light shoveling (less than 10 pounds per minute), or weeding while standing or bending
- Planting trees, trimming shrubs and trees, hauling branches, stacking wood
- Pushing a power lawn mower or tiller
- Shoveling light snow
- Moderate housework: scrubbing the floor or bathtub while on hands and knees, hanging laundry on a clothesline, sweeping an outdoor area, cleaning out the garage, washing windows, moving light furniture, packing or unpacking boxes, walking and putting household items away, carrying out heavy bags of trash or recyclables (for example, glass, newspapers, and plastics), or carrying water or firewood
- General household tasks requiring considerable effort
- Putting groceries away—walking and carrying especially large or heavy items less than 50 lbs.
- Actively playing with children—walking, running, or climbing while playing with children
- Walking while carrying a child weighing less than 50 pounds

- Walking while pushing or pulling a child in a stroller or an adult in a wheelchair

- Carrying a child weighing less than 25 pounds up a flight of stairs

- Child care: handling uncooperative young children (for example, chasing, dressing, lifting into car seat), or handling several young children at one time

- Animal care (shoveling grain, feeding farm animals, or grooming animals) or playing with or training animals

- Hand washing and waxing a car

- Occupations that require extended periods of walking, pushing or pulling objects weighing less than 75 pounds, standing while lifting objects weighing less than 50 pounds, or carrying objects of less than 25 pounds up a flight of stairs or performing tasks frequently requiring moderate effort and considerable use of arms, legs, or occasional total body movements (for example, cleaning services, waiting tables, institutional dishwashing, or moderate farm work).

Vigorous Activity: Greater Than 6.0 METs (more than 7 kcal/min)

- Racewalking and aerobic walking—5 mph or faster

- Jogging or running

- Wheeling your wheelchair

- Walking and climbing briskly up a hill

- Backpacking

- Mountain climbing, rock climbing, rappelling

- Roller skating or in-line skating at a brisk pace

- Bicycling more than 10 mph or bicycling on steep uphill terrain

- Stationary bicycling—using vigorous effort

- Aerobic dancing—high impact

- Step aerobics

- Water jogging

- Calisthenics—push-ups, pull-ups, vigorous effort

- Karate, judo, tae kwon do, jujitsu

- Jumping rope or performing jumping jacks
- Using a stair climber machine at a fast pace
- Using a rowing machine—with vigorous effort
- Using an arm cycling machine—with vigorous effort
- Circuit weight training
- Boxing—in the ring, sparring
- Wrestling—competitive
- Professional ballroom dancing—energetically
- Square or folk dancing—energetically
- Clogging
- Tennis—singles
- Most competitive sports, including football, basketball, soccer, rugby, kickball, field or rollerblade hockey, ice hockey, and lacrosse
- Beach volleyball—on sand court
- Handball—general or team
- Racquetball or squash
- Downhill skiing—racing or with vigorous effort
- Ice-skating—fast pace or speedskating
- Cross-country skiing
- Sledding or tobogganing
- Swimming—steady paced laps
- Synchronized swimming
- Treading water—fast, vigorous effort
- Water jogging
- Water polo
- Water basketball
- Scuba diving

- Canoeing or rowing—4 mph or faster

- Kayaking in whitewater rapids

- Horsebackriding—trotting, galloping, jumping, or in competition

- Playing polo

- Running and skipping

- Roller-skating or in-line skating—fast pace

- Playing a heavy musical instrument while actively running in a marching band

- Gardening and yard work: heavy or rapid shoveling (more than 10 pounds per minute), digging ditches, or carrying heavy loads

- Felling trees, carrying large logs, swinging an ax, hand-splitting logs, or climbing and trimming trees

- Pushing a nonmotorized lawn mower

- Shoveling heavy snow

- Heavy housework: moving or pushing heavy furniture (75 pounds or more), carrying household items weighing 25 pounds or more up a flight of stairs, or shoveling coal into a stove

- Standing, walking, or walking down a flight of stairs while carrying objects weighing 50 pounds or more

- Carrying several heavy bags (25 pounds or more) of groceries at one time up a flight of stairs

- Grocery shopping while carrying young children and pushing a full grocery cart, or pushing two full grocery carts at once

- Vigorously playing with children—running longer distances or playing strenuous games with children

- Racewalking or jogging while pushing a stroller designed for sport use

- Carrying a child weighing pounds or more up a flight of stairs

- Standing or walking while carrying a child weighing 50 pounds or more

- Animal care: forking bales of hay or straw, cleaning a barn or stables, or carrying animals weighing over 50 pounds

- Handling or carrying heavy animal-related equipment or tack

- Pushing a disabled car

- Occupations that require extensive periods of running, rapid movement, pushing or pulling objects weighing 75 pounds or more, standing while lifting heavy objects of 50 pounds or more, walking while carrying heavy objects of 25 pounds or more or performing tasks frequently requiring strenuous effort and extensive total body movements (for example, manually shoveling or digging ditches, using heavy nonpowered tools, heavy farm work, or loading and unloading a truck).

Part Four
Activities For Team Athletes And Individuals

Chapter 27

Choosing The Right Sport For You

Corey and Angie, twin brother and sister, enjoy playing all kinds of outdoor games and sports with their friends. They especially love playing pickup games of basketball and touch football. On particularly nice days, Corey and Angie have been known to kick around the soccer ball, toss around the baseball, or go on long runs.

In just a month the twins will be high school freshmen and neither can figure out which sport to try out for in the fall. Corey is deciding between football, soccer, and cross-country. Angie is debating whether to try her hand at a sport she has never played, like field hockey, or go with one she knows, like soccer or cross-country. They're facing a dilemma a lot of teens face—which sports to play and which sports to give up.

So Many Sports, Only One You!

For some people, choosing which sports to pursue throughout high school is hard because they have never really played an organized sport before and aren't sure what they'll most enjoy. For others it's a tough decision because their friends don't like to play the same sports.

No matter what your sports dilemma is, you have to make the decision that is best for you. If you're great at soccer but would rather play football because you think it's more fun, then give the pigskin a go (just make sure it's cool with mom and dad)!

Sports are meant to be fun. If there is a sport you really enjoy but you aren't sure if you can make the team, try out anyway. What's the worst that can happen? If you get cut you can always

About This Chapter: "Choosing The Right Sport For You," January 2011, reprinted with permission from www .kidshealth.org. This information was provided by KidsHealth®, one of the largest resources online for medically reviewed health information written for parents, kids, and teens. For more articles like this, visit www.KidsHealth .org or www.TeensHealth.org. Copyright © 1995-2012 The Nemours Foundation. All rights reserved.

try another sport. And sports like cross-country and track don't typically cut participants from the team. You can still participate even if you're not on the meet squad.

Every Now And Then There Is An "I" In Team

Some sports, like lacrosse or field hockey, require every person on the field to be on the same page. Sure, certain people stand out more than others but superstars don't necessarily make a good team!

Sports like tennis, track and field, cross-country, swimming, gymnastics, and wrestling are all sports where individual performances are tallied into team scores. Of course there are exceptions, like relays in track and swimming, but for the most part it's possible to win a solo event in these sports and still have your team lose or vice-versa.

No one knows you better than you do. Maybe you enjoy the spotlight. Maybe you get annoyed by the way teammates act when they are über-competitive. Or maybe you just don't like competing with friends for a spot in the starting lineup. For whatever reason, team sports might not be your thing—and that's fine. Luckily, there are many individualized sports to choose from.

If Your School Doesn't Have Your Sport

Some schools are limited in resources—a city school may not have a lot of fields, for

When Most Organized Sports Land On The School Calendar

Fall

- Cheerleading
- Cross-Country
- Dance Team
- Field Hockey (Girls)
- Football (Guys)
- Soccer
- Volleyball
- Water Polo

Winter

- Basketball
- Cheerleading
- Dance
- Gymnastics
- Ice Hockey
- Indoor Track and Field
- Swimming and Diving
- Wrestling

Spring

- Badminton
- Baseball (Boys)
- Golf
- Lacrosse
- Rugby
- Softball (Girls)
- Tennis
- Track and Field

example, while a rural school may not have enough students to make up a team for every sport.

A school's geographic region can also play a role. If you live in a climate where it snows from the fall to the spring, your school may not be able to participate in a lot of outdoor sports.

If your school doesn't have your sport, don't let it get you down. You can always try out for a different sport during the same season or look into whether your local town has a recreational league that you can join.

You Aren't Under Contract

If you try a sport for a season and you don't enjoy it, or it's not what you expected, it's OK to try out for another sport the next year. Don't let parents or coaches persuade you to stick with something you don't want to—ultimately it's your decision.

If Organized Sports Aren't Your Thing

Many people are attracted to the competition and popularity that can come with team sports. Others love the camaraderie and unity that are present in a team atmosphere. But for some people, teams are just frustrating and another form of cliques. If you're not the biggest fan of organized sports, where you have to follow someone else's schedule and rules, many other fun and exciting options are out there for you.

You might already have an exercise routine or activity you like to do in your free time, but if you're looking for something that will both keep you busy and allow you to blow off steam, try some of these activities:

If You Don't Have It, Start It!

If you are interested in a sport, and your school doesn't have it, maybe you and some friends can talk to the administration and start a club or intramural team. With enough willing participants and the school's permission, you could have a high school cricket team!

- **Climb To The Top.** Did you love scaling trees and walls when you were younger? Rock climbing offers participants one of the best all-around workouts possible. As a rock climber, you work your hands, arms, shoulders, back, stomach, legs, and feet—ALL AT ONCE!

- **Take A Hike** (and bring your bike). Hiking and trail biking are two great ways to learn about nature while still getting your heart rate up. Even if you're just going to a local trail, bring at least one other person along in case something happens. If you're going for an intense multiday hike, you should bring someone who is experienced and trained in hiking.

- **Water World.** The water is the perfect place to give yourself new challenges. There are plenty of water activities for all levels of difficulty and energy. Besides swimming, try canoeing, kayaking, fishing, rowing, sailing, wakeboarding, water skiing, windsurfing, and, if you're feeling particularly daring, surfing.

> ## Hiker's Gear List
>
> The American Red Cross has a huge list of supplies for hiking. Here are some of the basics you should throw in your bag:
>
> - Cell phone
> - Extra clothing
> - Compass
> - First-aid kit
> - Extra food
> - Flashlight
> - Bug spray
> - Maps
> - Any prescriptions
> - Radio with batteries
> - Sunscreen
> - Water
> - Whistle
> - Poncho or trash bag to make a poncho

Find Your Inner Self

Many activities can be relaxing and taxing at once. These three activities strengthen you physically and mentally:

- Yoga can improve flexibility, strength, balance, and stamina. In addition to the physical benefits, many people who practice yoga say that it reduces anxiety and stress and improves mental clarity.

- Pilates is a body conditioning routine that seeks to build flexibility, strength, endurance, and coordination without adding muscle bulk. Pilates also increases circulation and helps to sculpt the body and strengthen the body's "core" or "powerhouse" (torso). People who do Pilates regularly feel they have better posture and are less prone to injury.

- T'ai chi is an ancient Chinese martial art form that is great for improving flexibility and strengthening your legs, abdominal or core muscles, and arms.

Take An Off-Season—But Not A Season Off!

Whether you choose one sport or three, make sure you give yourself a break from intense competition with some cross-training activities. Through cross-training you can take a rest from your sport or sports while still getting a workout and staying in shape.

Two examples of cross-training are swimming and cycling. They not only help build cardio-vascular fitness, but also work your muscles. Swimming can really help tone your upper body, while cycling strengthens your legs.

You can also try outdoor bike rides and runs on nice days, stopping periodically to do sit-ups and push-ups. These simple exercises can work and tone your core muscles.

That time between seasons is also the perfect opportunity to get into a strength-training routine. Before starting strength training, consult your doctor and school's strength and conditioning coach. Your doc will be able to give you health clearance to participate in the different types of physical activities, and your strength coach can come up with a workout to help you prepare for your specific sports.

Chapter 28

Activities For Teens Who Don't Like Sports

Team sports can boost kids' self-esteem, coordination, and general fitness, and help them learn how to work with other kids and adults.

But some kids aren't natural athletes, and they may say that they just don't like sports. What then?

Why Some Kids Don't Like Teams

Not every child has to join a team, and with enough other activities, kids can be fit without them. But try to find out why you aren't interested. You might be able to address deeper concerns or steer yourself toward something else.

Your parents might like to help you work on a solution. This might mean making changes and sticking with the team sport or finding a new activity to try.

Here are some reasons why sports might be a turnoff for kids:

Still Developing Basic Skills

Though many sports programs are available for preschoolers, it's not until about age 6 or 7 that most kids have the physical skills, the attention span, and the ability to grasp the rules needed to play organized sports.

About This Chapter: "Fitness For Kids Who Don't Like Sports," October 2010, reprinted with permission from www.kidshealth.org. This information was provided by KidsHealth®, one of the largest resources online for medically reviewed health information written for parents, kids, and teens. For more articles like this, visit www.KidsHealth.org, or www.TeensHealth.org. Copyright © 1995-2012 The Nemours Foundation. All rights reserved.

Before beginning any sport or fitness program, it's a good idea for a child to have a physical examination from the doctor. Kids with undiagnosed medical conditions, vision or hearing problems, or other disorders may have difficulty participating in certain activities.

Kids who haven't had much practice in a specific sport might need time to reliably perform necessary skills such as kicking a soccer ball on the run or hitting a baseball thrown from the pitcher's mound. Trying and failing, especially in a game situation, might frustrate them or make them nervous.

What You Can Do: Practice at home. Whether it's shooting baskets, playing catch, or going for a jog, you'll get an opportunity to build skills and fitness in a safe environment. You can try—and, possibly, fail—new things without the self-consciousness of being around peers. If you practice with your parents or other family members, you're also getting a good dose of quality together time.

Coach Or League Is Too Competitive

A kid who's already a reluctant athlete might feel extra-nervous when the coach barks out orders or the league focuses heavily on winning.

What You Can Do: Investigate sports programs before signing up for one. Talk with coaches about the philosophy. Some athletic associations, like the YMCA, have noncompetitive leagues. In some programs, they don't even keep score.

As kids get older, they can handle more competitive aspects such as keeping score and keeping track of wins and losses for the season. Some kids may be motivated by competitive play, but most aren't ready for the increased pressure until they're 11 or 12 years old. Remember that even in more competitive leagues, the atmosphere should remain positive and supportive for all the participants.

Stage Fright

Kids who aren't natural athletes or are a little shy might be uncomfortable with the pressure of being on a team. More self-conscious kids also might worry about letting their parents, coaches, or teammates down. This is especially true if a child is still working on basic skills and if the league is very competitive.

What You Can Do: Keep your expectations realistic—most kids don't become Olympic medalists or get sports scholarships. The goal is to be fit and have fun. If the coach or league doesn't agree, it's probably time to look for something new.

Still Shopping For A Sport

Some kids haven't found the right sport. Maybe a child who doesn't have the hand-eye coordination for baseball has the drive and the build to be a swimmer, a runner, or a cyclist. The idea of an individual sport also can be more appealing to some kids who like to go it alone.

What You Can Do: Be open to your interests in other sports or activities. That can be tough if, for instance, your parents just loved basketball and wanted you to continue the legacy. But by exploring other options, you have a chance to get invested in something you truly enjoy.

Other Barriers

Different kids mature at different rates, so expect a wide range of heights, weights, and athletic abilities among kids of the same age group. A child who's much bigger or smaller than other kids of the same age—or less coordinated or not as strong—may feel self-conscious and uncomfortable competing with them.

Kids also might be afraid of getting injured or worried that they can't keep up. Kids who are overweight might be reluctant to participate in a sport, for example, while a child with asthma might feel more comfortable with sports that require short outputs of energy, like baseball, football, gymnastics, golf, and shorter track and field events.

What You Can Do: Give some honest thought to your strengths, abilities, and temperament, and find an activity that might be a good match. Some kids are afraid of the ball, so they don't like softball or volleyball but may enjoy an activity like running. If you are overweight, you might lack the endurance to run, but might enjoy a sport like swimming. A child who's too small for the basketball team may enjoy gymnastics or wrestling.

Remember that some kids will prefer sports that focus on individual performance rather than teamwork. The goal is to prevent you from feeling frustrated, wanting to quit, and being turned off from sports and physical activity altogether.

Try to think about your true concerns. By understanding yourself and your strengths, you'll help foster success in whatever activity you choose.

Fitness Outside Of Team Sports

Even kids who once said they hated sports might learn to like team sports as their skills improve or they find the right sport or a league. But even if team sports never thrill you, there's plenty a kid can do to get the recommended 60 minutes or more of physical activity each day.

Free play can be very important for kids who don't play a team sport. What's free play? It's the activity kids get when they're left to their own devices, like shooting hoops, riding bikes, playing whiffleball, playing tag, jumping rope, or dancing.

Kids might also enjoy individual sports or other organized activities that can boost fitness, such as:

- swimming
- horseback riding
- dance classes
- inline skating
- cycling
- cheerleading
- skateboarding
- hiking

- golf
- tennis
- fencing
- gymnastics
- martial arts
- yoga and other fitness classes
- Ultimate Frisbee
- running

Your Choices

Even if the going's tough, it's worth the effort to find something active that you like. Try to remain open-minded. Maybe you are interested in an activity that is not offered at school. If you want to try flag football or ice hockey, for example, look for a local league or talk to school officials about starting up a new team.

You'll need to be patient if you have difficulty choosing and sticking to an activity. It often takes several tries before kids find one that feels like the right fit. But when something clicks, you'll be glad you invested the time and effort. It's one big step toward developing active habits that can last a lifetime.

Chapter 29

Baseball And Softball

Baseball

How To Play

Baseball is known as America's favorite pastime. This sport uses many different skills from pitching, catching, and batting (which require lots of hand-eye coordination), to base running which means going from a standing start to a full sprint. To get started, you just need a bat and a ball.

How To Hit The Ball: First, get hold of that bat by stacking your hands on the handle (right hand on top if you're a righty, left hand on top if you're a lefty), making sure the curve of the bat is in the middle of your fingers and that your knuckles are in a straight line. Balance on the balls of your feet, with your weight on your back foot, and bend your knees slightly. Your hands should be shoulder height, elbows in, and keep your head in line with your torso, turned toward your front shoulder. As the pitcher throws, step toward the pitch, and swivel toward the ball with your hips, keeping your arms steady as you move toward the ball. Keep your eye on the ball, and complete your swing by pivoting forward and shifting your weight to your front foot, following through with the bat after you hit the ball.

How To Throw The Ball: Did you know that throwing the ball accurately requires a little footwork? First, step toward the target with the glove side foot, making sure the toe of your shoe is pointing directly to where you want the ball to go. Aim the leading shoulder at the target. Aim the bill of your hat (the duckbill) at the target and throw.

About This Chapter: This chapter includes excerpts from "Baseball Activity Card" and "Softball Activity Card," undated documents produced by BAM! Body and Mind, Centers for Disease Control and Prevention (CDC), available online at www.bam.gov; accessed May 19, 2012.

How To Catch The Ball: Keep your eye on the pitch and stay low with your feet apart and knees bent so you can move quickly in any direction. Have your glove ready at or below knee level, pocket side out. When scooping up a ground ball, bend down and use both hands to scoop it to the middle of your body so you have it securely.

Gear Up

All ball players will need a ball, a bat, and a glove. All baseballs are pretty much the same, but bats can be either wooden or aluminum. These days, only the pros use wooden bats full time. Aluminum bats are lighter and easier to handle and don't break as often. There are a couple of different types of gloves, depending on your field position.

All batters should wear a helmet while at the plate and on base to protect the head. For better base running, try wearing baseball cleats instead of sneakers.

Catchers have a special set of protective gear that includes a helmet, a mask, shin guards, and a chest protector. All of these pieces are very important to protect you if you play behind the plate.

Play It Safe

Wear your protective gear during all practices and games, especially if you're a catcher—those fast balls can pack a punch! Don't forget to warm up and stretch before each practice or game.

In the infield? Stay behind the base on any throw. You'll avoid hurting yourself—and the base runner. In the outfield? Avoid bloopers with your teammates by calling every fly ball loudly, even if you think nobody else is close by. And in the batters' box, wear a batting helmet and use a batting glove to protect your knuckles from those inside pitches. If you think a pitch is going to hit you, turn away from the ball and take it in the back.

Fun Facts

- There are exactly 108 stitches on a baseball.
- In 1974, girls started playing on Little League teams.
- A major league pitcher can throw a baseball up to 95 miles an hour—which takes less than 0.5 seconds for the ball to cross the plate.
- Softball, including slow pitch and fast pitch, is the #1 participation team sport in the United States with more than 40 million players.
- The U.S. won the gold medal in softball's first Olympic appearance in the 1996 Atlanta Games.

Throwing those fastballs can really take a toll, so if you're a pitcher, make sure to get plenty of rest between games, and don't pitch more than 4–10 innings per week.

Softball

How To Play

Softball is a game of speed, skill, and smarts. Whether you're looking to play in your backyard or at the state championships, softball is a great team sport that everyone can play.

Many of the skills in softball are similar to those in baseball, but there are some unique differences that make softball a game of its own.

Did you know that a softball isn't really soft at all, and that it's almost two times bigger than a baseball? Because a softball is big, it doesn't go as far when you hit it. But, keep your eye on the ball—a softball can sometimes cross the plate at a very fast speed. Even with their underhanded pitching style (unlike baseball's overhand style), softball pitchers can put a lot of heat on the ball. Most beginners play in slow pitch leagues where the hitting game is having a sharp eye and timing your swing. Keep your eyes peeled for pitches that are shoulder high and that drop right over the plate—they are perfect for driving into the field.

If you're interested in playing at a more competitive level, fast-pitch softball is what you'll see—you can steal bases and bunt, and you only need nine players to get a game going.

If you're playing a pickup game with your friends, you'll probably play slow pitch softball. You only need ten players to field a team, but invite as many people as you want—it's more fun that way.

Gear Up

You'll need a glove that fits your hand and skill level and is geared to the position you play. There's a lot of truth to the old saying, "Fits like a glove"—if your glove is too big, or small, you may have problems catching and fielding the ball. For beginners, gloves that are about 9½ to 11 inches long are a good start.

You can't play without a bat and ball! Try aluminum or other non-wooden bats—they are lighter and easier to handle. As for the ball, you can find softballs at most stores that sell sports equipment.

Also, for organized team play, you'll need a pair of shoes with rubber cleats—they dig into the ground and can give you more traction while running the bases or fielding a ball. If you're playing a pick-up game with your friends, a pair of sneakers will do. If you're a catcher, you'll need special protective gear like a helmet with a facemask, shin guards, and a chest protector.

And remember, always wear a helmet to protect your head while at the plate, or on base.

Play It Safe

Before you hit the field, warm up. Get all of your muscles ready to play by stretching before every game.

Whether you're in the field or up to bat, don't forget to wear your safety gear in games and in practices. A helmet is important when batting, waiting to bat, or running the bases. If you're a catcher, make sure you wear your protective gear during all practices and games, and wear it properly—have your coach or a parent check it out for you. Don't wear jewelry like rings, watches, or necklaces—they could cut you (or someone else), or get caught when you're running the bases.

Did you know that an umpire could call you out for throwing your bat? Well, they can! And, it's not just the out you have to worry about—it's your teammates' safety! Always drop your bat next to your side in the batter's box before you head for first base.

Be a team player—always know where your teammates are before throwing the ball or swinging your bat. Make sure they are ready and have their glove up as a target before you throw the ball to them. Call loudly for every fly ball or pop up in the field, even if you don't think any of your teammates are close by. Teams that play together win together.

Chapter 30

Basketball

How To Play

Basketball is fun to play in pick-up games in the yard with your pals, or you can join an organized league. Different positions rely on different skills—point guards should focus on their dribbling and passing, while centers and forwards should be powerful rebounders and shooters. Outside guards need to be quick and strong to make those 3-point shots. Want some basics?

How To Dribble: Bounce the ball on the floor with your strongest arm. When it bounces back, use your fingertips to stop the upward motion and push it back to the floor, keeping it about waist high when it bounces. Once you've mastered dribbling in place with one hand, switch to the other and begin to move around as you dribble. Practicing dribbling by moving the ball in a figure eight between your legs is one good way to build your skills.

How To Pass The Ball: Face the person you're passing to, with your head up and knees slightly bent. Spread your fingers wide and hold the ball at chest level, elbows out. Extend your arms, take a step toward the person you're passing to, and snap your wrists forward and up as you release the ball.

How To Shoot A Layup: Start about 10 feet in front of and to the right of the basket. Dribble toward the basket, timing it so that your last step is with your left foot. Holding the ball with both hands (left in front, right in back), jump off your left foot, let go with your left hand, and extend your right arm fully to release the ball at the top of your jump. Keeping your eyes on where you want the ball to go really helps land this shot.

About This Chapter: This chapter includes excerpts from "Basketball Activity Card," an undated document produced by BAM! Body and Mind, Centers for Disease Control and Prevention (CDC), available online at www .bam.gov; accessed May 19, 2012.

How To Cut, Stop, And Land A Jump: Ease up on your cuts or pivots by making them less sharp to avoid rotating your knees. When stopping, rather than coming to a sudden stop or bringing your weight down on one foot with a single step, use the "stutter step" to slow yourself down by taking two extra steps. When landing your jumps, do it softly by bending your knees over your feet (which should be pointed straight ahead) when you hit the ground. Instead of landing flat-footed, land on either the balls or toes of your feet and rock back toward your heels.

Gear Up

A Basketball: Basketballs come in different sizes depending on your age and whether you're a girl or boy. There are also different basketballs for inside and outside use. If you're buying a new basketball, make sure you ask the salesperson for help to figure out what size and type ball you need.

A Hoop: Basketball hoops are available in most gyms and in many parks. You can even buy a hoop and attach it to the side of your house or garage, if you have one. To create your own regulation court at your house, make sure you set your foul line 15 feet from the backboard.

Play It Safe

Basketball can really make you work, so make sure you stretch and warm up before playing. Because of all of the quick moves and jumping, it can put a lot of wear and tear on your ankles, so protect them by wearing the right pair of shoes—medium or high tops do the best job of supporting your ankles. Protect those knees by learning how to cut, stop, and land a jump safely.

Be careful not to misuse basketball equipment. It's great if you've got the skills to put up a mean slam dunk, but hanging on the rim is dangerous and could cause you to get hurt. Also, make sure the court and sidelines are clear of any obstacles such as other basketballs or water bottles. If you're playing outside, make sure the baskets and sidelines are not too close to walls, fences, or bleachers and there are no holes on your court.

If you're a serious player, you may want to invest in a mouth guard to keep your teeth safe from flying elbows; knee and elbow pads so you don't get scraped up (especially if you're playing on an outdoor court); and sports glasses to protect your eyes.

> ### Did You Know?
> Michael Jordan was cut from the varsity basketball team when he was in the 10th grade—and went on to be the NBA's Most Valuable Player for five seasons!

Chapter 31

Bicycling And Indoor Cycling

Bicycling

How To Play

Bicycling can be a great competitive sport, as well as a fun activity to do with your friends. And there are plenty of different types of bicycling depending on your personality. If you love to go fast-n-furious, bicycle racing is probably more your speed. If you like to hit the rocky road, mountain biking sounds more like your taste. And if you just like to pedal for pleasure, any kind of bicycling will do. Try riding to school or to a friend's house.

Gear Up

A Bike: Think of the type of riding you want to do before you buy one. Mountain bikes are strong and stable and built for gravel roads and tricky trails. Racing bikes are built to go super fast on pavement, and sport bikes, a combination of both, are good for many different purposes.

A Helmet: Your helmet should sit right above your eyebrows and be tightly buckled so it doesn't slip while you are riding.

Play It Safe

Use your head and wear a helmet! You should always wear a helmet when you ride—plus, it's the law in many states. It's also important that your helmet is approved by one of the groups

---

About This Chapter: This chapter begins with excerpts from "Bicycling Activity Card," an undated document produced by BAM! Body and Mind, Centers for Disease Control and Prevention (CDC), available online at www .bam.gov; accessed May 19, 2012. It continues with additional information from the American Council on Exercise, which is cited separately within the text.

who test helmets to see which ones are the best: the Consumer Product Safety Commission (CPSC) or Snell B-95 standards are best for bicycling helmets.

Try not to ride at night or in bad weather, and wear brightly colored, or reflective clothes whenever you ride so you can be seen. You can even put reflectors or reflective stickers on your bike—who knew being safe could look so cool? Also, watch out for loose pant legs and shoe laces that could get caught in your bike chain.

Be street smart. Ride on the right side of the road, moving with traffic, and obey all traffic signs and signals. Discuss the best riding routes with your parents—they'll help you determine safe places to ride near your home.

When you reach an intersection, be sure to stop and look left, right, and then left again to check for cars—then go. Use hand signals to show when you're going to turn, and be sure to keep an eye out for rough pavement ahead so you can avoid it. And although you may think you can't go out without your favorite tunes, never wear headphones when you're on your bike.

What You Need To Know About Group Indoor Cycling

"What You Need To Know About Group Indoor Cycling," American Council on Exercise (ACE) Fit Facts®. Copyright © 2009 American Council on Exercise. All rights reserved. Reprinted by permission. Fit Facts is a registered trademark of the American Council on Exercise.

Some call it torturous, others exhilarating. But there's no denying the popularity of group indoor cycling. What sets these classes apart from the usual boredom of stationary cycling is the visual imagery provided by instructors. Participants are led on a "virtual" outdoor road race complete with hills, valleys, straight-aways, and finish lines. But before you reserve your spot (many classes are so popular that reservations are a must) and start composing your victory speech, there are few questions to ask yourself, as well as a few precautions to take, to make your first ride a smooth and enjoyable one.

What Kind Of Shape Am I In?

This question is crucial. Despite its heavy promotion as a workout for even the most uncoordinated, indoor cycling is by no means for everyone. The intensity levels of many classes are far beyond what most novices or part-time exercisers can achieve and maintain, particularly for 40 minutes or more.

Physics And Bicycling

The faster you are going, the longer it will take you to completely stop your bike once you hit the brakes. Science says that if you are going 20 MPH and you hit the brakes, it will take 15 feet to stop if you are on dry pavement, and 23½ feet if you are on wet pavement, so make sure you brake early.

Source: Centers for Disease Control and Prevention (CDC).

It's easy to get caught up in an instructor's chant of "Faster RPMs!" and "Don't sit down!" even if your body is telling you otherwise. And because not all fitness facilities are able to offer classes tailored for beginning exercisers, it's important that participants either be in very good cardiovascular condition, or have the ability to monitor and adhere to their body's cries for moderation.

Get In Cycling Shape

Just because you may not be ready for a cycling class now doesn't mean you can't be in the very near future. Consider doing some cycling-specific training before you take your first indoor cycling class. Spend some time on a stationary bike, but make it interesting by creating your own virtual experience by "traveling" some of your favorite road trips in your mind as you listen to music. You can increase your endurance by interspersing periods of higher-intensity cycling (faster speed, greater tension) with more leisurely pedaling. In just a few short weeks you'll be ready to sign up for your first indoor cycling class.

Indoor Cycling Essentials

The following helpful tips can make your first cycling experience a positive one:

- Don't make the dreaded mistake of showing up in running shorts or heavy sweats there's no better way to make your ride unbearable. Opt instead for bike shorts, preferably padded ones like most outdoor cyclists wear. While this won't eliminate the possibility of chaffing and discomfort altogether, it helps a lot.

- Your second most important item: a full water bottle. Get ready to consume plenty of fluids before, during, and immediately following your workout.

- Adjust the seat to the appropriate height. If the seat is too low, you won't be able to get enough leg extension on the downstroke and your legs will tire out faster. If it's too high, you'll be straining to reach and might injure yourself. Here's a good rule to follow:

Your upstroke knee should never exceed hip level, while your downstroke knee should be about 85 percent straight. And don't grip the handlebars too tightly, as this will increase the tension in your neck and shoulders.

• Ask your instructor about his or her training. In addition to cycling knowledge, they should have experience teaching group exercise and have earned a primary certification from an organization such as the American Council on Exercise (ACE). Look for an instructor who encourages perceived exertion measures and/or heart-rate monitoring and is willing to get off their own bike to coach beginners.

• Above all, concentrate on exercising at your own pace. Don't be intimidated by the high speeds and furious intensity of your cycling mates. Listen to your body and adjust the tension and speed accordingly, and don't be afraid to slow down or take a break when necessary.

What A Workout!

An ACE-sponsored study revealed that exercisers in a typical group indoor cycling class reported an exertion level in the high teens (using Borg's Rating of Perceived Exertion, a scale from 6 to 20) throughout most of the class. In addition, heart-rate measurements indicated that participants were exercising close to their maximum heart rate, which validated their perceptions that they were working hard. Clearly, group indoor cycling classes provide a challenging, high-intensity workout.

Chapter 32

Football

How To Play

There are lots of skills needed to play football from throwing and catching the ball to blocking and tackling the other players. There's even a national Punt, Pass, and Kick contest devoted just to the main skills you need. League teams are a great way to learn all the rules and strategies of football. Pop Warner is the most popular youth football league, but there are many others nationwide. Want the basics?

Throwing The Ball: Grip the ball by placing each of your fingers between each lace of the ball. Bring your throwing arm back with your elbow bent. Extend your free arm (the one without the ball) in front of you and point to your target. Snap your throwing arm forward, releasing the ball, and follow through with your shoulders and hips. When you are finished, your throwing arm should be pointing toward your target with your palm facing the ground.

Catching The Ball: Hold your arms out with your elbows slightly bent in front of your chest. Bring your hands together, touching the thumbs and index fingers to make a triangle with your fingers. Catch the nose of the ball in the triangle, and use your chest to help trap the ball. Bring your arms in around the ball and hold it tight against you.

Punting The Ball: Place your feet shoulder-width apart with your kicking foot slightly in front. Slightly bend your knees and bend your body forward a little. Hold the ball out in front of you with the laces facing upward. Take two steps forward, beginning with your kicking foot

About This Chapter: This chapter includes excerpts from "Football Activity Card," an undated document produced by BAM! Body and Mind, Centers for Disease Control and Prevention (CDC), available online at www .bam.gov; accessed May 19, 2012.

and drop the ball toward your kicking foot. Kick the ball hard with the top of your foot and follow through with your leg as high as you can.

Gear Up

Obviously, you need a football to play, and you should choose the size based on your age. Always wear a helmet with a face mask and jaw pads and a mouthpiece to protect against those hard hits. Because football is a contact sport, there are many different pieces of gear you should wear to protect different areas of your body. For upper body protection, you should wear a neck roll to prevent whiplash, shoulder pads, rib pads, arm pads and elbow pads. For leg protection, you should wear hip pads, tailbone pads, thigh pads, and knee pads. Most leagues require all this, but it's a good idea to protect yourself even in backyard games.

Fun Facts

- The numbers worn on players' uniforms represent the positions they play. For example, wide receivers and tight ends have numbers between 80 and 89.
- A football field is 120 yards long (including the two end zones) and 53 1/3 yards wide.

Play It Safe

Be sure to stretch and warm up before every practice and game and always wear your protective gear. To avoid getting hurt, learn from your coaches how to block and tackle correctly. Don't tackle with the top of your head or helmet—not only is it illegal, but it can cause injury to both players. If you play in an organized league, there are lots of rules, and they are there for a reason—to keep you safe. If you break these rules, you risk not only getting hurt, or hurting someone else, but your team will be penalized. If you're playing in the backyard with your friends, stay safe by sticking to touch or flag football, and only play with kids who are around your age and size.

Chapter 33

Frisbee

How To Play

Frisbee is a great way to spend time outside on a beautiful day. Just grab your Frisbee and a few friends and you've got yourself a game.

One of the best parts about Frisbee is that you probably know more than you think about how to play. Like how to throw a backhand: Just stand with your feet shoulder-width apart, point yourself sideways, place your index finger on the outside rim with your middle finger extended along the top of the Frisbee and your thumb underneath and flick your wrist toward your throwing partner.

A forehanded Frisbee throw is more complicated, but just remember, practice makes perfect. Place your middle finger straight and flat against the inside rim of the Frisbee so that the outer rim is between your thumb and your index finger. If you are right handed, stand sideways with your left shoulder forward, pull your right arm back to your outer thigh, keeping the Frisbee at an angle, and flick your wrist forward, releasing the Frisbee about halfway across your body.

Now that you've perfected throwing the Frisbee, you've got to learn to catch it. There are two ways to catch a Frisbee. In one, called the Pancake, the palms of your hands face each other and are held close to your body. That way, if you can't catch the Frisbee with your hands, it hits your body, not the ground. Another catch style is called the Crocodile. This catch involves holding your arms out in front of your body and clapping your hands together just like a crocodile's mouth snapping shut.

About This Chapter: This chapter includes excerpts from "Frisbee Activity Card," an undated document produced by BAM! Body and Mind, Centers for Disease Control and Prevention (CDC), available online at www.bam.gov; accessed May 19, 2012.

Once you've mastered catching and throwing your Frisbee, grab some friends and organize a game of Ultimate. This is a team sport played on a 70-yard by 40-yard rectangular field with an end zone that stretches 25 yards deep. Two teams of seven people each are needed to play. A team scores when the Frisbee is thrown into the other team's end zone. Ultimate players referee their own games, making good sportsmanship the most important thing to remember.

The Spin

If you want to make your Frisbee soar, make sure you put lots of spin on it when you throw. Spinning helps keep the Frisbee from flipping over, which would put an end to your throw. Frisbee designers help you by making the edges thicker than the rest of the Frisbee and by putting tiny ridges on the top to help keep it balanced.

Gear Up

Of course the first thing you'll need is a Frisbee. The most common kinds are made of plastic and come in all sorts of cool colors. If you are planning to play a serious game, or want to play an organized game of Ultimate, you'll also need cleats or tennis shoes with good tread. Kneepads aren't a bad idea and are a great way to avoid scratching up your knees.

Play It Safe

When playing a game of Frisbee, just make sure that you don't throw too hard and always try and stay on your feet while playing. If you are playing a more intense game of Ultimate also make sure to avoid diving for the Frisbee.

It's important to warm up and stretch before any game. Listen to your body. Don't play through any pain. If you are injured, wait until you've healed before starting to play again. And if you have glasses or braces, wear protective eye or mouth guards.

Whether you're just tossing the Frisbee with friends or playing a competitive game of Ultimate, make sure to drink plenty of water before, during and after your game. It's also a good idea to wear sunscreen to keep from burning and bug repellent to keep the bugs where they belong—off of you.

Chapter 34

Golf

How To Play

Golf is played on a course with either nine or 18 different holes—a complete game of golf is called a round. It's important to know the basics of the game and how to use (and choose) your clubs. You may want to take a few lessons from the pro at your local golf course, or rent an instructional video to learn more about the proper swing, grip, and stance.

Check out these tips to get you swinging in the right direction.

The Clubs: If your clubs are too long or too short, you're likely to have problems. To find the right size clubs for you, try swinging with a few different lengths. A good rule of thumb is to choose clubs that are about as long as the distance from your belly button to the floor. You don't need to decide right away—lots of courses and driving ranges have sample clubs that you can practice with until you find the perfect fit.

The Swing: The key to the swing is to keep your eyes on the ball. Focus on the ball and keep your head down (and still) when you swing. Your eyes should stay on the ball through your entire swing.

Jack Nicklaus, one of the best players in golf, learned one basic thing from his father—hit the ball hard, and not worry about where it goes—you can always fix that later. By trying to hit the ball far, you'll naturally try to make the biggest swing with your arms that you can. Swing them back as far as you can—getting your hands behind your head, and follow through as far

About This Chapter: This chapter includes excerpts from "Golf Activity Card," an undated document produced by BAM! Body and Mind, Centers for Disease Control and Prevention (CDC), available online at www.bam.gov; accessed May 19, 2012.

as you can. You'll feel your body turn and you'll notice that while swinging back, your weight will shift to your right foot, and then to your left as you swing through the ball.

Tee It Up: If you're a beginner, hit the ball off of a tee every time—it's much easier to get under the ball. Put the tee into the ground at different heights to see where you like it best. If you're a more experienced player, only use a tee when using your drivers. Experiment with your irons once you're in the fairway to get the ball onto the green. Just remember that the iron you choose depends on how far (and high) you need to hit the ball. Use a 3 iron for long shots to the hole—a 9 iron can be used for those shorter shots.

Gear Up

Don't worry about buying an entire set of golf clubs right away. If you're just starting out, all you really need are the 5, 6, or 7 irons, a driver, and a putter. You'll use a driver off of the tee for long distance shots, followed up by your irons, which give more control for shorter shots. And don't forget your putter—the putter is used on the green.

Next on your list should be golf balls and tees. Tees look like a round peg with a flat top, and are used to raise the ball off of the ground so you can get your club under it better. Put the tee into the ground and sit your golf ball on top of it. Make sure you have plenty of tees on hand—they sometimes break when you hit the ball. Don't get overwhelmed by the number of golf balls there are to choose from. You don't have to use an expensive ball because a lot of them will probably end up in the woods or water anyway.

Fun Facts

- There are 336 dimples on a regulation golf ball. The dimples on a golf ball make it travel farther. It has to do with air flow. As air flows around a ball without dimples, it breaks away from the surface of the ball forming a pocket of swirling currents behind it—like the wake behind a speedboat. This creates a "drag" on the ball, slowing it down. Dimpled golf balls can easily sail two hundred yards from the tee, while a smooth one (with no dimples) would only go about fifty yards. Golfers discovered this about a hundred years ago, when they noticed their old golf balls, covered with scratches and nicks, sailed farther down the fairway than shiny new ones.
- When walking on the moon, astronaut Alan Sheppard hit a golf ball that went 2,400 feet, nearly one-half a mile.

Also, don't forget that some courses have a dress code. This means that they can ask you to wear certain types of clothing like shirts with collars and shorts or pants without holes in them. As a rule of thumb, keep your clothing simple. Dress in comfortable, loose fitting shirts, pants, or shorts. Sneakers are fine for beginners. And don't forget a hat and sunscreen. On those hot, sunny days, it's important to protect yourself from the sun.

Once you've got all of your gear, hit the links and have some fun.

Play It Safe

It's important to warm-up and stretch before you step onto your local golf course. Before swinging, make sure that no one is standing too close—it's a good rule of thumb to stand at least four club lengths away from the person swinging the club. Don't play until the group in front of you is out of the way. Stand still and stay quiet while others are in play. If your ball lands in the rough of the course (in high grass, brush, or trees), watch out for creepy, crawly animals and poisonous plants.

Check the weather forecast before going out onto the course. The general rule for avoiding storms is: If you can see lightning, flee it, if you can hear thunder, clear it. Get away from small metal vehicles like golf carts, and put your clubs away. Stay away from trees because they attract lightning, and avoid small on-course shelters—they are made to protect you from rain showers and provide shade.

Whether you're walking the course or riding in a cart, don't forget your water bottle. It's important to drink plenty of water before, during, and after your round. Need a rest? Sit down in a shady area, or under a tree—put a cold towel around your neck to keep you cool.

Chapter 35

Gymnastics, Cheerleading, And Ballet

Gymnastics

How To Play

Gymnastics is known as the sport of all sports. It's a great way to improve strength, flexibility, balance, and coordination for other types of physical activities, and it's a great way to meet new people and have fun.

It doesn't matter if you're a guy or a girl—gymnastics has a few different categories to choose from so you can find your favorite. Artistic gymnasts use lots of skills to perform on many different kinds of apparatuses (pieces of equipment). Boys participate in six events (floor, vault, parallel bars, high bar, still rings, and pommel horse) and girls in four (floor, vault, uneven parallel bars, balance beam). Gymnasts who participate in rhythmic gymnastics jump, tumble, flip, and dance to music while using rope, hoops, bars, or ribbons as part of their routines. In gymnastics, there's something for everyone.

Gear Up

Unlike some other sports, gymnastics doesn't require a lot of equipment, but there are certain things you'll need for specific events, and some standard gear that all gymnasts should have.

Female gymnasts usually wear leotards (one or two piece outfits that fit snuggly to the body). Boys can wear running shorts or sweatpants with fitted tops, or with your shirt tucked in. Just make sure you don't wear clothing that is too loose—it could get caught on the equipment when

About This Chapter: This chapter includes excerpts from "Gymnastics Activity Card," "Cheerleading Activity Card," and "Ballet Activity Card," undated documents produced by BAM! Body and Mind, Centers for Disease Control and Prevention (CDC), available online at www.bam.gov; accessed May 19, 2012.

you are performing your tricks and cause you serious problems. For those of you with long locks, you'll need to pull it back with a hair band or in a braid—this will prevent it from getting in your face during your routine which could cause you to lose concentration and sight.

Gymnasts also wear hand guards and use chalk to prevent their hands from slipping when working on the floor mats, rings, or bars. The hand guards help prevent blisters and make it easier to swing around on the bars.

Play It Safe

The most important gymnastics rule to remember is to know what you're doing. Never attempt a trick you are not familiar with. Make sure you always have a trained spotter (someone who stands near you in case you need help while doing your tricks) just in case you lose your balance on the beam, or attempt a wobbly handstand.

Before you attempt any trick or stunt, always make sure the equipment is sturdy and has been set up properly (always ask a coach or another grown-up for help). Floors should be padded with mats that are secured under every piece of equipment. Also, make sure there is enough distance between each piece of equipment before you start swinging. Collisions can cause you, or others around you, to get hurt if you don't watch out. Use your head. Pay attention and be serious about your practice—horseplay and goofing around can get you into trouble. Always know what your teammates are doing and where they are.

And last but not least, never eat or chew gum while doing gymnastics—the moment you become unaware of what is in your mouth, it can easily become lodged in your throat and you could choke.

Fun Facts

- The first large-scale gymnastics competition was during the 1896 Olympics in Athens, Greece.
- About 98% of all female college cheerleaders are former gymnasts. Madonna, Halle Berry, Kim Basinger, Cameron Diaz, and Kirsten Dunst were all cheerleaders. Male celebrities who were cheerleaders include Samuel L. Jackson, Steve Martin, and Aaron Spelling.
- Ballet is often thought of as artistic and beautiful. However, out of the 61 most common sports, only professional football is more physically demanding. Like football, dance is not an endurance sport. Dancers experience short bursts (1–2 minutes) of serious cardiac activity followed by periods of rest or easier dancing. A 120 pound dancer burns almost 1,000 calories per performance.

Cheerleading

How To Play

When you hear the word cheerleading, what do you think of? How about a fast-paced competitive sport for both guys and girls that involves a high level of endurance, strength, and precision? For many cheerleaders, that is exactly what cheering is. Cheerleading is coming into its own as a competitive sport. Cheer squads compete up to the national level, developing cheer and dance routines that include complex pyramids, lifts and tosses.

If you're just starting out, here are some basic cheerleading arm motions:

- **Goal Post:** Arms should be above your head, straight up in the air, and touching the side of your head. Your fists should be closed with your thumbs facing each other.

- **High V:** From the goal post position, move your arms out slightly wider to form a high V. Fists should be closed and thumbs facing away from your body. Your arms should be slightly in front of you so that you can see your fists out of the corner of your eyes.

- **Low V:** For this motion, the opposite of a high V, move your arms down into a v-like position by your sides. Keep your fists closed with your thumbs facing away from your body.

- **Basic T:** Your arms should be straight out on each side, in line with your shoulders. Keep your fists closed with your thumbs facing down, and your arms straight and level. Your body should look like a T.

Gear Up

You'll need a good comfortable pair of sneakers that provide a lot of support and cushion for your feet. Also, many cheerleaders use spirit-raising tools such as pom-pons and megaphones.

Play It Safe

Today's cheerleading is super fun, but it's risky too, especially if you perform stunts. On this team sport, each squad member's position is key to completing the stunts safely and dazzling the crowd.

Make sure you're well conditioned for all those kicks, jumps, and splits. Warm up before each practice and game, and do lots of stretching. Focus on stretching your legs and back. If you do stunts and build pyramids, make sure you stretch your arms and shoulders too.

Practice safe stunts. If your squad does lifts, tosses, or builds pyramids, make sure you follow these important safety rules.

- Always practice stunts on mats or pads.

- Never attempt a stunt unless a coach is there.

- Always use spotters for each and every stunt.

- If you are new to stunting, start with easier stunts and gradually move up to harder ones.

- Remember that if someone in the stunt yells "Down," the stunt should come down immediately.

Ballet

How To Play

Confidence, good posture, balance, self-discipline, concentration, flexibility, endurance, speed, strength, and power. Would you believe there's a single activity that promotes all these things at the same time? Well, believe it or not, there is—ballet.

There are two types of classic ballet, which is an art form that tells stories through characters in costume. Pointe is one type, where dancers wear a special type of shoe so that they can move on the tips of their toes. Since Pointe is really advanced, we'll just be focusing on demi-ballet. In this type, dancers dance on the balls of their feet.

There's a whole lot to remember when dancing ballet—things like how important it is to find the right studio. Because when you're learning the basics, it's important to make sure you learn correctly.

There are five basic positions for ballet. All classic dance steps start or end in one of these five positions:

- **First Position:** The heels are together, legs stretched straight. Turn your toes outward to form a straight line. Your arms should form a curve raised right above your waist. Your hands should be between your waist and the level of your chest.

- **Second Position:** Separate your feet to the side about 1½ feet apart. Your feet should be well turned out. Open your arms, rounding them slightly. Your elbows should be slightly lower than your shoulders.

- **Third Position:** Put the heel of your right foot against the middle of your left foot. Bring your right arm up so that a semicircle forms above your head. Your left arm should remain in the second position.

- **Fourth Position:** Slide your right foot forward so that it is parallel to your left foot with about 12 inches in between. Place your right arm overhead in a vertical position. Your left arm should be in the first position.

- **Fifth Position:** Place your right foot close up in front of your left foot. The toes of your left foot should touch the heel of your right foot. Both arms should be overhead and form a round shape. There is a small space between hands.

In addition to the dancing done with their legs and feet, dancers use their hands and arms to express themselves. Showing expression through the hands and arms is always very important, especially since it can be difficult to see a dancer's face from a distance.

But the most important thing to remember—always respect the instructor.

Gear Up

Tutus and toe shoes are a classical dancer's standard costume. When trying to figure out what to wear, keep in mind the following tips:

A simple leotard with tights is best for class—wearing them allows the instructor to see that all muscles are moving correctly. Boys often wear black tights and a white T-shirt.

In order to keep their muscles warm and help prevent injuries, sometimes dancers wear legwarmers for warming up and doing exercises at the barre. A barre is a handrail that dancers use to steady themselves during the first part of a ballet class. ("Barre" is also a shorthand term for exercises done at the barre, and you might hear a dancer say they are "doing a barre" before performing which means they are warming up).

Ordinary ballet shoes have paper-thin soles, no heals, are held on the foot with elastic and come in different colors (but usually black or pink). The right and left foot shoes are identical and take on the shape of each foot through use.

Pointe shoes have re-enforced toes that help the toes bear the weight of the body and provide extra support for dancers going up on Pointe. Pointe places a lot of force on the toes, and the re-enforcements also help distribute this pressure over the entire tip of the foot. But even then, dancers usually add padding inside the shoe to cushion their feet further. It's important that dancers don't wear toe or point shoes until their ankles, back, and other supporting muscles are strong enough for this type of exercise—remember that Pointe is not for beginners. It's always best to go to a store that specializes in dancewear to have shoes fitted properly. A dancer's toes should be able to move freely inside while the shoe is snug and secure on the outside.

It's usually best to leave jewelry like watches, necklaces, and dangling earrings at home. They could scratch another dancer or snag a leotard or tights, and might turn out to be a hassle.

Wearing your hair up for class allows your instructor to fully see how your muscles are aligned—and it helps you see where you are going.

Play It Safe

Stretching is one of the most important things a dancer can do. Stretching makes the muscles stronger and more flexible, so make sure you warm up and stay focused while stretching.

To prevent toe trouble, wear toe pads and tape around tender and tight parts of your feet like your toes and heals.

Learn the proper technique. To ensure correct technique, make sure you are being taught by a qualified teacher with proper credentials and that you practice under supervision.

Eat healthy in order to keep your energy and attention levels up so that you can perform at your best. Some dancers confuse healthy eating with not eating enough and develop eating disorders. It's never a good idea to try and make yourself skinny by hurting your body.

Ballet is more than just physical exertion. It's the total process of expressing yourself through creative movement—have confidence in your self expression and in everything else you do.

Simple crunches, lunges, and bike riding are good ways to strengthen back muscles. You can also stretch your back muscles by laying on your stomach, slightly lifting both arms and legs, and holding them in place for a few seconds.

Chapter 36

Martial Arts

How To Play

Martial arts—a special type of defense skills—started in the Orient (East Asia). Today, they're taught all over the world for self-defense and avoiding conflict, too. Body and mind control, discipline, and confidence are key. There are a lot of martial arts styles, but since certain types rough up the joints (like knees) more than others, these are some of the best for kids your age:

- Judo comes from Japan and means "gentle way." It's like Jujitsu, one of the oldest martial arts, but not as hard core. Judo has lots of wrestling moves. It also teaches participants how to make good decisions and be mentally strong. Judokas (judo players) focus on competition.

- Karate comes from Japan, and means "empty hand." It's Japan's most popular martial art. Feet, legs, elbows, head, and fists get used for kicking, punching, defensive blocks, and more. Karate stresses defense and uses weapons.

- Tae Kwon Do comes from Korea and means "the way of the foot and fist." It's famous for high kicks. Tae Kwon Do became Korea's national sport in 1955 and is now the world's most popular martial art.

Other martial arts include Aikido, Hwarang Do, Kung Fu, Jujitsu, Kendo, Ninjutsu, Northern and Southern Shaolin Boxing, Tai Chi, and T'an Su Do.

About This Chapter: This chapter includes excerpts from "Martial Arts Activity Card," an undated document produced by BAM! Body and Mind, Centers for Disease Control and Prevention (CDC), available online at www .bam.gov; accessed May 19, 2012.

Interested? The first thing you need to do is to decide on the style you want to study. Do you want to enter tournaments, or simply know how to defend yourself? After that, just get into a good class.

Gear Up

Most martial arts students wear white pants, a white jacket, and a cloth belt. For some martial arts, the belt color shows the student's skill level and personal development—from white (beginner) to black (expert). The colors reflect nature. For example, the white belt that students start out with stands for a seed. The yellow belt that they get next stands for the sunshine that opens the seed. To advance from one grade level to another, you have to pass loads of tests—five for the green belt, nine for the brown belt, and 10 for the black belt. You can get a first-degree black belt in two to four years, but after that, there's still more to learn—there are 10 black belt levels.

For sparring (practice fighting), go for full gear, including a mouthpiece and padding on your head, hands, feet, and shins.

Play It Safe

Look for an instructor who's into respect and discipline, but still has plenty of patience. The class area should have lots of space and a smooth, flat floor with padding. The fewer students the better—more attention for you.

Wear all the right gear. Warm up and stretch so you're loose and ready to go. You need good instruction before launching into any moves. And when you do learn the moves, remember your limits. For example, white belt students shouldn't spar (practice fight). When you are ready for matches, you must have an instructor around to regulate.

Chapter 37

Skating: Inline Skates And Skateboards

Inline Skating

How To Play

If you're just beginning inline skating, here are some tips to get you rolling.

Practice balancing on your skates by walking in them on a flat, grassy area. As you move to the pavement, balance yourself without trying to move. Gradually begin to skate by moving forward, but not too fast. Keep your knees bent and flexible when you skate—it will keep you more stable. And if you fall—fall forward. Then you will fall on your kneepads—they're there to protect you.

It's also a good idea to take lessons from a certified instructor—you can find one through the International Inline Skating Association. As you get more skilled on your skates, there are several types of competitive inline skating activities—like speed skating and aggressive skating, which includes events like those at the X Games. There are also sports leagues just for those who play on wheels, such as roller hockey, roller soccer, and roller basketball.

Gear Up

There are several different types of inline skates, depending on the type of skating you do. Recreational skates have a plastic boot and 4 wheels. These skates are best for beginners. Hockey skates have laces and are made of leather with small wheels for quick movement. Racing skates have 5 wheels and, usually, no brake. Freestyle skates have three wheels and a pick stop for tricks. Fitness skates have larger wheels and are used for cross-training. Aggressive

About This Chapter: This chapter includes excerpts from "Inline Skating Activity Card" and "Skateboarding Activity Card," undated documents produced by BAM! Body and Mind, Centers for Disease Control and Prevention (CDC), available online at www.bam.gov; accessed May 27, 2012.

skates, the kind worn by X Games competitors, are made of thick plastic with small wheels for quick movement, and grind plates to protect the skate when doing tricks. No matter what kind of skates you wear, always wear a helmet, as well as wrist guards, elbow pads, and knee pads.

Play It Safe

Avoid getting hurt by making sure your helmet and pads are on correctly. Your helmet should be tightly buckled, with the front coming down to right over your eyebrow, and your pads should be on tight, so they don't slip while you are skating. It's also important that your helmet is approved by one of the groups who test helmets to see which ones are the best: the Consumer Product Safety Commission (CPSC), or Snell B-95 standards are best for inline skating helmets. Make sure you are always in control of your speed, turns, and stops, and be careful of cracks in the pavement where you are skating—they can be dangerous if your wheels get caught in them. It's best to go skating out of the way of traffic and other people (skating rinks are great places to skate).

Fun Facts

- Inline skates were invented by a Minnesota hockey player so that he could skate during the off-season.
- Many professional skiers use inline skating to train during the off-season, because some of the skills of each activity are the same.
- While skateboarding, if you ride with your right foot forward, you have what's called a goofy stance. If you ride with your left foot forward, you have a regular stance.
- The first X Games competition was held in June 1995 in Rhode Island.

Skateboarding

How To Play

If you're just starting out, follow these steps to develop your skateboarding skills. Put one foot on the board, toward the front, with the other on the ground. Push off the ground with your foot and put it on the rear of the board while you glide. Push again when you slow down. If you start going too fast, step off the board with your back foot. To turn, shift your weight to your back foot so that the front truck lifts off the ground and then move your body in the direction you want to go—the board will go with you.

If you want to find half pipes, vert ramps, and skate courses near you to practice your moves, look for a nearby skate park, designed to give skateboarders a great ride.

There are several different styles of skateboarding:

- Street skating is skateboarding on streets, curbs, benches, and handrails—anything involving common street objects. Street skating is best left to the pros though—it's very dangerous.
- Downhill skating is racing down big hills, usually on a longer skateboard called a longboard.
- Freestyle skating is more artistic, involving a series of tricks and stunts.
- Vert skating is skateboarding on mini-ramps and half pipes, which are U-shaped ramps.

Gear Up

Skateboards can be bought pre-assembled, or you can buy all of the pieces and put it together yourself. Pre-assembled boards are best for beginners, until you decide if skateboarding is really for you. If you are putting your own board together, you'll need a deck (the board itself), grip tape for the top of the deck so your feet don't slip, two trucks (the metal parts that are the axles of the wheels), four wheels, and two bearings per wheel (these keep the wheels spinning on the truck's axle).

Before each time you ride, make sure your trucks are tightened and your wheels are spinning properly. Don't forget to wear a helmet, knee and elbow pads, and wrist guards. It's important that your helmet is approved by one of the groups who test helmets to see which ones are the best: the Snell B-95 standard is best for skateboarding helmets. Non-slippery shoes are a good idea too, so you can have better control of your board.

Play It Safe

Before you ride, make sure you give your board a safety check to make sure everything is put together right. Always wear all of your protective gear including a helmet, knee and elbow pads, and wrist guards. If you do tricks with your board, you may also want to wear gloves to protect your hands from the pavement. If you're just starting out, skate on a smooth, flat surface so you can practice keeping control of your board.

And no matter how experienced you are—never hold on to the back of a moving vehicle. It's best to skate out of the way of traffic and other people (skate parks are great places to skate). But if you are skating in streets near your house, be aware of cars and people around you, and stay out of their way. Also, once the sun sets, it's a good idea to put up your board for the night, since skating in the dark can be dangerous.

Chapter 38

Soccer

How To Play

In addition to a good strong kick, you'll want to master basic skills like passing (moving the ball to a teammate with a controlled kick), dribbling (tapping the ball with your feet to move it down the field), trapping (stopping the ball with your feet, legs, or chest), and heading (using your head to stop or pass the ball). Once you get these skills down, you'll be unstoppable.

Here are some great passing and trapping tips.

Passing: Pick your target out before you start the pass. Keep your head down to make sure you kick the ball correctly. Plant your non-kicking foot next to the ball and kick the ball right in the center using the inside of your foot and follow through with your leg.

Chest Trap: As the ball comes toward you, get in front of it and let it hit your chest. Bring your shoulders around and slightly inward, creating a cavity for ball. Make sure you keep your arms down, so the ball doesn't accidentally hit your hands and cause a foul. When the ball hits your chest, arch your back, so your chest pops the ball upward before the ball lands at your feet.

Gear Up

You'll need a ball. Soccer balls come in different sizes depending on how old you are. Kids 8–12 should use a size 4 ball, and kids 13 and over should use a size 5 ball. Synthetic leather balls are best for beginners, because they don't absorb water and get heavy.

About This Chapter: This chapter includes excerpts from "Soccer Activity Card," an undated document produced by BAM! Body and Mind, Centers for Disease Control and Prevention (CDC), available online at www.bam.gov; accessed May 19, 2012.

If you play in a league, a goal will usually be provided for you, and you can buy a smaller goal if you want to play in your backyard—just make sure it is anchored to the ground. No goal? No problem. Just set up any two objects (cones or water bottles are good) to shoot between.

Two pieces of equipment you need to wear at all times when playing soccer are shin guards and cleats. Shin guards are designed to protect your legs from the ball, and from being kicked by other players. They are required in most leagues. The right cleats to wear for soccer are ones that are plastic or rubber—they'll help you with your quick starts, stops, and turns.

Did You Know?

- Soccer players can run as many as six or seven miles during the course of a game.
- If you played soccer on top of a mountain, you'd be able to kick the ball much further. Why? The air pressure on top of a mountain is lower than at the bottom. When a soccer ball is kicked into the air, the air pressure pushes against the ball and slows it down. Since the air pressure on top of a mountain is much lower, there is less pressure to push against the ball and slow it down. As a result, the ball will go further.

Play It Safe

Be sure to wear shin guards and appropriate soccer cleats during games as well as practices. Warming up, especially your leg muscles, is very important. To avoid headaches and dizziness, use your head and learn the proper technique for heading a ball in a game. Many leagues have strict rules about wearing jewelry, watches, and barrettes during games. Since any of these items can cause you to get hurt if you're hit with a ball, it's a good idea to not wear them when you play. Also, to protect your mouth from collisions (especially if you have braces), wear a mouthguard.

Chapter 39

Tennis, Table Tennis, And Volleyball

Tennis

How To Play

Tennis is a fun activity that two people (a singles match) or four people on two separate teams (doubles) can play. You can play with friends at your local tennis courts or join an organized team. When you start playing tennis, some of the key strokes you should learn are: serve, forehand, backhand, two-handed backhand, volley, and smash. But first, check out these basic skills to get you started:

Holding The Racquet: The racquet handle has eight sides—four are flat and four are angled. Take the racquet handle between your thumb and index finger of your dominant hand (the one you write with) as if you were shaking hands. The knuckle on your index finger should be on the top right angle. Then, grip and make sure it feels comfortable. Separate your third and fourth fingers slightly.

Serving: Hold the ball with the thumb, index finger, and middle finger of your free hand (hand not holding the racquet). Extend the arm with the ball just in front of you and then raise it above your head. Toss the ball gently, so it goes a few inches higher than the full height of the racquet extended above your head. Keep your eye on the ball. Bring the racquet around above your shoulder and hit the ball while it's in the air. Try to use the same toss every time.

About This Chapter: This chapter includes excerpts from "Tennis Activity Card," "Table Tennis Activity Card," and "Volleyball Activity Card," undated documents produced by BAM! Body and Mind, Centers for Disease Control and Prevention (CDC), available online at www.bam.gov; accessed May 27, 2012.

Receiving And Returning The Ball: Stand in the middle of the court and hold the racquet gently with both hands so you can run in either direction when the ball comes over the net. When the ball is hit to your forehand side (on the right if you're right-handed), step toward the ball with your opposite leg and swing. If the ball comes to your backhand side (on the left if you're right-handed), go for the ball with your dominant arm in front of your chest and your other hand holding the racquet as well. Swing without moving your wrists.

Scoring: In tennis, "love" means that your opponent has not scored any points yet and has a score of zero. One point = 15, two points = 30, three points = 40, and usually, 4 points = a win.

Why are tennis balls so fuzzy?

The fuzz increases the wind resistance, which slows down the ball and helps the players to volley (hit the ball back and forth without stopping) longer. Without it, the ball would fly off the court after every serve. The fuzz also helps players control the ball, by keeping it stuck to their racquet strings for just a little longer when they hit it.

Gear Up

What's all the racket about racquets? Well, you can't play tennis without one. If you're buying a junior racquet, choose the longest one that you can comfortably use. If you weigh more than 85 pounds you should look for an adult racquet.

When you have a racquet, you'll need to find a court. Look around at school or at parks in your neighborhood. Then, put on socks (if they're not cotton, they'll help you avoid blisters) and sneakers with good ankle support. Don't forget the tennis balls!

Play It Safe

Tennis is an activity that forces you to turn your body quickly in many different directions, so make sure you warm up and stretch before playing. Wear tennis shoes with good support to protect your ankles and thick (not cotton) socks that fit well to prevent blisters on your feet. To prevent hand blisters, keep your racquet handle dry by using sawdust or hand chalk. Always bend your arm when you swing, or else it might start to hurt—a problem known as tennis elbow. Clip your toenails and make sure there is extra room in your shoes, because tennis toe can be nasty too.

To protect other players, never throw your racquet or tennis balls, and try to keep loose balls off the courts. Be courteous and keep yourself and others safe by staying off courts where other people are playing.

When you're outside waiting to play, sit in the shade and drink lots of water—that way you'll stay cool and won't get sunburned. While you are playing, take a break between games or sets to cool off. And you may want to keep a wet towel around your neck while you wait. Also, you can look and feel cool by wearing a cold, wet bandana on your head while you play. And always wear sunscreen.

Table Tennis

How To Play

First, you'll need to know how to stand and hold your paddle. Hold your arm out in front of you—like you're about to shake hands. Then extend your fingers but keep your thumb pointing up. The paddle's handle should rest between your thumb and forefinger, and its face should point up like your thumb. Close your fingers around the handle, and use your forefinger and thumb for control. You'll want to grip the handle firmly, but keep it relaxed. Simply tighten your grip for more powerful shots.

Stand far enough from the table so that your arm and paddle can be fully extended. Shift your weight to the balls of your feet, and keep your knees slightly bent. Lean forward a bit using your non-paddle hand to keep balance.

There are a variety of ways to score a point. You'll score when a server makes a bad serve or when a player isn't able to hit the ball back to the other player. Points are also scored if the ball bounces two or more times on one player's side, or if the player touches the net or table.

Gear Up

You'll need the right equipment to get started. First, you'll want a table. The tables that are used look a lot like a tennis court—they are usually rectangular and green with white lines. A six-inch net is used to divide the table in half.

Next, you'll need a ball and paddles. The balls used in tournaments and during professional competitions are made of plastic and are hollow inside. Paddles, sometimes called rackets, are mostly made of wood. Each side is covered with a sheet of rubber. Often times the rubber sheets are made with different textures. This allows players to hit the ball at different speeds and with different types of spin. Even if a player chose different textures for each side of the paddle, official regulations require one side to be red and one side to be black. This way, players can always tell which side of the paddle their opponent is using.

Games

Chances are, you've played table tennis at school or at a friend's house. But did you know table tennis, also called Ping-Pong, is one of the most popular competitive sports in the world? It can be very different from what you might play at school or at home with friends. Table tennis is played at a very fast pace—some people even say it's the fastest ball sport in the world. This makes it really challenging and requires athletes to be in great shape. And, they have to have super hand-eye coordination.

Table tennis is a pretty new when you compare it to sports like running or soccer. In fact, it started at the end of the 19th century. It's believed that table tennis began in England where people used common household objects like corks and box lids to play. Once hollow, plastic balls replaced the cork and rubber balls originally used, the game became popular in North America too. These new balls allowed people to play with more bounce and at a much faster pace which helped to turn the game into a competitive sport.

Volleyball

How To Play

Volleyball was invented by William G. Morgan in 1895. He blended ideas from basketball, baseball, tennis, and handball to create the game, which he originally called "mintonette." It is fun to play because everybody gets involved. The game is unique because the same player isn't allowed to hit the ball twice in a row, so everyone takes turns serving, passing, and setting the ball. A team can hit the ball up to three times before they get it over the net. Before you play, check out these moves:

Serving The Ball: Stand at the back of the court and face the net. Hold the ball in the palm of your non-dominant hand (for example, left if you're right-handed) and stretch out your arm at waist level. Lean forward and swing your dominant hand (the one you write with) up toward the bottom of the ball. Now, drop the ball and hit it with your fist or the bottom of your hitting hand. Follow through, pointing your hitting arm toward your target. After you have practiced this underhand for a while, you can try a powerful overhead serve. Only the team that's serving can score points.

Passing The Ball: Move to the place where you think the ball will land and stand with your feet shoulder-width apart. Bend your knees and put your arms straight out in front of you.

Lock your hands together with your thumbs pointed forward. Watch the ball make contact with your arms and then push it forward with your forearms. Aim with your shoulders and straighten your legs, using the force from your legs to move the ball where you want it to go.

Setting The Ball: Stand with your feet shoulder-width apart, facing your target. Bend your knees and raise your hands above your head with your elbows bent. Put your hands together about six inches above and in front of your forehead, and make a diamond shape with your thumbs and pointer fingers. When the ball comes to you, use only your thumbs and the tops of your fingers to push the ball up in the direction you want it to go. Your palms should not touch the ball.

Gear Up

Volleyballs are about 26 inches around and weigh a bit more than half a pound. The net is stretched across the middle of the court and adjusts to different heights—7½ feet for girls and 8 feet for guys.

When you're playing volleyball, you're probably going to hit the ground a few times. Protect yourself with elbow and knee pads.

The bottoms of volleyball shoes are made of special rubber to keep you from slipping as you move around the court. Your shoes should also give you good ankle support and have lots of cushioning to protect your feet while you're jumping.

Play It Safe

Be sure to wear knee and elbow pads when you're playing on a hard court to protect you when you dive for the ball. When you go up for the ball, try landing on the balls of your feet with your knees bent and your hips lowered a little. Also, warm up and stretch before you play, and take off any jewelry.

Communicate with your teammates while you're playing to keep from running into each other. Make sure everyone on the team knows to "call" the ball by saying "got it" or "mine" if they plan to go for it.

If you're playing outside, find a soft court made of sand or grass, and clean up any sharp objects that you see. Be sure that there aren't any trees or basketball hoops in your way. And, wear sunscreen and always drink plenty of water. If you're playing inside, the court should be made of wood.

If your volleyball net is held up by wires, make sure they are covered with soft materials. That way you won't get hurt if you accidentally jump or run into the net.

Chapter 40

Walking And Hiking

Walking

How To Play

You've probably been walking for about as long as you've been talking. But walking isn't just a way to get from here to there, it's also a great physical activity. Walking doesn't require a lot of equipment, you can do it anywhere, it is always available by just walking out your front door, and it's a great way to relax and refresh. It's also something you can do alone or with your friends and family.

Check out these tips for how to walk and breathe correctly so your walk will be safer and easier.

Posture: How you hold your body is important. Stand up straight and tall. This means putting your shoulders back and relaxing them (no slouching), and keeping your chin up and stomach in. It's a good idea to look 20 feet ahead—about the lengths of two cars. This keeps your chin up and your eyes on your path.

Steps: Start out your first step with the heel first. Then roll your foot from heel to toe and push off the toes with the next step. Bringing the opposite leg forward, repeat this again. (This may feel a little funny at first but as your muscles get stronger it gets easier.)

Arm Motion: Moving or swinging your arms when you're walking can give you power, and it balances what your legs are doing. Bend your elbow 90 degrees (so your arm looks like the

---

About This Chapter: This chapter includes excerpts from "Walking Activity Card" and "Hiking Activity Card," undated documents produced by BAM! Body and Mind, Centers for Disease Control and Prevention (CDC), available online at www.bam.gov; accessed May 27, 2012.

letter "L"), while keeping your hands slightly curled. When you step, one foot moves forward and the arm opposite this foot should come forward too. As your foot goes back, bring back the opposite arm with it. Keep your elbows close to the body.

Breathe: Your breathing should have a rhythm. Inhale one deep breath for four steps and then hold that breath for two steps. Then exhale to the count of four steps, and hold it for two steps before beginning all over again. So the rhythm is—breathe in (step 1, 2, 3, 4), hold (step 1, 2) breathe out (step 1, 2, 3, 4) hold (step 1, 2). Everyone's stride is different, so if you feel that four steps are too long or too short, adjust it to what is comfortable for you.

Gear Up

Shoes are the most important part of your walking gear. Good walking shoes are generally flat, but flexible, so your foot rolls with each step. They should fit well, but leave enough room for your feet to spread out while walking. Wear socks that are comfortable. Try socks made of cotton or other sweat-wicking materials—they will keep your feet drier and help prevent blisters. Running shoes are okay to use for walking. Don't forget to trade in the old shoes when the treads start wearing out—which is about 500 miles.

Wear comfortable clothing when walking. Try to dress in layers, so you can always take off something as you warm up. Layering with a t-shirt, sweatshirt, or windproof jacket is a good idea if it's windy or chilly outside.

Two other essentials: sunscreen and a hat. The sunscreen protects your skin from the sun. In the summer, a hat keeps the sun out of your face, and in the winter it helps to keep you warm by trapping the heat that is lost from the top of your head. A bright colored hat will also make it easy for drivers to see and avoid you.

Play It Safe

Before you walk out the door, talk about the best walking routes with your parents so you know your safety zones and how to avoid traffic. And, only walk in those areas so your parents will know where you are.

It's always best to walk where you can avoid traffic—like parks or even the mall. Or try to find an area where there are sidewalks. If you have to walk on a street without sidewalks, walk close to the curb facing traffic. Remember to cross the street only at marked crosswalks or at corners, keep your ears and eyes open, and watch out for traffic in front and back of you. Wear bright-colored clothing or reflectors so drivers can see you. If you are walking alone, don't wear headphones—if they are too loud, they can keep you from hearing any oncoming traffic.

It's also a good idea to drink some water before you head out to walk, while you are walking, and when you get back—even if it's cold outside or you don't feel thirsty. In the summer, late afternoons (not nights) and mornings are the best times to walk to avoid the midday heat and humidity.

It is best to warm up your muscles before stretching them. So warm up for five minutes at an easy walking pace before stretching. Then stretch by starting at the top of your body and working your way down. Make sure to cool down and stretch after your walk too.

Remember—start out slowly and gradually increase the speed and distance you walk—don't try walking a marathon your first time out. And no matter where you are walking, be aware of what is going on around you.

Hiking

How To Play

Hiking with your friends or family is a great chance to get outdoors, breathe some fresh air, and get active. It's easy to get started. Just look for a trail in a national park near you.

For your first day hike (hiking for a day or less without camping overnight), choose a safe, well-marked trail that doesn't have too many steep climbs. Otherwise, you'll get tired too early and won't make it as far as you want to go. Each time you go hiking, try going a little farther and take a slightly steeper trail.

Gear Up

First, you'll need a good pair of shoes and thick socks designed for this type of activity. You can start with some sturdy sneakers with thick bottoms. When you begin to take on more difficult trails, try a pair of hiking boots, and make sure they fit. Also, get a backpack or fanny pack to carry all of your hiking supplies. Dress in layers and bring along a waterproof jacket with a hood in case you get caught in the rain. And don't forget a hat, sunscreen, and sunglasses because the higher you hike, the more dangerous the sun's rays become.

To keep hiking fun, you always need to be prepared to beat problems that could happen while you're out, like finding the trail if you get lost or stuck in bad weather. Make sure you bring a map of the area you'll be hiking in and a sturdy compass. You'll also need to bring plenty of water and extra food, like sports bars or trail mix, in case you have to stay out late and get hungry. The adults on your hike should bring a box of waterproof matches and an Army-style knife. A flashlight and extra batteries will help you find your way if you end up out after dark. Finally, you'll need to bring a first aid kit, in case someone gets hurt during your hike.

Play It Safe

Get in shape before you head out on your hike. Try walking around your neighborhood with your pack loaded with five pounds more gear than you'll actually carry on your hike. If that goes well, plan a short hike to test your abilities on the trail.

Take a friend and an adult along on your hike. That way you can look out for each other and you'll have people to talk to. Also, be sure to let someone who's not going know where you'll be hiking and what time you'll be back.

Carry lots of water even if you are only planning a short hike. For warm-weather hikes, bring six to eight quarts of water per day. In the cold weather or higher elevations, you can be safe with half that amount. Whenever you are near water, make sure you wet yourself down. Dampen a bandana and wipe your face, neck, and arms or wrap it around your head while you hike.

To prevent blisters, try spraying your feet with an antiperspirant before heading out. Bring extra pairs of socks that you can change into if your feet get wet or sweaty—if they aren't made of cotton, they'll keep your feet drier. Once you're on the trail, stop as soon as you feel a "hot spot" on your feet and apply special type of bandage called "moleskin" to the sore area. Also, try using a hiking stick to keep some pressure off of your legs and knees.

Don't get bugged by bugs. Protect yourself from bites and stings by using a bug repellant that includes DEET. Repellents that contain DEET are the most effective, but make sure you rub them on according to the directions. A good rule of thumb from the experts is that kids should use repellents with less than 10% DEET. Get your parents to help you put it on your face so you don't get it in your mouth or eyes. And wash your hands after you apply it. Remember that stuff that smells good to you smells good to bugs too, so don't use scented shampoos or lotions before hiking.

Watch the weather. When it's hot, pick trails that are shaded and run near streams. If you need to hike uphill in the sun, first soak yourself down to stay cool. You can also try wearing a wet bandana around your head or neck. Also, try to stay out of cotton clothes. Keep yourself out of bad weather by checking forecasts before you hike and watching the skies once you're out on the trail. During lightning storms, head downhill and away from the direction of the storm, and then squat down and keep your head low.

Chapter 41

Water Sports

Canoeing And Kayaking

How To Play

Paddlers (people who canoe or kayak) really know how to have fun on the water—just a boat, a paddle, nature, and you. Here's how to paddle:

- **Canoeing:** Hold the paddle with your inside hand on top and your water-side hand two to three feet down. Your knuckles should be facing out. Without stretching, insert the blade of the paddle all the way in the water as far forward as you can reach. Push your top hand forward and pull your bottom hand back, turning your shoulders to move the paddle blade straight through the water to your hip. Keep the top of the paddle handle lower than your eyes and don't follow the curve of the canoe. Again. Have a friend paddle on the other side of the canoe, or switch sides as you paddle, to keep the boat gliding along straight.

- **Kayaking:** Kayak paddles have a blade on each side. Lift your paddle with both hands and hold it across your chest. Place your hands the same distance from each blade, just outside your shoulders. Hold the paddle out in front of you, just a few inches above the kayak. Keeping your left elbow straight, bring your right hand straight back, letting your right elbow bend back toward your body. Your body will twist to the right a bit. Paddle. Now, use the other arm

About This Chapter: This chapter includes excerpts from "Canoeing/Kayaking Activity Card," "Diving Activity Card," "Fishing Activity Card," "Snorkeling Activity Card," "Surfing Activity Card," "Water Skiing Activity Card," and "White-Water Rafting Activity Card," undated documents produced by BAM! Body and Mind, Centers for Disease Control and Prevention (CDC), available online at www.bam.gov; accessed May 27, 2012.

Kayakers and canoers follow these tips so they don't annoy other people or the environment.

- Only get to the water through marked paths—not through someone else's property. Take your paddling breaks in public places too.

- Keep your lunch spots and campsites clean—don't leave garbage in the water or lying around. If there's nowhere to put your trash, take it with you and dump it when you get home.

- Give people fishing plenty of room and try not to disturb the water too much where they are—it'll scare the fish off.

- Keep away from the wildlife.

Gear Up

You'll need a kayak (boat that's almost completely closed on top with space for just one person) or a canoe (open boat that can fit you and a friend or two) plus the right kind of paddle. Kayak paddles have a blade on both sides, but canoe paddles have one blade. Be sure to pick the right size paddle—the stick part of a canoe paddle should be about six to eight inches longer than the length of your arm with your fingers out.

Don't forget another essential: the life vest. Water shoes or sneakers—not sandals—that grip on the bottom will help your feet stay put when you are pulling the paddle through the water. Keep a whistle attached to your life vest so you are always ready to get attention if trouble strikes.

Play It Safe

You need to be a strong swimmer because you might have to swim underwater, or in moving water. Always go paddling with another person.

Make sure your life jacket fits. Since paddling is an activity that you can do all through the year, leave enough room to put clothes under it when it is cold out. Be prepared to get wet. Take along extra dry clothing, just in case. Remember to keep sun proof with sunscreen.

Save paddling for good weather days. Since you don't know what mother nature will throw at you, know where your float trip will take you, spots where you can get out or camp for the night, and different ways to go in case unexpected trouble strikes your route. Avoid whitewater rapids, dams, and falls—only experienced whitewater paddlers should take these on.

Sure, you want all your friends and their stuff to come along, but don't put too much weight in the boat—you should have more than six inches of side between the top of the fully loaded boat and the water. Spread out the weight (including people) so the boat will stay balanced.

Take lessons to help you learn ways to get yourself back in your boat if it tips over—before you take your first trip. And then practice them. The main thing to remember is: Don't panic. If you can't get back in, stay with your boat and flip it back over—it'll float—and try to swim the boat to shore. (Remember, you're wearing a life jacket, right?!)

Diving

How To Play

Diving is about precision, flexibility, and strength. Experienced divers leap 5–10 meters (about 16–33 feet) into the air from a springboard or platform, do stunts like somersaults or twists, and then plunge into the water below. Divers hit the water at speeds of up to 34 miles per hour.

Be water wise. Check the depth before you dive.

A certified diving instructor can help you master the diving board, but for now, try this beginners' dive: Point your arms straight over your head, with your shoulders by your ears. Keep your head between your arms and tuck your chin to your chest. Bend at the waist, but don't bend the knees. Keep your legs straight. Fall towards the water, making sure not to lift your head or shoulders. Follow through with your fingers into the water. That's it—you've made the plunge.

Gear Up

It's simple—all you need is a swimsuit and a pool with a diving board. Check out your neighborhood or a community center in your area for a pool you can use.

Play It Safe

Here's the deal: Know how to swim well before stepping on the board. Always dive with someone else. And protect your head and spinal cord. You must know the water depth before you dive, and never ever dive into shallow water. Check around for signs or ask a lifeguard. Diving areas are usually marked. In case you haven't figured this out yet, above-ground pools are not designed for diving. They're way too shallow! (Lots of in-ground pools aren't deep enough either, so check out the water before you dive.)

When you are on the board, enter the water straight on and make sure there's nothing in your way before you leap. If people come into the diving area from other parts of the pool, wait until they're gone, or just ask the lifeguard to clear the area for you. If you jump when there is someone else in the diving area, or even just mess around while diving, you could land on top of someone and get hurt.

Don't run up to a dive. Always stand at the edge of the board or pool and then dive. And dive straight ahead—not off to the side. Most of all, only try dives that are in your comfort zone. Leave those fancy or stunt leaps to experienced divers. An adult can help you decide which dives are safe to try.

Fishing

How To Play

Fishing is a great way to spend some nature time—and maybe even get dinner while you're at it. Fish live in all sorts of water—ponds, rivers, lakes, oceans—and there are tons of ways to catch 'em. But let's start with the basics:

Take your rod and stick the hook at the end of the line (plastic string) through something fish think they want to eat: bait. Fish love real, squirmy worms, but you can also use plastic bait or other tasty things like crickets, night crawlers, or little minnows (kind of fish).

Grip your rod like you're shaking hands with it. Keep your thumb on top of the release button. Make sure no one is near you—you're trying to hook fish, not people. Put your weight on the balls of your feet and keep your wrist straight. Bring the rod back just behind your head, hold the handle tight, and quickly move the rod forward as you press the release button to let go of the line. The hook and bait should fly out far in front of you and drop into the water. Relax and wait until you see a tug on the line.

Fun Facts About Fishing

- The world's largest fish is a whale shark. It grows to be more than 50 feet long and weighs several tons. The world's smallest fish is a goby. It only grows to be a ½ inch long.
- Check out how old a fish is by looking at the growth rings on its scales. They're similar to rings found on tree trunks, except fish get a new growth ring every summer and every winter. Every two rings represent one year.
- A bass (kind of fish) brain has two memory centers—one for each eye. That's why it's possible to catch the same bass twice. The bass sees the bait out of one eye the first time it gets caught. If it is thrown back into the water, it can see the same bait out of the other eye and not remember it. So, it may decide to go in for a bite anyway.
- Fish swim by contracting their muscles (making them smaller)—first on one side of their body and then on the other—to whip their tails from side to side. The fins pointing straight up help the fish keep its balance, and fins on the belly help the fish hang out in one place, as well as move forward.

Gear Up

You'll need a fishing rod and reel. Look for a rod that's about as tall as you are and has a push button reel. You can also use a cane pole (no reel) and tie your own line to the end. You'll need bait too—earthworms rule for most fish. You can buy them, dig for them, or find them lying around after a rainstorm. A net will help you scoop the fish out of the water once you've brought them in. You'll also want a basic tackle box to hold your stuff.

Play It Safe

Make sure someone knows where you are and how long you will be gone. Check out all the signs where you'll be fishing and stick to what they say. Pick the right spot—stay away from tree branches that hang over the water, power lines, or strong currents. Look before you sit, step, or touch—you don't want to get near animals, or slip on wet rocks. Be careful if you're fishing off a dock or pier so you don't fall in. Check the weather report before going fishing and if a storm sneaks up on you, head for home.

Wear a life jacket if you are anywhere near deep water, running water, or on the ice. Wear a hat and sunscreen to shield you from the rays, and make sure you have your shades on to fight the glare off the water.

Fishing hooks are sharp, so be careful not to hook yourself, or someone else. Keep a first aid kit handy in case you get stuck. Carry a whistle to get help if you need it.

If you want to ice fish (fishing through a hole drilled in the ice), wait until the ice is at least 4 inches thick. For fly fishing (special type of fishing in moving water with bait handmade to look like bugs), shuffle into the flowing current sideways. If you're fishing in the waves, shuffle your feet along to scare away fish and other sea creatures.

Snorkeling

How To Play

Before heading out to explore the water, it's important to know how to swim. Snorkeling is like swimming, but with fins, a mask, and a tube called a snorkel for breathing underwater. It's easy and fun and you can do it in an ocean, lake, or even at your neighborhood pool. Snorkeling is also a great starting point if you want to get involved in scuba diving. It teaches you the basics of breathing and exploring underwater, but it doesn't have an age limit or require expensive equipment like scuba diving. So strap on your fins and dive in.

Learning to use a snorkel is easy. You may want to practice in a swimming pool (or shallow water where you can stand) until you get the hang of it. First, put your mask on—it should have a small rubber strap that attaches the snorkel to your mask, and the snorkel should pass just above your left ear. Take a deep breath, bite down on the mouthpiece and slowly place your head into the water (make sure to breathe through your mouth). Breathe out through your mouth once to clear any water out of the snorkel—this is called blasting. Inhale slowly in case there's water in your tube, then blast your snorkel again just to make sure you get as much water out as you can. Swim along the surface of the water at a slow pace. If you swim too fast, or make lots of sudden movements with your arms and legs, you can scare the fish and other sea creatures away.

After you get the hang of using your snorkel and mask, you may want to take a dive. Try some shallow dives to get an idea of how long you can hold your breath. It's important to know your limits.

Gear Up

To snorkel you don't need a lot of complicated equipment—a mask, snorkel, fins, and swimsuit or swimming trunks are all you need.

It's important to buy a good mask that's the right size for your face and has a tight-fitting seal. The easiest way to test how well your mask fits is to lift the strap over the top of the mask and press the mask to your face without breathing in. If it stays tight to your face (without you holding it on), you've got the right fit. If not, keep looking until you find one that seals properly. You'll want to get a mask that has a glass face (not plastic) to keep it from fogging up or making the sights below look weird.

There are many different sizes and designs of snorkels—find one that is comfortable, and allows you to clear water easily. It's important that you find the right snorkel for you—it's what helps you breathe while you're cruising along in the water checking out the sites below.

There are a few different types of fins to choose from—full-foot fins fit like a slipper around your heel, while open-heel fins fit your feet and have a strap that fits around your heel. Your fins should be snug, but not too tight (if your fins are too tight or loose, they may cause blisters). They should be flexible and lightweight—to give you speed and mobility. You may also want to get diving booties to prevent blisters and protect your feet.

If you're swimming in salty water, make sure to rinse all of your equipment with fresh water. If you don't, salt crystals can form causing the straps to stiffen and crack, and the fabric may tear. So, keep your equipment clean.

234

Play It Safe

Always make sure your snorkel, fins, and mask are in good working order before taking the plunge. It's also important to know the basics like how to clear water from your snorkel (blasting), and how to put your mask back on while treading water. Until you get more experienced, you may want to wear a life jacket—it will help you stay afloat if you need a rest, or if you get into trouble in the water.

Most importantly, never snorkel alone. Always swim with a buddy and keep them close by so you can help each other out—and, it's more fun with a friend.

Check out the weather forecast and the water's visibility before you jump in. And don't forget, coral reefs are fun to explore, but don't go too close to them until you've learned how to steer your body in the water. Never touch a reef—they are sharp and some have ocean life that may be poisonous. Always be considerate of the places you are snorkeling in, they may be another animal's home.

Finally, watch out for the sun. Wear a t-shirt and sunscreen to make sure you don't get sunburned.

Surfing

How To Play

Surfing takes lots of practice, but when you're riding that wave, it's incredible. Here's how to start:

Which Foot? Put your best foot forward—find out whether you are regular or goofy-footed. Try sliding across a smooth floor with socks on. If you lead with your left foot, you're "regular," and the left foot goes near the front of the board when you're surfing. If your right foot goes first, you're "goofy," and the right foot goes up front.

Paddling: To get around in the water, lay chest-down on your board, keeping your legs straight behind you. With each arm, make an overhand swimming stroke that starts at the front of the board and finishes under the board near your legs. (It's like swimming the crawl stroke, except you're on top of the board.) As you finish the stroke with one hand, the other hand is just starting. Try practicing in shallow water or a pool first.

Catching The Wave: When you see white water (breaking waves) coming, turn around to face the shore, aim your board the direction the wave is coming, and start to paddle in. When the wave reaches you, it will push you forward. Stop paddling, grab the side of the board, push up your body, and quickly get your feet under you. Both should land at the same time, toes pointing sideways. Move your lead (regular or goofy) foot in front. You're surfing.

Gear Up

All you really need is a bathing suit or a wetsuit (for cold water or if it's cold out), and of course, a surfboard. Here are some tips: You may want to get a used or inexpensive board at first. It wouldn't be smart to mess up a cool, new board making beginner's mistakes. The fins should be in good condition, and it should have a place to attach a leash (cord that hooks your ankle to the board so it doesn't get away). Long boards are easier to ride and control. Your board should be 12 to 14 inches taller than you. Also, put two coats of wax on your board if the deck (top) doesn't have a pad that keeps you from slipping.

Play It Safe

First things first: You must be a strong swimmer. As a beginner, you are going to be in the water more than riding your board. And always surf with someone else. Always leash your board to control it. When you begin the wipeout (fall at the end of a ride), kick your board out and away from you.

While you're a beginner, stick to waves no bigger than three feet. If you are a real beginner, surf only broken (white) waves. Never paddle out farther than you can swim back with your board. Most of all, if it doesn't feel right or you are too scared, just don't go.

Finally, make sure to wear sunscreen. And always remember, bad weather means no surfing.

Who Owns The Wave?

Did you know that surfers have rules for who "owns" a wave? Surfers riding waves have to get out of the way of those paddling out, and everyone has to stay clear of swimmers. A surfer who is standing and riding a wave gets to keep it—no one should "drop in" (try to catch the same wave).

Water Skiing

How To Play

Want to walk on water? Try water skiing! Water skiers hold onto a rope and are pulled on their skis behind a boat going fast. They glide across the water with the wind in their faces. It's a great activity that you can do with your family or friends, and it can be competitive. Check out these tips and you'll be skiing in no time:

Getting Started: Before you get in the water to ski, make sure you're wearing a life vest that is the right size and is on the right way. Get in the water with your skis. Wet your ski bindings before you put on your skis, and keep the bindings loose enough that the skis will come off if you fall. Bend your knees up towards your chest with your arms straight out in front of you. As the boat pulls the rope toward you, grab the rope handle with both hands and hold it between your knees. You should almost be sitting on the skis. Facing the boat, lift the tips of your skis a bit above the water, keep your skis shoulder width apart, and keep your arms straight. Nod your head to let the boat driver know you are ready to go, and begin straightening your legs as you are pulled out of the water. If you stand too soon you'll fall down, so take it slow and be patient.

Steering: To turn, just lean in the direction you want to go. Move your weight to the edge of the skis on the side you want to turn toward while you keep the skis pointed forward. If you want to turn faster, crouch down while you lean.

Gear Up

First you'll need water skis. There are four types: combination pairs, slalom, tick, and jump skis. New skiers should start with combination pairs, since they are wider and easiest to learn on. Make sure your skis have been checked and that they fit properly. You will also need a flexible towrope that has a floating handle.

All water skiers wear life vests (also called personal floatation devices or PFDs). You should wear a special water skiing life vest that is approved by the Coast Guard. You and your parents should check this out to get the official word on which life vest is right for you.

Finally, since you're outside, you need to guard against the sun.

Play It Safe

Water skiers need to be good swimmers and always wear a life jacket that fits properly.

Safe water skiing requires three people: the skier, an experienced boat driver, and the spotter to look out for the skier's signals. Since the noise from the boat is so loud, it's important that everyone agrees on and understands the hand signals to use so you can talk without saying a word. Remember, you need to master hand signals before you begin cutting across the water on your skis.

When you're out on the water, be sure you're in a safe area to ski. Don't ski near docks, boats, rocks, or in shallow water. The only place to start is in the water—dock or land starts should be left to the pros.

If you start to lose your balance while skiing, just bend your knees and crouch down so you don't fall. If you do fall—and everyone does—remember to let go of the rope. Then, find your skis and hold one of them up to signal you're okay and to let other boaters know you're in the water.

White-Water Rafting

How To Play

White-water rafting takes place on a river, but not just any river will do—it has to have rapids. Rapids occur where the water moves very quickly downhill over rocks or boulders. To the experts, rapids are classified on a scale of 1–6. Class 1 rapids are small with low waves, a slow current, and no obstructions in the water, while Class 6 rapids can have large, frequent waves that are often unavoidable, and in some cases, you may even have to navigate a waterfall. Class 6 rapids are extremely difficult and almost impossible to pass. Beginners should stick to Class 1 and 2 rapids—they're exciting, extreme, and safe. If you have questions about rapid classifications, river guides are always glad to explain the rating system.

White-water rafting is definitely a team effort—so understanding the basics of paddling are important. If everyone in the raft gives it their all, it's much easier to guide the raft down the river and through the rapids.

Once you're in the raft, sit facing downriver with your back to the stern (back of the raft). Hold the paddle with your inside hand (the hand farthest away from the paddle) on top and your outside hand, knuckles facing out, gripping the paddle low on the stem. Lean forward from your hips, straighten your arms out in front of you, and keep your back straight. Straighten your wrists and put the paddle into the water—make sure the blade is completely under the surface of the water. Straighten your top arm while pulling back the paddle with your lower arm guiding the paddle. Reverse this motion to back paddle. If you want to turn the raft right, the right side of your rafting team needs to paddle backward while the left side paddles forward. The same goes for turning left except the members on the left side of the raft need to paddle backward and the right side forward. Rafting is all about communicating and working as a team.

Gear Up

You'll need a raft and paddles (usually eight people per raft) to navigate the rapids, as well as a good life jacket and helmet. If you're heading out into cooler temperatures, wear warm, waterproof clothing and wool socks—these will keep you warm and dry while splashing down the river. If it's warm outside, nylon shorts, a bathing suit or swim trunks, a t-shirt, or a tank top are all good choices—just make sure to lather on that sunscreen to protect yourself from the sun. As for shoes, your best bet is to wear a pair with rubber soles or slip-on water shoes that you don't mind getting wet—because even during a good run, you're sure to get wet.

Some rafting trips can take a few hours (or even an entire day), so pack plenty of drinking water and food—just make sure to pack it up tight to keep the water out.

Play It Safe

Before jumping into that raft, it's important to know how to swim. Even if you're a strong swimmer, always wear a life jacket. It should fit snugly and have back and shoulder protection as well as floatation to help you swim safely in white water. Also, don't forget to wear your helmet—it should be designed for water sports, fit properly and snugly on your head, and allow for water to drain from the helmet. It should also cover your ears, temples, and the back of your neck. Once you have the proper gear and are sure it's all in working order, you're ready to run the river.

It's also really helpful if you've done a little exploring first. Make sure you know the river you are rafting on—check out the rating of the rapids and what the current is like. It's best to a have a trained, experienced guide on your team and in your raft. The guide will know the best course and the safest passage. Don't enter a rapid unless you're sure you can run it safely or swim it without getting hurt. If you fall out of the raft, position your body so that you are on your back with your feet facing down river—try to keep your feet and legs up.

Usually a group of three boats is the minimum on a river—but only one boat should run the rapids at a time. Safe rafting is all about teamwork, so pick a captain to call out directions so everyone can work together.

Most importantly, be prepared. Get a first aid and survival kit, and include extra ropes, a raft repair kit, and extra life vests. Better safe than stranded.

Chapter 42

Winter Sports

Figure Skating

How To Play

Did you ever watch the figure skaters in the Olympics wondering how the heck they did all those jumps and spins? Well, according to the experts, the key to becoming a successful skater is one simple thing—balance. Good posture is an important part of balance, because it helps even out your weight over the skates. This keeps you from falling and helps you glide smoothly and work up some speed. Keep your head and chin up and imagine that they are connected with an imaginary line that runs down the center of your chest and connects with the toes of both of your feet.

It's also important to know how to stop. The basic stop is called a snowplow. Keeping both knees bent, shift your weight to one foot, then turn the other foot inward at an angle. Gradually shift your weight to the angled foot, which will slow you down and eventually bring you to a stop. A hockey stop is a more advanced move. To do it, quickly turn your feet sideways until they are perpendicular to the direction you were moving, putting more weight on your back foot.

Gear Up

Figure skates are very thick and heavy and have a toe pick attached for tricks. Figure skates are made up of two parts, the boot and the blade. If you are just starting out, you can buy skates

About This Chapter: This chapter includes excerpts from "Figure Skating Activity Card" and "Snow Skiing Activity Card," undated documents produced by BAM! Body and Mind, Centers for Disease Control and Prevention (CDC), available online at www.bam.gov; accessed May 27, 2012. It also includes excerpts from "Snowboarding," a document produced by the President's Council on Sports, Fitness, and Nutrition (www.fitness.gov), January 2012.

with both a boot and a blade, but more advanced skaters can buy each separately. The boot should be snug in the heel and supportive of the ankle. The blade is attached to the boot with screws, and it is wider than the blade on an ice hockey skate, so that the edge grips the ice. You should not use figure skates to play ice hockey, because the blades extend past the boot and can cause other players to get injured.

If you are a beginning skater, along with your skates, you may want to wear a helmet to protect your head against any falls.

Be sure to wear layers so that you can put on or take off clothes depending on whether you are cold or warm. It's important to be able to move, so sweatpants or warm-up pants are perfect. You should only wear one pair of lightweight socks inside your skates, though, and remember to wear mittens and a hat to keep warm.

Play It Safe

Be a courteous skater—always be aware of other skaters and follow the traffic flow of the rink. Be careful not to get too close to other skaters with your exposed blades. And keep your skate laces tied tightly so that you don't trip yourself or anyone else up.

If you feel yourself beginning to fall, bring your hands, arms, and head into your body to absorb the shock of hitting the ice. And make sure you hop up quickly so that you are not in the way of other skaters.

Skating can be hard work, and puts a lot of stress on your leg and back muscles, so be sure to warm up before you skate and stretch those muscles well.

Snow Skiing

How To Play

Skiing can be done as a fun activity with your family or friends, and as your skills increase, you might even want to ski competitively There are several main skiing categories including alpine skiing, which is the fast-n-furious downhill skiing; freestyle skiing, in which skiers perform jumps and tricks over moguls (large bumps on the ski slope) while skiing downhill; and cross country skiing, where skiers race long distances over flatter land.

Here are some key tips to get you started:

To get on a lift, put both your poles in your inside hand. Turn to the outside and watch for the next chair. As it gets to you, grab the outside pole and sit normally on the chair. Keep your skis apart, with the tips up, as you're lifted off the ground.

To get off the lift, grab a pole in each hand, but don't put on your wrist straps. Point the pole tips toward the outside of the chair, and hold them up so they don't catch on the snow. Hold the bar on the outside of the chair for balance, relax your legs, and ease yourself forward, pushing off once your skis touch the snow. Don't stand up until the chair has passed over the top of the mound, and move away from the chairlift before you prepare to ski so that others can get off behind you.

You'll also need to know how to get up after a fall. Make sure your skis are below you on the hill. Grab the top of both poles in one hand, grab the bottom of both with the other, and plant your poles in the snow just above your hip. Push up with both arms to shift yourself forward and over your skis. Make sure your weight is forward and over your skis before you stand up.

Gear Up

Are your skis the right size? If the tip of your upright ski reaches your face between your nose and chin, they are. If you're a beginner, shorter skis will be easier to control. The bindings (the part that holds your boot to the ski) are the most important parts of the ski—to make sure they don't break, get them tested regularly by a pro.

Make sure your boots fit and are comfortable. In general, ski boots are ½ size smaller than your normal shoe size.

Ski poles are used to give you balance and help you get up if you fall, or need to side-step up a hill.

Goggles are important to protect your eyes from flying dirt or snow, as well as stopping the sun's glare while whooshing down the slopes. Some goggles come with fun tinted lenses. If you don't have goggles, you can use sunglasses instead.

Be a trendsetter by picking up the helmet habit. Choose an ASTM approved model that fits right, is ventilated, and doesn't affect your hearing or field of vision.

If you are renting equipment, the staff at the ski shop can help you find all the right stuff.

Here are some tips about what to wear to help you stay warm on the slopes:

- Long underwear to keep you warm and absorb sweat
- Insulated tops and pants such as sweaters and leggings—this layer should be warm, but not baggy
- Ski pants and jackets to protect you from snow and wetness
- A hat, because 60 percent of heat loss is through the head

Play It Safe

If you can, sign up for lessons from a ski school, even if you've taken lessons before—your instructor can teach you all the right moves, for beginners as well as for more advanced students.

The key to skiing is control of your equipment and your speed. If you feel yourself start to lose control, fall onto your backside or your side and don't attempt to get up until you stop sliding.

The easiest way to get hurt while skiing is to try a run or a move that is too hard. Always ski on trails that match your skill level and never attempt a jumping move, or other trick, unless taught by an instructor.

Did you know that it is just as important to drink water when you are active in the cold as in the heat? Why? Higher altitudes and colder air can cause your body to lose water. If you experience dizziness or have dry mouth, headache, or muscle cramps, take a water break. A good rule would be to drink water or sports drinks before, during, and after your ski runs.

Always check the snow conditions of the slope before you go up—you'll need to ski differently in icy conditions than you would if you were on wet snow or in deep powder.

Altitude can zap your energy. Don't push it. Ski the easier runs later in the day when you are tired. Most importantly—know when to quit.

While on the slopes, set a meeting time and place to check in with your parents or friends. And always ski with a buddy. And wear plenty of sunblock, because those rays are strong on the mountain due to high altitude and reflection off the snow.

Be sure to keep the Responsibility Code for Skiers in mind:

- Always stay in control and be able to stop or avoid other people or objects.

- People ahead of you have the right of way. It is your responsibility to avoid them.

- Do not stop where you obstruct a trail or are not visible from above.

- Whenever starting downhill or merging into a trail, look uphill and yield to others.

- Always use devices to help prevent runaway equipment.

- Observe all posted signs and warnings. Keep off closed trails and out of closed areas.

- Before using any lift, you must have the knowledge and ability to load, ride, and unload safely.

Snowboarding

History

Snowboarding is an American original. As one story goes, Sherman Poppen invented the snowboard for his daughter in 1965 when he braced a pair of skis together and tied a rope to the front to help steer. The "snurfer," as it was called when it debuted a year later, is said by some to be the world's first production snowboard. Others credit snowboarding's origins to creative efforts by surfers and skateboarders to adapt their activities, techniques and equipment to winter recreation over the last few decades. No matter how snowboarding got started, there's no doubt—it's a native-born American sport, one that has taken the world by storm.

Snowboarding competition began in the 1980s. The United States held its first national championships in 1982 and hosted the first World Championships in 1983. Snowboarding made its Olympic debut in 1998 at Nagano, where its two events—the giant slalom and the halfpipe—were introduced to the world.

There are four snowboard events at the Olympics: men's halfpipe, women's halfpipe, men's parallel giant slalom, and women's parallel giant slalom.

The halfpipe competition takes place in a half-cylinder-shaped course dug deep into the hill. The pipe is generally 3 to 4 meters deep and 110 meters long with an 85-degree pitch and high vertical walls on each side. Using speed gained on the slope, snowboarders come up over the rim of the pipe and perform acrobatic aerial tricks. The object of the halfpipe is to perform difficult tricks with perfect form. The halfpipe is judged on rotations, amplitude, and overall impression.

The parallel giant slalom is an exciting version of alpine snowboarding, It features head-to-head match ups on the mountain. After the qualification round, a 16-person tournament is established and competitors battle it out on two side-by-side courses until there is a winner.

How To Play

Learning snowboarding can be humbling but fun. It's sometimes said that "snowboarding is hard to learn but easy to master, and skiing is easy to learn but hard to master." Snowboarding requires more balance than skiing in the beginning. Just remember—you have to learn to walk before you run.

Wearing The Right Clothing

Wearing the right clothing is extremely important when participating in cold weather sports. Dress in layers, wearing warm, waterproof/resistant clothing. Clothing for snowboarding should protect the participant from cold, wind, and precipitation and should also provide ventilation—be breathable. To reduce wind resistance, the clothing should fit snugly to the body. Pay special attention to protecting feet, hands, face, and head. Up to 40 percent of body heat can be lost when the head is exposed. Footgear should be insulated to protect against cold and dampness.

Wearing multiple layers of varying thickness allows you to regulate your body temperature. You should flexibly layer the clothing and use proper materials so you will stay warm and still not restrict your movement. Many peel off layers when snowboarding, then replace those layers when stopping to rest and rehydrate.

Wear at least three layers of clothing:

- A water-resistant outer layer to break the wind and allow some ventilation (nylon or other water-resistant synthetic fabric)

- A middle layer of wool or wool-like synthetic fabric to absorb sweat and retain insulation

- An inner layer close to the skin. It's important to keep moisture away from your skin—avoid cotton, which clings to perspiration. Synthetic materials such as supplex and coolmax are ideal because they keep you warm and dry.

Equipment

- **Helmet:** A hard plastic helmet is essential to prevent head injuries; helmets manufactured for ski sports are required for snowboarding competition.

- **Board:** For the halfpipe, a wide flexible board; for the parallel giant slalom, a stiff, narrower board to allow for turns and high speed.

- **Boots:** For the halfpipe, most participants use soft boots with foot and ankle support and lace-up inner boots; for the parallel giant slalom, you'll need alpine boots with a hard plastic exterior for extensive foot and ankle support, similar to alpine ski boots.

Snowboarding Basics

When you're ready to head for the snow, the best way to get started is to sign up for snowboarding lessons at a ski resort. Classes exist for all ages and styles, from the free rider, who just wants to whoosh down the hill, to the freestyle artist, who wants to perform the dangerous jumps to thrill the audience below. Keep your expectations realistic the first day or two. Pace yourself, and commit to keep trying to learn snowboarding for at least three days. Then you'll start to gain confidence and feel more control. Once you are comfortable with momentum and controlling speed, it becomes easier to balance.

Snowboarding Glossary

Backside: The side of the snowboard on which the athlete's heels rest; the side of the snowboard to which the athlete's back faces.

Duckfoot: A snowboard stance in which the toes point outward.

Fakie: Riding backwards.

Fall Line: An imaginary line that combines the steepest pitch and most direct line, from top to bottom, of any slope.

Flex: The stiffness of the snowboard.

Freeriding: Snowboarding for fun, not in a competition.

Freestyle Snowboarding: The type of snowboarding that includes tricks; halfpipe is a type of freestyle snowboarding.

Frontside: The side of the snowboard on which the toes rest; the side of the snowboard the athlete's chest faces.

Goofy-Footed: Riding a snowboard with the right foot forward.

Halfpipe: The snow structure on which the halfpipe competition is contested. It is made up of two walls of the same height and size and a transition area in between.

Nose: The front tip of the snowboard.

Ollie: A method to obtain air without jumping. It is performed by first lifting the front foot, then lifting the rear foot as the rider springs off the tail.

Regular-Footed: Riding on a snowboard with the left foot forward.

Revert: To switch from riding fakie (backwards) to forward, or from forward to fakie.

Stance: The position of the feet on the snowboard.

Step-In Binding: Binding system in which no major manual adjustment is needed to attach and detach the boot from the binding.

Traverse: To ride perpendicular to the fall line; to ride across the halfpipe.

Vertical: The top portion of the wall in a halfpipe that allows the snowboard to fly straight up in the air.

180 Air: An aerial maneuver in which the snowboard rotates 180 degrees—a half of a spin.

360 Air: An aerial maneuver in which the snowboard rotates 360 degrees—one full spin.

540 Air: An aerial maneuver in which the snowboarder rotates 540 degrees—one and a half spins.

720 Air: An aerial maneuver in which the snowboarder rotates 720 degrees—two full spins.

900 Air: An aerial maneuver in which the snowboarder rotates 900 degrees—two and a half spins.

Source: President's Council on Sports, Fitness, and Nutrition (www.fitness.gov), January 2012.

Before going out on the snow, you might consider dry land training—practicing with the snowboard on a carpet indoors to help you become oriented and introduce you to the proper primary body alignment. The goal is an efficient foundation/stance. You should be balanced and relaxed, maintaining an athletic stance over the edge you are riding on—the heel edge (back) or the toe edge (front). You should minimize tension or twist up at the waist, and your upper body should align with the angle of your feet. Remember: You're not skiing. You'll need to keep the upper body in somewhat of an alignment with the lower body. Your shoulders should be parallel with the board to assure that you are weighting and balancing on both feet evenly (50–50) and staying on the "sweet spot" (center) of the board.

When you are ready to take your first run down the hill, you will have to decide how you want to stand on the board. Most people stand or "board" with their left foot forward, much like sliding into home plate. Others prefer to lead with their right foot. Your choice may depend on whether you are left- or right-handed. Some "boarders" can do it either way. You'll quickly discover which side is more comfortable for you.

Next, strap your front leading foot onto the board. Your toes will inch over the edge of the board a bit, your heel against the toes of the other foot as you balance precariously for a second or two. Strap your other foot in, and start slowly down the mountain side (or bunny hill). Make sure you're facing forward, hands in front; keep your weight low and your knees bent. Try to maintain an even keel in the snow without catching the front or back end of your board in the snow.

- **Turns:** Turns are made by leaning forwards or backward and from side to side, using the toe edge (front) and the heel edge (back) of the board for steering and speed control. Similar to inline skating, the back of your board will slow you down if you press it into the snow. Many new riders find it disconcerting to travel facing the trees or the side of the slope while going down the mountain, but after a few gentle turns and twists you'll be thrilled as you gingerly pick up speed and enjoy the powder under your feet.

- **Stopping:** Stopping a snowboard is much like coming to a stop on ice skates—bring both feet perpendicular to the slope, then scrape to a stop. Be prepared to fall more than a few times while learning this skill. Just as in ice skating, you have to learn how to balance your weight to scrape the snow/ice just enough to stop but not so much that you upset your position and fall. These maneuvers will take time and practice to learn, but they are necessary skills to acquire and are fun once you master them.

Finally, unbuckle your back foot from the board and push off with your foot, sliding easily to the lift for your next ride up to the top to continue snowboarding. Hands free and fancy free, you're on your way to becoming a great snowboarder.

Part Five
Sports Safety

Chapter 43

Fitness Safety Tips

There are many things you need to do to stay safe and injury-free during exercise. Review these items so that you don't get hurt!

Warming Up And Cooling Down

Before you start exercising, you need to warm up your muscles. It is best to warm up your muscles before stretching them. You can warm up by walking at an easy pace before stretching. Then stretch by starting at the top of your body and working your way down. Slowly stretch your calf, quad, groin, and hamstring muscles (you can view sample stretches online at http://www.girlshealth.gov/fitness/exercise/stretching.cfm). Warming up can also include jogging slowly, doing knee lifts, and arm circles.

Make sure to cool down and stretch after exercising, too! A cool-down is a gentle exercise or stretch that helps the body return to its normal state after vigorous exercise. Cool-downs help your pulse (or heart rate) return to normal and can help prevent your muscles from feeling stiff after a workout.

Important Exercise Safety Tips

- See your doctor for a sports physical before you start a sport.
- Don't exercise when it is really hot and humid out. You do not want your body to overheat or get dehydrated. If it's very hot or humid outside, try moving your exercise indoors that day. Also, if you live in an area with high air pollution, exercise early in the day or at night and avoid congested streets and rush hour traffic.

About This Chapter: Text in this chapter is from "Fitness: Keeping Safe and Injury-Free," Office on Women's Health (www.girlshealth.gov), October 9, 2009.

- Drink water before, during, and after exercise or sports competitions.

- Make sure you warm up and stretch your muscles for five minutes before and after workouts to make your muscles more flexible. It is easier to get hurt if your muscles are not stretched. It is also important to increase the intensity of your workout gradually. If you exercise intensely right away, you could risk getting hurt.

- See a doctor or let your parents/guardian know if: 1) You are in severe pain, 2) you see swelling around where you got hurt, or 3) The pain gets in the way of sleep and activities. Don't jump back to your regular exercise after getting hurt because you could get hurt again. Follow your doctor's orders for how to care for your injury and when you can be active again.

- Follow the rules of the game! The rules are there, in part, to keep you safe.

Using The Right Equipment

When you exercise or play sports, it is important to use the right safety equipment.

Helmets

Helmets are needed for sports such as baseball, softball, biking, snow skiing, and inline skating. Make sure you wear the right helmet for the sport you are playing and that it fits well. Also make sure that the helmet you wear for biking has a sticker from the Consumer Product Safety Commission (CPSC), which means that it is safe for this activity.

Mouth Guards

Mouth guards protect your mouth, teeth, and tongue. You should wear a guard if there's a chance you could get hit in the head while taking part in activities such as volleyball, basketball, or martial arts. You can find mouth guards at sport stores or your dentist. It will also help keep your mouth safe to take out your retainer.

Eye Protection

Special eye protection is needed for sports such as ice hockey, soccer, and basketball. Goggles and face masks should fit snugly and have cushion for a comfortable fit. If you wear glasses, you need to get fitted for guards that fit over your glasses. You could also buy special prescription goggles, which cost about $60 or more. These guards and goggles are made with a special plastic called polycarbonate. This special plastic will not hurt your eyes.

Shoes

It is important to wear the right footwear for your sport. Check with your coach or an athletic shoe salesperson about what shoes to wear.

Protective Pads

Wrist, knee, and elbow pads can help prevent broken bones when you are inline skating, skateboarding, snowboarding, or playing sports such as hockey.

Female Athlete Triad

Some girls who play sports or exercise intensely are at risk for a problem called female athlete triad. Female athlete triad is a combination of three conditions: disordered eating, amenorrhea (or missed periods), and osteoporosis. A female athlete can have one, two, or all three parts of the triad.

Eating Disorders

Most female athletes who develop an eating disorder are trying to lose weight so they can be better at their sport. This kind of eating disorder can range from avoiding certain types of food the athlete thinks are "bad" (such as foods containing fat) to serious eating disorders like anorexia nervosa or bulimia nervosa.

Menstrual Dysfunction

A missed period is a concern for girls and women who over-exercise. Your body needs a certain amount of fat to function and to have regular periods. Eating right and exercising is important for having a healthy body, but some girls take it too far. Too much exercising or very strict dieting can use up your body fat and delay your period, or cause it to stop until you gain some weight back. Not having menstrual periods is called amenorrhea—a sign that hormone patterns have changed. Oligomenorrhea is having very few periods, usually with cycles that last longer than 35 days.

Low Bone Mineral Density

Osteopenia and osteoporosis is when your bones become weak. If a female athlete doesn't eat a balanced diet that includes plenty of calcium, she can develop osteopenia or osteoporosis. This can ruin a female athlete's career because it may lead to stress fractures and other injuries. Usually, the teen years are a time when girls should be building up their bone mass to their highest levels—called peak bone mass. Not getting enough calcium during the teen years can also have a lasting effect on how strong a girl's bones are later in life.

Over-Exercising Can Actually Be Harmful

Sometimes you really can have too much of a good thing. If you over-exercise your emotional health can suffer. It is linked to depression and eating disorders.

Sometimes, teens over-exercise along with having an eating disorder such as anorexia. People with anorexia take extreme steps to lose weight, including not eating at all. This combination puts your health in danger.

Sports Safety Tips

When playing baseball or softball, what kind of safety equipment should be used?

In baseball and softball, the use of safety balls, breakaway bases, protective helmets, and face-guards can help reduce the risk injuries. Reduced-impact balls, which are softer than traditional baseballs, are designed to protect players who are still developing fielding skills. These balls come in a variety of materials and impact levels (the higher the level, the harder the ball). The American Academy of Orthopaedic Surgeons recommends using breakaway bases at all levels of baseball and softball to reduce the risk of injury. Wearing a hard-shell helmet while batting and running bases can reduce the risk of sustaining a head injury. Proper instruction in sliding techniques should be taught and practiced before using any bags, including breakaway bases. Strict rules against headfirst sliding should be enforced.

When playing football, what kinds of equipment should be used?

According to the Pop Warner Football, Official Rule Book, youth football players should wear the following protective gear:

- Helmet
- Pads (shoulder, hip, tail, and knee)
- Pants (one piece or shell)
- Thigh guards
- Jersey
- Mouthguard (a "keeper strap" is required to safely secure the mouthguard to the face mask)

If you think that you may be over-exercising or have an eating disorder, talk about it with someone you can trust. Talk to a school counselor or nurse. The longer you wait, the harder it will be to bring it up. If you think that your friend may have one of these problems, help them find someone to talk to. Be supportive and let them know you care about them.

Knee Injuries

It's fairly common for teens to develop knee injuries, especially if you're very active in sports. If your knee hurts so much that it affects your usual routine, you can't put weight on it, or is red or swollen, you should see a doctor.

- Athletic supporter
- Shoes (Depending on the league, players can wear sneakers or rubber cleat shoes.)
- Eyeglasses worn by football players should be made of shatter-proof glass (safety glass), or, as an alternative, these athletes should wear contact lenses.

When playing ice hockey, what kinds of equipment should be used?

All hockey players should wear the following protective equipment:

- Helmet/face mask with strap properly fastened
- Body padding (shoulder, shin, elbow, hip, and tendon)
- Padded hockey pants
- Gloves
- Jersey
- Mouthguard
- Athletic supporter
- Eyeglasses worn by hockey players should be made of shatter-proof glass (safety glass), or players should wear contact lenses.

What are some important safety rules that should be followed when playing ice hockey and football?

Strict rules against body checking (using the body to knock an opponent against the boards or to the ice) and spearing (the use of a helmet to butt or ram an opponent) should be enforced.

Source: Excerpted from "Team Sports Safety, Children Ages Six to 19 Years," © June 2010 New York State Department of Health; reprinted with permission.

You can help prevent knee injuries by following these steps:

- Wearing the correct protective equipment for your sport (for example, knee pads and shin guards)

- Warming up and cooling down before exercise

- Stretching regularly

- Bending your knees when you land from a jump

- Using correct technique for your sport, like cutting and pivoting

Osteoporosis

Osteoporosis is when your bones become weak and break easily. If a female athlete doesn't eat a balanced diet that includes plenty of calcium, she can develop osteoporosis. This can ruin a female athlete's career because it may lead to stress fractures and other injuries.

The teen years are the most important time for girls to build up their bone mass to their highest levels—called peak bone mass. Not getting enough calcium, vitamin D, and physical activity during the teen years can have a lasting effect on how strong a girl's bones are later in life.

Chapter 44

Safety Tips For Runners

Whether it's as part of a high school track program or cross-country team or just a way of getting in shape, running is a wonderful sport. It's great exercise, virtually anyone can do it, and all you really need to get started is a good pair of sneakers.

But running is not without its risks. Injuries—from sprained ankles and blisters to stress fractures and tendonitis—are commonplace. And runners need to be aware of potential hazards (from vehicles to wild animals) when choosing a place to run.

To keep things safe while running, follow these tips:

Avoiding Running Injuries

Statistically speaking, you're more likely to be injured when running than you are while skiing or bicycling. Granted, running-related injuries are typically less severe than those suffered by skiers and cyclists. But the odds are good that at some point in your running career you will get injured.

Running, especially on asphalt or other hard surfaces, generates a tremendous amount of stress on the legs and back. This can lead to all manner of lower-body problems. The most common running injuries include sprained ankles, blisters, Achilles tendonitis, chondromalacia (runner's knee), iliotibial band (ITB) syndrome, plantar fasciitis (heel pain), and shinsplints.

Runners also often get groin pulls, heel spurs, and hamstring pulls.

About This Chapter: "Safety Tips: Running," May 2010, reprinted with permission from www.kidshealth.org. This information was provided by KidsHealth®, one of the largest resources online for medically reviewed health information written for parents, kids, and teens. For more articles like this, visit www.KidsHealth.org or www.TeensHealth.org. Copyright © 1995-2012 The Nemours Foundation. All rights reserved.

Two steps can help you avoid serious injuries from running:

1. Try to prevent injuries from occurring in the first place. Use the right gear, warm up your muscles before you start, and take precautions to deal with weather conditions—like staying well hydrated in hot weather and keeping muscles warm in the cold.

2. Stop running as soon as you notice any symptoms. Ignoring the warning signs of an injury will only lead to bigger problems down the road.

Gear Guidelines

Running might require less gear than other sports, but it is still vitally important to get the right equipment to minimize the stresses it puts on your body. Anyone who has ever run in the wrong shoes can tell you what a painful experience it can be, and anyone who has run in the wrong socks probably has blisters to prove it.

Here are a few tips to make sure you get the right footwear before you start running:

Shoes

Before you buy a pair of running sneakers, know what sort of foot you have. Are your feet wide or narrow? Do you have flat feet? High arches? Different feet need different sneakers to provide maximum support and comfort. If you don't know what sort of foot you have or what kind of sneaker will work best for you, consult a trained professional at a running specialty store.

All running shoes should provide good support, starting with a thick, shock-absorbing sole. Runners with flat feet should choose shoes that advertise "motion control" or "stability." Runners with high-arched feet should look for shoes that describe themselves as "flexible" or "cushioned."

Getting shoes that fit correctly is more important in running than in virtually any other sport. As you rack up the miles, any hot spots or discomfort will become magnified and lead to blisters and stress-related leg problems.

If you plan on running on trails or in bad weather, you'll need trail-running shoes with extra traction, stability, and durability. Whichever type of shoes you end up purchasing, make sure they are laced up snugly but not so tight that they cause discomfort.

Socks

Running socks come in a variety of materials, thicknesses, and sizes. The most important factor is material. Stay away from socks made from 100% cotton. When cotton gets wet, it stays wet, leading to blisters in the summer and cold feet in the winter. Instead, choose socks made from wool or synthetic materials such as polyester and acrylic.

Some runners like thicker socks for extra cushioning while others prefer thin socks, particularly in warm weather. Make sure you wear the socks you plan to wear when running while you try on sneakers to ensure a proper fit.

Choose Where To Run

One of the nice things about running is that you can do it almost anywhere. In most cases, it will be possible to simply step out your front door and begin. That being said, there are definitely safer places to run and places that you might want to avoid.

Road Runners

Look for streets that have sidewalks or wide shoulders. If there are no sidewalks or shoulders, and you find yourself having to run in the street, try to find an area with minimal automobile traffic. Always run toward oncoming cars so you can see any potential problems before they reach you.

Avoid running routes that take you through bad neighborhoods. If you're running in an unfamiliar area, be prepared to change your route or turn around if you sense that the area you're headed toward may not be safe. Trust your intuition.

Find someone to run with if you can—there's safety in numbers. Can't find a running partner? Consider joining a running club through your school or the local parks and recreation department. When running in a group, be sure to run single file and keep to the side of the road. Always yield the right-of-way to vehicles at intersections. Don't assume that cars will stop or alter their paths for you. Obey all traffic rules and signals.

Trail Runners

Choose well-maintained trails. Steer clear of trails that are overgrown or covered with fallen branches—you don't want to trip or encounter ticks or poison ivy! Also, you should avoid trails that travel through deserted areas or take you far away from homes and businesses. Know the location of public phones and the fastest way back to civilization in the event of an emergency.

Watch for dogs or wild animals. If you encounter a mountain lion, bear, or other dangerous animal stop running and face it. Running may trigger the animal's instinct to attack. Make yourself look larger by raising your hands over your head. Give the animal plenty of room to escape. If the animal appears to be acting aggressively, throw rocks, sticks, or whatever is read-ily available at it. Stay facing the animal.

If you run into an aggressive dog, don't make eye contact—the dog might see this as a threat. The dog may be trying to defend its territory, so stop running and walk to the other side of the street. If the dog approaches, stand still. In a firm, calm voice, say "No" or "Go home." If you keep running into the same dog, choose a new route or file a report with animal control.

Plan for Weather

Rain And Snow

If you intend to run in rain or snow, make sure you dress for the conditions (windproof jacket, hat, gloves, etc.). Wear synthetic fabrics that will help wick away moisture from your body. Consider putting Vaseline or Band-aids on your nipples to keep them from being chafed by a wet shirt.

Wind

If it's windy, run more slowly than you normally would when facing into the wind. This will help you keep from overexerting yourself while still giving you the same amount of exercise. Try to start your run by heading into the wind so that you will have the wind at your back later in the run when you are tired.

Heat

On hot days, drink plenty of water before your run and bring extra water with you. Heat prostration can be a very serious problem for runners. Wear white clothing to reflect the sun's rays and a hat to shade your head from the sun, and stop running if you feel faint or uncom-fortable in any way.

Before You Start

Before you begin, warm up. Jog in place for a minute or two or do some jumping jacks to get the blood flowing. Then be sure to stretch well, with a particular focus on your calves, hamstrings, quadriceps, and ankles.

Carry a few essentials with you. These include some form of identification, a cell phone or change for a pay phone, and a whistle. Don't wear headphones or earbuds or anything else that might make you less aware of your surroundings while you run.

Tell a friend or family member your running route and when you plan to return. If no one is available, write down your plans so you can be located in the event of an emergency.

While Running

Try to run only during daylight hours, if possible. If you must run at night, avoid dimly lit areas and wear bright and/or reflective clothes so that others can see you clearly.

When you begin, have a definite idea of how far you intend to go. Less experienced runners should start by running short distances until they build up their stamina and get a better idea of how far they can run safely. For younger teens, the body is still developing and can easily be stressed by running long distances. As a general guideline, a 10K race is the upper limit of what a 13-year-old should attempt, and no one under 18 should try to run a marathon. (Most marathons will limit their entries to people 18 and older.)

Stay alert. The more aware you are of your surroundings and the other people around you, the less vulnerable you will be. Staying safe while running involves the same common sense you use to stay safe anywhere else, like avoiding parked cars and dark areas, and taking note of who is directly behind you and ahead of you. If a car passes you more than once or seems suspicious, try to note the license plate number, and make it clear that you are aware of the vehicle. Most runners don't get attacked, especially if they take precautions like running in populated areas. You just need to use common sense.

Chapter 45

Helmets

Which Helmet For Which Activity?

Why are helmets so important?

For many recreational activities, wearing a helmet can reduce the risk of a serious head injury and even save your life. During a fall or collision, most of the impact energy is absorbed by the helmet, rather than your head and brain.

Are all helmets the same?

No. There are different helmets for different activities. Each type of helmet is made to protect your head from the impacts common to a particular activity or sport. Be sure to wear a helmet that is appropriate for the particular activity you're involved in (see Table 45.1 for guidance). Other helmets may not protect your head as effectively.

How can I tell which helmet is the right one to use?

Bicycle and motorcycle helmets must comply with mandatory federal safety standards. Many other recreational helmets are subject to voluntary safety standards.

Helmets certified to a safety standard are designed and tested to protect the user from serious head injury while wearing the helmet. For example, all bicycle helmets manufactured after 1999 must meet the U.S. Consumer Product Safety Commission (CPSC) bicycle helmet standard. Helmets meeting this standard provide substantial head protection when the helmet

About This Chapter: The main text in this chapter begins with "Which Helmet for Which Activity," U.S. Consumer Product Safety Commission, 2006. It continues with information from "Hard Facts about Helmets," BAM! Body and Mind, Centers for Disease Control and Prevention, 2003. Reviewed by David A. Cooke, MD, FACP, April 2012.

is used properly. The standard requires that chin straps be strong enough to keep the helmet on the head and in the proper position during a fall or collision.

Helmets specifically marketed for exclusive use in an activity other than bicycling (for example, go-karting, horseback riding, lacrosse, and skiing) do not have to meet the requirements of the CPSC bicycle helmet standard. However, these helmets should meet other federal and/or voluntary safety standards.

Don't rely on the helmet's name or claims made on the packaging (unless the packaging specifies compliance with an appropriate standard) to determine if the helmet meets the appropriate requirements for your activity. Most helmets that meet a particular standard will contain a special label that indicates compliance (usually found on the liner inside of the helmet). See Table 45.1 for more information on what to look for.

Are there helmets that I can wear for more than one activity?

Yes, but only a few. You can wear a CPSC-compliant bicycle helmet while bicycling, recreational roller or in-line skating, and riding a nonpowered scooter. Look at Table 45.1 for other activities that may share a common helmet.

Are there any activities for which one shouldn't wear a helmet?

Yes. Take off your helmet before playing on playgrounds or climbing trees. If a person wears a helmet during these activities, the helmet's chin strap can get caught on the equipment or tree and pose a risk of strangulation. The helmet itself may present an entrapment hazard.

How can I tell if my helmet fits properly?

A helmet should be both comfortable and snug. Be sure that it is level on your head—not tilted back on the top of the head or pulled too low over your forehead. It should not move in any direction, back-to-front or side-to-side. The chin strap should be securely buckled so that the helmet doesn't move or fall off during a fall or collision.

When buying a helmet, be sure to try it on so that the helmet can be tested for a good fit. Carefully examine the helmet and accompanying instructions and safety literature.

What can I do if I have trouble fitting the helmet?

You may have to apply the foam padding that comes with the helmet and/or adjust the straps. If this doesn't work, consult with the store where you bought the helmet or with the helmet manufacturer. Don't wear a helmet that doesn't fit correctly.

Facts For Athletes About Concussions

A concussion is a brain injury that is caused by a bump or blow to the head. It can change the way your brain normally works. A concussion can occur during practices or games in any sport. You can have a concussion even if you haven't been knocked out. They can be serious even if you've just been "dinged."

Concussion Symptoms

- Headache or "pressure" in head
- Balance problems or dizziness
- Bothered by light
- Feeling sluggish, hazy, foggy, or groggy
- Memory problems
- Does not "feel right"

- Nausea or vomiting
- Double or blurry vision
- Bothered by noise
- Difficulty paying attention
- Confusion

If You Think You Have A Concussion

- Tell your coaches and your parents. Never ignore a bump or blow to the head even if you feel fine. Also, tell your coach if one of your teammates might have a concussion.
- Get a medical checkup. A doctor or health care professional can tell you if you have a concussion and when you are OK to return to play.
- Give yourself time to get better. If you have had a concussion, your brain needs time to heal. While your brain is still healing, you are much more likely to have a second concussion. Second or later concussions can cause damage to your brain. It is important to rest until you get approval from a doctor or health care professional to return to play.

Preventing Concussions

Every sport is different, but there are steps you can take to protect yourself. Follow your coach's rules for safety and the rules of the sport. Practice good sportsmanship at all times, and use the proper sports equipment, including personal protective equipment (such as helmets, padding, shin guards, and eye and mouth guards).

Remember, in order for equipment to protect you, it must be the right equipment for the game, position, or activity. It must be worn correctly and fit well, and it must be used every time you play.

Source: "Heads Up: Concussion in Youth Sports," Centers for Disease Control and Prevention (www.cdc.gov), July 2007. Reviewed by David A. Cooke, MD, FACP, May 2012.

Will I need to replace a helmet after an impact?

That depends on the severity of the impact and whether the helmet can withstand one impact (a single-impact helmet) or more than one impact (a multiple-impact helmet). For example, bicycle helmets are designed to protect against a single severe impact, such as a bicyclist's fall onto the pavement. The foam material in the helmet will crush to absorb the impact energy during a fall or collision and can't protect you again from an additional impact. Even if there are no visible signs of damage to the helmet, you must replace it.

Other helmets are designed to protect against multiple moderate impacts. Two examples are football and ice hockey helmets. These helmets are designed to withstand multiple impacts of the type associated with the respective activities. However, you may still have to replace the helmet after one severe impact, or if it has visible signs of damage, such as a cracked shell or permanent dent in the shell or liner. Consult the manufacturer's instructions for guidance on when the helmet should be replaced.

Where can I find specific information about which helmet to use?

Look at the information in Table 45.1 and follow these easy steps:

- Find the activity of interest in the first column (Activity).

- Read across the row to find the appropriate helmet type for that activity listed in the second column (Helmet Type).

- Once you've found the right helmet, look for a label or other marking stating that it complies with an applicable standard listed in the third column (Applicable Standard(s)).

Hard Facts About Helmets

Your helmet should sit flat on your head—make sure it is level and is not tilted back or forward. The front of the helmet should sit low—about two finger widths above your eyebrows to protect your forehead. The straps on each side of your head should form a "Y" over your ears, with one part of the strap in front of your ear, and one behind — just below your earlobes. If the helmet leans forward, adjust the rear straps. If it tilts backward, tighten the front straps. Buckle the chinstrap securely at your throat so that the helmet feels snug on your head and does not move up and down or from side to side.

Helmets: Fact Or Fiction?

Fiction: Helmets aren't cool.

Table 45.1. Helmet Types For Common Activities

❶ Activity	❷ Helmet Type	❸ Applicable Standard(s)
Individual Activities — Wheeled		
Bicycling (including low speed, motor assisted) Roller & In-line Skating — Recreational Scooter Riding (including low speed, motor assisted)	Bicycle	**CPSC**, ASTM F1447, Snell B-90/95, Snell N-94†
BMX Cycling	BMX	**CPSC**, ASTM F2032
Downhill Mountain Bike Racing	Downhill	**CPSC**, ASTM F1952
Roller & In-line Skating — Aggressive/Trick Skateboarding	Skateboard	ASTM F1492†, Snell N-94†
Individual Activities — Wheeled Large Motor		
ATV Riding Dirt- & Mini-Bike Riding Motocrossing	Motocross or Motorcycle	DOT FMVSS 218, Snell M-2005
Karting/Go-Karting	Karting or Motorcycle	DOT FMVSS 218, Snell K-98, Snell M-2005
Moped Riding Powered Scooter Riding	Moped or Motorcycle	DOT FMVSS 218, Snell L-98, Snell M-2005
Individual Activities — Non-Wheeled		
Horseback Riding	Equestrian	ASTM F1163, Snell E-2001
Rock- & Wall-Climbing	Mountaineering	EN 12492†, Snell N-94†
Team Sport Activities ‡		
Baseball, Softball & T-Ball	Baseball Batter's	NOCSAE ND022
	Baseball Catcher's	NOCSAE ND024
Football	Football	NOCSAE ND002, ASTM F717
Ice Hockey	Hockey	NOCSAE ND030, ASTM F1045
Lacrosse	Lacrosse	NOCSAE ND041
Winter Activities		
Skiing Snowboarding	Ski	ASTM F2040, CEN 1077, Snell RS-98 or S-98
Snowmobiling	Snowmobile	DOT FMVSS 218, Snell M-2000
Although a helmet has not yet been designed for the following two activities, until such helmets exist, wearing one of the three listed types of helmets may be preferable to wearing no helmet at all.		
Ice Skating Sledding	Bicycle	**CPSC**, ASTM F1447, Snell B-90/95 or N-94†
	Skateboard	ASTM F1492†, Snell N-94†
	Ski	ASTM F2040, CEN 1077, Snell RS-98 or S-98

The federal CPSC Safety Standard for Bicycle Helmets is mandatory for those helmets indicated by **CPSC**.

† This helmet is designed to withstand more than one moderate impact, but protection is provided for only a limited number of impacts. Replace if visibly damaged (e.g., a cracked shell or crushed liner) and/or when directed by the manufacturer.

‡ Team sport helmets are designed to protect against multiple head impacts typically occurring in the sport (e.g., ball, puck, or stick impacts; player contact; etc.), and, generally, can continue to be used after such impacts. Follow manufacturer's recommendations for replacement or reconditioning.

Definitions: ASTM - ASTM International; CEN - European Committee for Standardization; DOT – Dept. of Transportation; EN - Euro-norm or European Standard; NOCSAE - National Operating Committee on Standards in Athletic Equipment; Snell - Snell Memorial Foundation.

Fact: Who says helmets can't be cool? If you're shopping for a helmet, there are lots of options, so you can pick out your favorite color. Or decorate your helmet with stickers and reflectors to show your personal style. Helmets are designed to help prevent injuries to your head, because a serious fall or crash can cause permanent brain damage or death. And that's definitely not cool.

Fiction: Helmets just aren't comfortable.

Fact: Today's helmets are lightweight, well ventilated, and have lots of padding. Try on your helmet to make sure it fits properly and comfortably on your head before you buy it.

Fiction: Really good riders don't need to wear helmets.

Fact: Crashes or collisions can happen at any time. Even professional bike racers get in serious wrecks. In three out of four bike crashes, bikers usually get some sort of injury to their head.

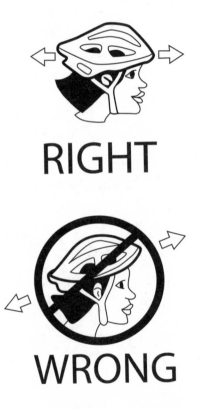

RIGHT

WRONG

Figure 45.1. The right way and the wrong way to wear a bicycle helmet.

Chapter 46

Clothes And Shoes For Workout Comfort And Safety

What To Wear For Winter Exercise

Winter-weather exercise clothing has technologically advanced fabrics. Manufacturers produce clothes in a variety of natural and synthetic materials that wick moisture, insulate the body and protect skin from cold temperatures, and these clothes often block both wind and precipitation while remaining highly mobile and comfortable.

Before you challenge the elements, it is important to know the current weather conditions and if they may change as your exercise session progresses. Being underprepared or underestimating the elements is unwise, and there are days when the best option is finding an indoor alternative. Keep in mind that definitions of winter weather will vary based on geographical location, personal experience, and personal tolerances. When you begin your exercise session, your body should feel cold, but you will warm up quickly and begin to feel more acclimated to the winter weather. Your body will sweat; thus, skin exposure and moisture management are key to remaining warm, safe and comfortable.

Skin exposure can create dangerous—even deadly—circumstances if you are unprepared for cold temperatures and wind chill factors. Keeping the outside "out" is important, and many materials made of both synthetic and natural fibers keep the elements away from your skin.

About This Chapter: This chapter includes text excerpted and reprinted with permission from "What to Wear for Winter Exercise," by Thomas Altena, Ed.D., FACSM, *ACSM Fit Society Page*, Winter 2011, pp 3–4, © 2011 American College of Sports Medicine; and "Preparing for and Playing in the Heat," by Mary Nadelen, M.A., ATC, *ACSM Fit Society Page*, Summer 2009, p. 3, © 2009 American College of Sports Medicine. For additional information, visit www.acsm.org.

Winter Weather Materials

A few manufacturers make windproof materials that completely block the wind from penetrating the fabric, which is typically incorporated at the specific locations of jackets, pants, tights, and gloves that face the wind. The downside of windproof material is that it does not allow sweat to escape, so plan to accumulate sweat under the shell. A shell like GORE-TEX is great for winter because the material is waterproof to precipitation yet allows sweat to escape. But GORE-TEX is not windproof. If your choice is to not wear a synthetic material or a windproof fabric, wool or wool blend (50 percent wool) are amazing natural fiber alternatives that provide excellent breathability, mobility, wind prevention, and insulation. Unlike synthetic materials that do not accumulate moisture, sweat and precipitation will pass through natural wool-blended fabrics and will freeze on the outer part of the fabric. This freezing effect may seem detrimental, but the ice formed on top of the fabric creates a natural wind barrier effective for keeping a person warm. Many of these high-tech fabrics, including hats, socks, and gloves, have special washing and drying instructions. Washing these items on delicate or hand-wash cycle and drying them on low heat or line-drying will make sure the fabrics continue to be high performers with longevity for many winter seasons.

Moisture Management

Moisture management might be the single most important factor for keeping the body warm during winter exercise. Even in the coldest of temperatures, the body will produce sweat and, if that moisture is not removed from the skin, feel chilled. Exercise experts recommend avoiding cotton and cotton blends because they absorb sweat. Instead of cotton, a better choice is known as base layers, a moisture-wicking synthetic fabric that moves sweat from the skin. Base layers are a blend of nylon, Lycra, elastane, polyester, and acrylic. A good base layer fits snugly against the skin and moves as your body moves because it is skin-tight and elastic. When selecting a base layer, make sure that you explore different fabric thicknesses for different temperatures. As an added bonus, layering two or three base layers can provide added insulation for very cold conditions (approximately 10° F or lower) and will increase moisture management. Running and cycling tights also come in a variety of material thickness, just like base-layer shirts. The Lycra-spandex tights of old are still available, but now tights incorporate windproof front panels or a polyurethane coating that feels like thin neoprene in the front of the legs to prevent wind and water from reaching the skin.

Layering 101

Concerning layers, the goal is to keep the core of your body warm, so upper-body layering is more important than lower-body layering. However, layering tights in the most extreme combinations of cold temperatures and wind chills is recommended, though it may compromise mobility. What you wear under your tights is a personal preference; one option preferred by some is tri-shorts (minimal chamois bike shorts).

Protecting Your Extremities

Hands: Gloves with a GORE-TEX lining are a great choice for moisture management, but windproof gloves might be an advantage in a cold wind. These gloves may fail after about 90 minutes of exercise, as sweat production exceeds the material's ability remove moisture. The thin, stretchy knit gloves are a low-cost option for gloves in moderately cold weather. These are easy to layer for variety. Plus, losing one glove won't break the bank.

Choosing The Right Fitness Shoe

If you've been walking, running, or high-stepping in the same pair of sneakers since last year, you're probably due for a change. By now, those well-cushioned athletic shoes that felt so comfy on the first day you wore them have given you all they've got.

As startling as it sounds, if you weigh 150 pounds and walk one mile, you've exerted 63.5 tons of force on each foot, according to a study from the American Podiatric Medical Association. No wonder that the average life span for fitness shoes is only the equivalent of 200 to 400 miles. For those of us who break the rules and use the same shoes we exercise in for daily wear, that mileage can be reached in as little as two months (figuring roughly 2,000 steps per mile).

Yet choosing a new pair of athletic shoes can feel like an overwhelming task. The selection is often vast, with models designed and marketed for varying activities. Follow these tips to help you get the pair that's best for you:

- It helps to shop at an athletic shoe store (avoid the chains if you can), where the salespeople know how to measure and fit your feet and advise about shoe features.
- For feet with a low or flat arch, choose rigid shoes that control motion and resist bending.
- Normal feet, with a medium arch, do well in slightly curved shoes designed for stability.
- High-arched feet need curved shoes that twist and bend easily.
- You can walk in running shoes, but never run in walking shoes (they're too rigid).
- Be practical about the fancy stuff. That shoe with the built-in pedometer or music chip might have a big "cool factor," but you'll be paying a lot for equipment you might already have in another form. Sneakers with pump-up tongues or shock-absorbing inserts might be worth the extra cost if they help the shoes fit your foot better.
- If you get frequent leg pains, have foot problems or have a chronic condition such as diabetes or arthritis, see a podiatrist for advice before selecting your next pair of athletic shoes.

Feet: If you exercise in ice and packed snow, trail running shoes have an aggressive tread pattern. To improve grip even more, fit your running shoes with crampons.

Face: Face covering is important to some people, but a facemask can capture humidity in breathing and impair vision by fogging up sunglasses or prescription lenses. Instead of a facemask, try using petroleum jelly on exposed skin in extreme cold. Petroleum jelly creates a thin barrier between your skin and the elements, but it will increase the risk of sunburn.

Cell Phones For Emergencies

As you consider exercising in the cold weather, carry a cell phone in case of emergency. But remember that sweat ruins cell phones. You can protect your cell phone with simple a zipper-locked plastic bag.

What To Wear In The Summer

When athletes train during the warm summer months, it is important for them to be prepared for the environment in which they will be training and playing.

Heat acclimatization or practicing in the environment the athlete will be playing in will allow the body to adapt to the warm environment, which will improve performance and heat tolerance. Athletes should progressively increase the intensity and duration of their training sessions over a 10–14 day period to become fully acclimated to their environment. Initially, training sessions should last 15–40 minutes for the first couple of days and can progress to a two- to four-hour training session by day 14. An individual properly acclimated should be able to train in the warm environment for one to two hours at an intensity equal to competition.

Choosing clothing and equipment that is light-colored, loose-fitting, and moisture-wicking will help keep an athlete cool. As the temperature increases, athletes should minimize the amount of clothing and equipment (helmet, shoulder pads) worn. The body's ability to cool itself through the evaporation of sweat decreases significantly as the amount of equipment worn increases. Athletes who must wear protective equipment should allow time to start training in shorts and T-shirt and gradually add equipment each day as their bodies acclimate.

Chapter 47

Increasing Activity Safely

Although physical activity has many health benefits, injuries and other adverse events do sometimes happen. The most common injuries affect the musculoskeletal system (the bones, joints, muscles, ligaments, and tendons). Other adverse events can also occur during activity, such as overheating and dehydration. On rare occasions, people have heart attacks during activity.

The good news is that scientific evidence strongly shows that physical activity is safe for almost everyone. Moreover, the health benefits of physical activity far outweigh the risks.

Still, people may hesitate to become physically active because of concern they'll get hurt. For these people, there is even more good news: They can take steps that are proven to reduce their risk of injury and adverse events.

The guidelines in this chapter provide advice to help people do physical activity safely. Most advice applies to people of all ages.

Physical Activity Is Safe For Almost Everyone

Most people are not likely to be injured when doing moderate-intensity activities in amounts that meet the *Physical Activity Guidelines for Americans*. However, injuries and other adverse events do sometimes happen. The most common problems are musculoskeletal injuries. Even so, studies show that only one such injury occurs for every 1,000 hours of walking for exercise, and fewer than four injuries occur for every 1,000 hours of running.

About This Chapter: Excerpted from "Chapter 6: Safe and Active," *2008 Physical Activity Guidelines for Americans*, U.S. Department of Health and Human Services (www.health.gov/paguidelines), 2008.

Both physical fitness and total amount of physical activity affect risk of musculoskeletal injuries. People who are physically fit have a lower risk of injury than people who are not. People who do more activity generally have a higher risk of injury than people who do less activity. So what should people do if they want to be active and safe? The best strategies are to be regularly physically active to increase physical fitness; and follow the other guidance—especially increasing physical activity gradually over time—to minimize the injury risk from doing medium to high amounts of activity.

Following these strategies may reduce overall injury risk. Active people are more likely to have an activity-related injury than inactive people. But they appear less likely to have non-activity-related injuries.

Choose Appropriate Types And Amounts Of Activity

People can reduce their risk of injury by choosing appropriate types of activity. The safest activities are moderate intensity and low impact, and don't involve purposeful collision or contact.

Key Guidelines For Safe Physical Activity

To do physical activity safely and reduce risk of injuries and other adverse events, people should follow these guidelines:

- Understand the risks and yet be confident that physical activity is safe for almost everyone.

- Choose to do types of physical activity that are appropriate for their current fitness level and health goals, because some activities are safer than others.

- Increase physical activity gradually over time whenever more activity is necessary to meet guidelines or health goals. Inactive people should "start low and go slow" by gradually increasing how often and how long activities are done.

- Protect themselves by using appropriate gear and sports equipment, looking for safe environments, following rules and policies, and making sensible choices about when, where, and how to be active.

- Be under the care of a health-care provider if they have chronic conditions or symptoms. People with chronic conditions and symptoms should consult their health-care provider about the types and amounts of activity appropriate for them.

Walking for exercise, gardening or yard work, bicycling or exercise cycling, dancing, swimming, and golf are activities with the lowest injury rates. In the amounts commonly done by adults, walking (a moderate-intensity and low-impact activity) has a third or less of the injury risk of running (a vigorous-intensity and higher impact activity).

The risk of injury for a type of physical activity can also differ according to the purpose of the activity. For example, recreational bicycling or bicycling for transportation leads to fewer injuries than training for and competing in bicycle races.

People who have had a past injury are at risk of injuring that body part again. The risk of injury can be reduced by performing appropriate amounts of activity and setting appropriate personal goals. Performing a variety of different physical activities may also reduce the risk of overuse injury.

Increase Physical Activity Gradually Over Time

Scientific studies indicate that the risk of injury to bones, muscles, and joints is directly related to the gap between a person's usual level of activity and a new level of activity. The size of this gap is called the amount of overload. Creating a small overload and waiting for the body to adapt and recover reduces the risk of injury. When amounts of physical activity need to be increased to meet the Guidelines or personal goals, physical activity should be increased gradually over time, no matter what the person's current level of physical activity.

Scientists have not established a standard for how to gradually increase physical activity over time. The following recommendations give general guidance for inactive people and those with low levels of physical activity on how to increase physical activity:

- Use relative intensity (intensity of the activity relative to a person's fitness) to guide the level of effort for aerobic activity.

- Generally start with relatively moderate-intensity aerobic activity. Avoid relatively vigorous-intensity activity, such as shoveling snow or running. Adults with a low level of fitness may need to start with light activity, or a mix of light- to moderate-intensity activity.

- First, increase the number of minutes per session (duration), and the number of days per week (frequency) of moderate-intensity activity. Later, if desired, increase the intensity.

- Pay attention to the relative size of the increase in physical activity each week, as this is related to injury risk. For example, a 20-minute increase each week is safer for a person who does 200 minutes a week of walking (a 10 percent increase), than for a person who does 40 minutes a week (a 50 percent increase).

The available scientific evidence suggests that adding a small and comfortable amount of light- to moderate-intensity activity, such as 5–15 minutes of walking per session, two to three times a week, to one's usual activities has a low risk of musculoskeletal injury and no known risk of severe cardiac events. Because this range is rather wide, people should consider three factors in individualizing their rate of increase: age, level of fitness, and prior experience.

Age

The amount of time required to adapt to a new level of activity probably depends on age. Youth and young adults probably can safely increase activity by small amounts every week or two. Older adults appear to require more time to adapt to a new level of activity, in the range of two to four weeks.

Level Of Fitness

Less fit adults are at higher risk of injury when doing a given amount of activity, compared to fitter adults. Slower rates of increase over time may reduce injury risk. This guidance applies to overweight and obese adults, as they are commonly less physically fit.

Prior Experience

People can use their experience to learn to increase physical activity over time in ways that minimize the risk of overuse injury. Generally, if an overuse injury occurred in the past with a certain rate of progression, a person should increase activity more slowly the next time.

Take Appropriate Precautions

Taking appropriate precautions means using the right gear and equipment, choosing safe environments in which to be active, following rules and policies, and making sensible choices about how, when, and where to be active.

Use Protective Gear And Appropriate Equipment

Using personal protective gear can reduce the frequency of injury. Personal protective gear is something worn by a person to protect a specific body part. Examples include helmets, eyewear and goggles, shin guards, elbow and knee pads, and mouth guards.

Using appropriate sports equipment can also reduce risk of injury. Sports equipment refers to sport or activity-specific tools, such as balls, bats, sticks, and shoes.

For the most benefit, protective equipment and gear should be the right equipment for the activity, appropriately fitted, appropriately maintained, and used consistently and correctly.

Be Active In Safe Environments

People can reduce their injury risks by paying attention to the places they choose to be active. To help themselves stay safe, people can look for places with these characteristics:

- Physical separation from motor vehicles, such as sidewalks, walking paths, or bike lanes

- Neighborhoods with traffic-calming measures that slow down traffic

- Places to be active that are well-lighted, where other people are present, and that are well-maintained (no litter, broken windows)

- Shock-absorbing surfaces on playgrounds

- Well-maintained playing fields and courts without holes or obstacles

- Breakaway bases at baseball and softball fields

- Padded and anchored goals and goal posts at soccer and football fields

Follow Rules And Policies That Promote Safety

Rules, policies, legislation, and laws are potentially the most effective and wide-reaching way to reduce activity-related injuries. To get the benefit, individuals should look for and follow these rules, policies, and laws. For example, policies that promote the use of bicycle helmets reduce the risk of head injury among cyclists. Rules against diving into shallow water at swimming pools prevent head and neck injuries.

Make Sensible Choices About How, When, And Where To Be Active

A person's choices can obviously influence the risk of adverse events. By making sensible choices, injuries and adverse events can be prevented. Consider weather conditions, such as extremes of heat and cold. For example, during very hot and humid weather, people lessen the chances of dehydration and heat stress by taking these steps:

- Exercising in the cool of early morning as opposed to mid-day heat

- Switching to indoor activities (playing basketball in the gym rather than on the playground)

- Changing the type of activity (swimming rather than playing soccer)

- Lowering the intensity of activity (walking rather than running)

- Paying close attention to rest, shade, drinking enough fluids, and other ways to minimize effects of heat

Exposure to air pollution is associated with several adverse health outcomes, including asthma attacks and abnormal heart rhythms. People who can modify the location or time of exercise may wish to reduce these risks by exercising away from heavy traffic and industrial sites, especially during rush hour or times when pollution is known to be high. However, current evidence indicates that the benefits of being active, even in polluted air, outweigh the risk of being inactive.

Advice From Health-Care Providers

The protective value of a medical consultation for persons with or without chronic diseases who are interested in increasing their physical activity level is not established. People without diagnosed chronic conditions (such as diabetes, heart disease, or osteoarthritis) and who do not have symptoms (such as chest pain or pressure, dizziness, or joint pain) do not need to consult a health-care provider about physical activity.

Inactive people who gradually progress over time to relatively moderate-intensity activity have no known risk of sudden cardiac events, and very low risk of bone, muscle, or joint injuries. A person who is habitually active with moderate-intensity activity can gradually increase to vigorous intensity without needing to consult a health-care provider. People who develop new symptoms when increasing their levels of activity should consult a health-care provider.

Health-care providers can provide useful personalized advice on how to reduce risk of injuries. For people who wish to seek the advice of a health-care provider, it is particularly appropriate to do so when contemplating vigorous-intensity activity, because the risks of this activity are higher than the risks of moderate-intensity activity.

The choice of appropriate types and amounts of physical activity can be affected by chronic conditions. People with symptoms or known chronic conditions should be under the regular care of a health-care provider. In consultation with their provider, they can develop a physical activity plan that is appropriate for them. People with chronic conditions typically find that moderate-intensity activity is safe and beneficial. However, they may need to take special precautions. For example, people with diabetes need to pay special attention to blood sugar control and proper footwear during activity.

Selected Examples Of Injury Prevention Strategies For Common Physical Activities and Sports

This list provides examples of various evidence-based injury prevention strategies compiled by one group of safety and injury prevention experts (Source: Adapted from Gilchrist, J.,

Saluja, G., and Marshall, S. W. (2007). Interventions to prevent sports and recreation-related injuries. In L. S. Doll, S. E. Bonzo, J. Mercy, & D. A. Sleet (Eds), *Handbook of injury and violence prevention* (pp. 117–136). New York: Springer.). It is provided as a resource for readers and is not a product of the Physical Activity Guidelines Advisory Committee.

Proven interventions have strong evidence of effectiveness in preventing injuries. Promising/potential interventions have moderately strong evidence of effectiveness from small studies or have been tested only under laboratory conditions.

Baseball/Softball

- **Proven:** Breakaway bases; Reduced impact balls; Faceguards/protective eyewear
- **Promising/Potential:** Batting helmets; Pitch count

Basketball

- **Proven:** Mouth guards
- **Promising/Potential:** Ankle disc (balance) training; Semi-rigid ankle stabilizers/braces[1]; Protective eyewear.

Bicycling

- **Proven:** Helmet use. Helmets worn while bicycling reduce the risk of death and injury. Educational campaigns, laws/legislation, and financial subsidy programs all increase use of helmets.
- **Promising/Potential:** Bike paths/lanes; Retractable handle bars

Football

- **Proven:** Helmets and other personal protective equipment; Ankle stabilizers/braces[1]; Minimizing cleat length; Rule changes (no spearing, clipping, etc.); Playing field maintenance; Preseason conditioning; Cross-training (reduce overuse injuries); Coach training and experience
- **Promising/Potential:** Limiting contact during practice

Ice Hockey

- **Proven:** Helmets with full face shield; Rule changes (fair play, no checking from behind, no high sticking, etc.); Increased rink size
- **Promising/Potential:** Enforcement of rules; Discouraging fighting

In-Line Skating/Skateboarding

- **Proven:** Wrist guards; Knee/elbow pads
- **Promising/Potential:** Helmets

Playgrounds

- **Proven:** Shock-absorbing surfacing; Height standards; Maintenance standards

Running/Jogging

- **Proven:** Altered training regimen
- **Promising/Potential:** Shock-absorbing insoles

Skiing/Snowboarding

- **Proven:** Training to avoid risk situations; Adjustable bindings; Wrist guards in snowboarding
- **Promising/Potential:** Helmets

Soccer

- **Proven:** Anchored, padded goal posts; Shin guards; Neuromuscular training programs. Neuromuscular training programs consist of four elements: (1) muscle strengthening, (2) balance training, (3) jump training, and (4) learning proper mechanics (pivoting, landing, etc.); Strength training.

1. Semi-rigid ankle stabilizers and braces have been shown to be most effective for persons with a previous history of ankle sprain. Stabilizers and braces are recommended for persons who have a previous ankle injury and are participating in all activities with a risk of ankle injury, for example jumping, running, twisting, etc.

Chapter 48

Tips For Exercising Safely In Adverse Weather

How To Exercise Safely In Cold Weather

Winter weather means taking special precautions when you exercise outside. Cold exposure can make outdoor activity uncomfortable or even dangerous for anyone unprepared for extreme weather. It's important to be aware of the early warning signs and symptoms of cold exposure and how to prevent problems.

Shivering

Shivering is usually the first sign of dangerous cold exposure. As the body is trying to generate its own heat you will develop uncontrolled muscle contraction. Shivering should be your first warning to seek shelter and warm up your core temperature.

The two most dangerous conditions that can result from cold weather exposure include frostbite and hypothermia.

Frostbite

Frostbite describes the freezing of superficial tissues of the face, ears, fingers and toes.

Signs And Symptoms Of Frostbite

- Pain

About This Chapter: This chapter begins with "How to Exercise Safely in Cold Weather," © 2012 About.com. Used with permission of About, Inc. which can be found online at www.About.com. All rights reserved. It continues with "Exercising in Hot Weather," by CDR Scott Gaustad, U.S. Public Health Service Commissioned Corps, August 2007. Reviewed by David A. Cooke, MD, FACP, May 2012. Additional information from the New York State Department of Health is cited separately within the chapter.

- Burning

- Numbness

- Tingling

- Skin turns hard and white

- Skin starts to peel or get blisters

- Skin starts to itch

- Skin gets firm, shiny, and grayish-yellow

Frostbite Treatment

To help a frostbite victim, get the person to a warm, dry place and remove constrictive clothing. Raise affected areas and apply warm, moist compresses to these areas. Do not rub frostbitten areas or apply direct heat.

Hypothermia

Hypothermia is a more severe response to cold exposure that is defined as a significant drop in body core temperature.

Signs And Symptoms Of Hypothermia

- Shivering

- Cold sensation, goose bumps, confusion, numbness

- Intense shivering, lack of coordination, sluggishness

- Violent shivering, difficulty speaking, mental confusion, stumbling, depression

- Muscle stiffness, slurred speech. and trouble seeing

- Unconsciousness

Hypothermia Treatment

At the first sign of hypothermia take the person to a dry, warm place or warm the victim with blankets, extra dry clothing or your own body heat.

Hypothermia Prevention

The first line of defense against cold exposure is dressing in layers that are appropriate for the conditions. Layers should include a combination of clothing (base, mid, and outer) that help regulate your temperature and keep you warm and dry. Other factors that can negatively affect your ability to handle cold temperatures can include inadequate winter hydration and nutrition, dehydration, alcohol consumption, certain medications and health conditions such as diabetes and heart disease, which can significantly decrease a person's ability to exercise outdoors in the cold.

To improve your comfort and safety while exercising in the cold, the American College of Sports Medicine recommends the following:

- *Layer Clothing:* Several thin layers are warmer than one heavy layer. Layers are also easier to add or remove and thus, better regulate your core temperature. The goal is to keep the body warm and minimize sweating and avoid shivering.

- *Cover Your Head:* Your head should be covered while exercising in the cold, because heat loss from the head and neck may be as much as 50 percent of the total heat being lost by your body.

- *Cover Your Mouth:* To warm the air before you breathe it, use a scarf or mask. Do this especially if breathing cold air causes angina (chest pain) or you are prone to upper respiratory problems.

- *Stay Dry:* Wet, damp clothing, whether from perspiration or precipitation, significantly increases body-heat loss.

- *Keep Your Feet Dry:* Use a fabric that will wick perspiration away from the skin. Polypropylene, wool, or other fabrics that wick moisture away from the skin and retain insulating properties keep the body warm when wet.

- *Stay Hydrated:* Dehydration affects your body's ability to regulate body heat and increases the risk of frostbite. Fluids, especially water, are as important in cold weather as in the heat. Avoid consuming alcohol or beverages containing caffeine, because these items are dehydrating.

- *Avoid Alcohol:* Alcohol dilates blood vessels and increases heat loss so the odds of experiencing a hypothermic event increase. Alcohol can also impair judgment to the extent that you may not make the best or brightest decisions in a cold weather emergency. It's best to leave the alcohol behind when you head out into the cold.

Source: "Extreme Cold: A Prevention Guide to Promote Your Personal Health and Safety," Centers for Disease Control and Prevention, http://www.bt.cdc.gov/disasters/winter/guide.asp. last accessed 12-09-2009.

Lightning Safety Tips

Lightening kills more people in this country than tornadoes, floods, or hurricanes. Thunderstorm activity is greatest during July and August. These simple precautions can save lives during a lightning storm.

Stay Alert

- Monitor local weather conditions regularly with a special weather radio or AM/FM radio.

- Recognize the signs of an oncoming thunder and lightning storm—towering clouds with a "cauliflower" shape, dark skies, and distant rumbles of thunder or flashes of lightning. Do not wait for lightning to strike nearby before taking cover.

Seek Shelter

- Look for a large, enclosed building when a thunder or lightning storm threatens. That's the best choice.

- If you are in a car and it has a hard top, stay inside and keep the windows rolled up.

- Avoid small sheds and lean-tos or partial shelters, like pavilions.

- Stay at least a few feet away from open windows, sinks, toilets, tubs, showers, electric boxes and outlets, and appliances. Lightning can flow through these and "jump" to a person.

- Do not shower or take a bath during a thunder or lightning storm

- Avoid using regular telephones, except in an emergency. If lightning hits the telephone lines, it could flow to the phone. Cell or cordless phones, not connected to the building's wiring, are safe to use.

Exercising In Hot Weather

Summer is the time when many amateur, recreational, and elite athletes transition from indoor programs to outdoor warm or hot weather exercise regimens. As the temperature and humidity rise, so does the incidence of environmental heat-related exertional illnesses. Understanding warm and/or hot weather definitions is very important for an athlete or just an exerciser for fitness so that they may better comprehend heat illness, preventative measures, and treatment options if necessary. Of the many relevant heat related definitions, the heat index is one of the most important.

If you are caught outside: (If you are unable to reach a safe building or car, knowing what to do can save your life.)

- If your skin tingles or your hair stands on the end, a lightning strike may be about to happen. Crouch down on the balls of your feet with your feet close together. Keep your hands on your knees and lower your head. Get as low as possible without touching your hands or knees to the ground. DO NOT LIE DOWN!
- If you are swimming, fishing or boating and there are clouds, dark skies, and distant rumbles of thunder or flashes of lightning, get to land immediately and seek shelter.
- If you are in a boat and cannot get to shore, crouch down in the middle of the boat. Go below if possible.
- If you are on land, find a low spot away from trees, metal fences, pipes, or tall or long objects.
- If you are in the woods, look for an area of shorter trees. Crouch down away from tree trunks.

Helping someone who is struck by lightning

When someone is struck by lightning, get emergency medical help as soon as possible. If more than one person is struck by lightning, treat those who are unconscious first. They are at greatest risk of dying. A person struck by lightning may appear dead, with no pulse or breath. Often the person can be revived with cardiopulmonary resuscitation (CPR). There is no danger to anyone helping a person who has been struck by lightning—no electric charge remains. CPR should be attempted immediately.

Treat those who are injured but conscious next. Common injuries from being struck by lightning are burns, wounds, and fractures.

Source: "Lightning Safety Tips," reprinted with permission of the New York State Department of Health (www.health .ny.gov). © 2007. Reviewed by David A. Cooke, MD, FACP, May 2012.

Steadman Or Heat Index

The heat index uses on combination of air temperature and humidity to give a description of how the temperature feels. This is not the actual air temperature. When the heat index is at or over 90 degrees Fahrenheit, extreme caution should be considered before exercising outdoors. A heat index chart can be found at http://www.nws.noaa.gov/om/heat/index.shtml.

Heat Illness

Heat illness or exertional heat illness progresses along a continuum from the mild (heat rash and/or heat cramps and/or heat syncope) through the moderate (heat exhaustion) to the life-threatening (heatstroke). Anyone is susceptible to a heat-related exertional illness. It is very important that the athlete or exerciser understand that the presentation of signs and symptoms associated with heat exertional illness does not necessarily follow this continuum. A dehydrated, non-acclimated or deconditioned individual may right away present with signs and symptoms consistent with heat stroke and not the milder symptoms first.

Heat Cramps: Heat cramps are associated with excessive sweating during exercise and are usually caused by dehydration, electrolyte (primarily salt) loss, and inadequate blood flow to the peripheral muscles. They usually occur in the quadriceps, hamstrings, and calves.

Treatment for heat cramps is rehydration with an electrolyte (salt) solution and muscle stretch.

Heat Syncope: Heat syncope results from physical exertion in a hot environment. In an effort to increase heat loss, the skin blood vessels dilate to such an extent that blood flow to the brain is reduced causing symptoms of headache, dizziness, faintness, increased heart rate, nausea, vomiting, restlessness, and possibly even a brief loss of consciousness.

Treatment for heat syncope is to sit or lie down in a cool environment with elevation of the feet. Hydration is very important so there is not a possible progression to heat exhaustion or heat stroke.

Heat Exhaustion: Heat exhaustion is a shock-like condition that occurs when excessive sweating causes dehydration and electrolyte loss. A person with heat exhaustion may have headache, nausea, dizziness, chills, fatigue, and extreme thirst. Signs of heat exhaustion are pale and clammy skin, rapid and weak pulse, loss of coordination, decreased performance, dilated pupils, and profuse sweating.

Treatment for heat exhaustion is to immediately stop the activity and properly hydrate with chilled water and/or an electrolyte replacement sport beverage. The exerciser should be cleared by his/her physician before resuming sport or other strenuous outdoor activities.

Exertional Heat Stoke (Hyperthermia): Hyperthermia, also called exertional heat stroke, is a life-threatening condition in which the body's thermal regulatory mechanism is overwhelmed. There are two types heat stroke—fluid depleted (slow onset) and fluid intact (fast onset). Fluid depleted means that the individual is not hydrating at a rate sufficient to function in a heat challenge situation. Fluid intact means that the extreme heat overwhelms the individual even though the fluid level is sufficient. Key signs of heat stroke are hot skin (not necessarily dry skin), peripheral vasoconstriction (pale or ashen colored skin), high pulse rate, high respiratory rate, decreased urine output, and a core temperature (taken rectally) over 104 degrees Fahrenheit, and pupils may be dilated and unresponsive to light.

Treatment for heat stroke is to move the person to a cool shaded area and reduce the body temperature immediately. If immediate medical attention is not available, immerse the person in a cool bath while covering the extremities with cool wet cloths and massaging the extremities to propel the cooled blood back into the core.

Exercise-Induced Hyponatremia: Water intoxication, which is known as exercised-induced hyponatremia (low sodium), is most commonly associated with prolonged exertion during sustained, high-intensity endurance activities such as marathons or triathlons. In most cases, it is attributable to excess free water intake, which fails to replenish the sometimes massive sodium losses that result from sweating. Symptoms of hyponatremia can vary from light-headedness, malaise, nausea, to altered mental status. Risk factors include hot weather, female athletes/exercisers, poor performance, and possibly the use of nonsteroidal anti-inflammatory medications.

As a treatment for hyponatremia, new guidelines advise runners to drink only as much fluid as they lose due to sweating during a race. The International Marathon Medical Directors Association recommends that, during extended exercise, athletes drink no more than 31 ounces (or about 800 milliliters) of water per hour. Individuals involved in strenuous exercise in warm or hot weather should consider the sodium (salt) concentration of the beverage being consumed.

Preventing Exertional Heat-Related Illnesses

The North American Society for Pediatric Exercise Medicine and the National Athletic Trainers' Association developed an Inter-Association Task Force on Exertional Heat Illnesses position statement (for more details, visit http://www.naspem.org). Some recommendations on how to prevent exertional heat related illness include the following:

- When exercising in high heat and humidity, rest 10 minutes for every hour and change wet clothing frequently.

- Avoid the midday sun by exercising before 10 a.m. or after 6 p.m., if possible.

- Use a sunscreen with a rating of SPF-15 or lower dependent upon skin type. Ratings above SPF-15 can interfere with the skin's thermal regulation.

- Wear light-weight and breathable clothing.

- Weigh yourself pre and post exercise. If there is a less than a 2% weight loss after exercise, you are considered mildly dehydrated. With a 2% and greater weight loss, you are considered dehydrated.

- During hot weather training, dehydration occurs more frequently and has more severe consequences. The American College of Sports Medicine recommends that you drink early and at regular intervals. The perception of thirst is a poor index of the magnitude of fluid deficit. Monitoring your weight loss and ingesting chilled volumes of fluid during exercise at a rate equal to that lost from sweating is a better method to preventing dehydration.

- Rapid fluid replacement is not recommended for rehydration. Rapid replacement of fluid stimulates increased urine production, which reduces the body water retention.

- Individuals involved in a short bout of exercise are generally fine with water fluid replacement of an extra 8–16 ounces. A sports drink (with salt and potassium) is suggested for exercise lasting longer than an hour, such as a marathon, and at a rate of about 16 to 24 ounces an hour depending upon the amount you sweat and the heat index.

- Replace fluids after long bouts of exercise (greater than an hour) at a rate of 16 ounces of fluid per pound of body weight lost during exercise.

- Avoid caffeinated, protein, and alcoholic drinks (for example, colored soda, coffee, tea).

- Acclimate to exercising outdoors, altitude, and physical condition. The general rule of thumb is 10–14 days for adults and 14–21 days for children (prepubescent) and older adults (> 60 years). Children and older adults are less heat tolerant and have a less effective thermoregulatory system.

- Educate and prepare yourself for outdoor activities. Many websites offer heat index calculations for your local weather conditions. One website that will calculate the heat index for you is http://www.erh.noaa.gov/box/calculate2.html.

Summer weather does not have to sideline your outdoor exercise regimen. The above suggestions can help you plan and find ways to modify your routine to exercise safely in warm, hot, and humid weather.

References

Arnheim DD. Prentice WE (editors). Environmental Considerations. *Principles of Athletic Training, 9th ed.* New York, NY, McGraw Hill, 1997, pp. 263–271.

Reamy, BV. Environmental Injuries, O'Connor FG, Sallis RE, Wilder RP, Pierre PS (editors): *Sports Medicine, Just the Facts, 1st ed.* New York, NY, McGraw Hill, 2005, pp. 235-237.

Whaley, MH. Appendix E: Environmental Considerations. *American College of Sports Medicine Guidelines for Exercise Testing and Prescription, 7th Edition.* Baltimore: Lippincott Williams and Wilkens, 2006, pp. 300–304.

Chapter 49

Understanding Hydration For Fitness

Selecting And Effectively Using Hydration For Fitness

Water is the most essential component of the human body as it provides an important role in the function of cells. Important functions of water include transportation of nutrients, elimination of waste products, regulation and maintenance of body temperature through sweating, maintenance of blood circulation and pressure, lubrication of joints and body tissues, and facilitation of digestion. More than half of the human body is composed of water, and it is impossible to sustain life without it.

Water Loss

Exercise produces an elevation in body temperature, which depends on the intensity and duration of exercise, environmental conditions, clothing worn, and metabolic rate. In order to get rid of the excess heat, your body secretes sweat, which is primarily composed of water and electrolytes such as sodium. The evaporation of sweat is the primary mechanism of heat loss during exercise.

Exercise can lead to substantial water and electrolyte loss from sweat leading to dehydration and, in cases of excessive fluid intake, hyponatremia (low sodium in the blood). However, considerable variability exists from person to person with regard to sweat loss. Therefore, the fluid and electrolyte requirements needed for the athlete are variable from person to person as well. If water and electrolytes are not replaced from these losses, the athlete will have a decrease in performance and perhaps an adverse effect on his or her overall health.

About This Chapter: "Selecting and Effectively Using Hydration for Fitness." Reprinted with permission of the American College of Sports Medicine (ACSM). Copyright © 2011 American College of Sports Medicine. This brochure is a product of ACSM's Consumer Information Committee. Visit ACSM online at www.acsm.org.

A Complete Physical Activity Program

A well-rounded physical activity program includes aerobic exercise and strength training exercise, but not necessarily in the same session. This blend helps maintain or improve cardiorespiratory and muscular fitness and overall health and function. Regular physical activity will provide more health benefits than sporadic, high intensity workouts, so choose exercises you are likely to enjoy and that you can incorporate into your schedule.

ACSM's physical activity recommendations for healthy adults, updated in 2011, recommend at least 30 minutes of moderate-intensity physical activity (working hard enough to break a sweat, but still able to carry on a conversation) five days per week, or 20 minutes of more vigorous activity three days per week. Combinations of moderate- and vigorous-intensity activity can be performed to meet this recommendation.

Examples of typical aerobic exercises are:

- Walking
- Stair climbing
- Rowing
- Swimming

- Running
- Cycling
- Cross country skiing

In addition, strength training should be performed a minimum of two days each week, with 8–12 repetitions of 8–10 different exercises that target all major muscle groups. This type of training can be accomplished using body weight, resistance bands, free weights, medicine balls or weight machines.

Fluid Balance

Thirst is a signal that your body is headed toward dehydration. Therefore, it is important to drink before you feel thirsty and to drink throughout the day. Thirst is not a good indicator of hydration and should not be used to monitor hydration status.

One way to check your hydration status is to weigh yourself before and after exercise. The before-exercise measurement is best as a nude weight first thing in the morning after urinating. Comparing your body weight before and after exercise can be used to estimate your sweat loss and your fluid requirements. Any weight loss is likely from fluid loss, so drinking enough to replenish these losses will maintain hydration. The Table 49.1 shows us that over a one percent loss in body weight indicates dehydration and over five percent indicates serious dehydration. These fluid losses need to be replaced.

Table 49.1. % Body Weight Change

Well Hydrated	-1 to +1%
Minimal Dehydration	-1 to -3%
Significant Dehydration	-3 to -5%
Serious Dehydration	> -5%

Another way to check hydration status is the urine color test. A large amount of light-colored urine means you are well hydrated. The darker the color, the more dehydrated you are (see Figure 49.1).

Figure 49.1. Hydration Status: The darker the urine color, the more dehydrated you are.

Dehydration

Dehydration is the loss of fluids and salts essential to maintain normal body function. Dehydration occurs when the body loses more fluids than it takes in. Dehydration can lead to:

- Muscle fatigue
- Loss of coordination
- Inability to regulate body temperature
- Heat illness (e.g., cramps, heat exhaustion, heat stroke)
- Decreased energy and athletic performance

Moderate caffeine intake does not affect hydration status or urine output. However, alcohol will increase your urine output and decrease hydration.

Enhancing palatability of a fluid will help to encourage fluid consumption. This can be done with proper flavoring, proper salt (sodium) content, and drinking a cold beverage (15–21 degrees Celsius).

Sports Beverages

Carbohydrates within a sports beverage help to replenish your sugar (glycogen) stores and electrolytes help to accelerate rehydration. Sports beverages for use during prolonged exercise should generally contain four to eight percent carbohydrate, 20–30 meq/L [milliequivalents per liter] of sodium, and 2–5 meq/L of potassium. The need for carbohydrates and electrolytes within sports beverages increases with prolonged activity.

Carbohydrate consumption helps to sustain and improve exercise performance during high-intensity exercise longer than one hour as well as lower-intensity exercise for longer periods. You should ingest one-half to one liter of a sports drink each hour to maintain hydration. Also, sports drinks should not exceed a carbohydrate concentration of eight percent.

Hydration Before Exercise

Check your hydration status before exercise because there is a wide variability in fluid needs for each person.

- Drink 16–20 fluid ounces of water or sports beverage at least four hours before exercise.
- Drink 8–12 fluid ounces of water 10–15 minutes before exercise.

Consuming a beverage with sodium (salt) and/or small meal helps to stimulate thirst and retain fluids.

Hydration During Exercise

- Drink 3–8 fluid ounces of water every 15–20 minutes when exercising for less than 60 minutes.
- Drink 3–8 fluid ounces of a sports beverage (5–8 percent carbohydrate with electrolytes) every 15–20 minutes when exercising greater than 60 minutes.

Do not drink more than one quart/hour during exercise.

Hydration Guidelines After Exercise

Obtain your body weight and check your urine to estimate your fluid losses. The goal is to correct your losses within two hours after exercise.

Staying Active Pays Off!

Those who are physically active tend to live longer, healthier lives. Research shows that moderate physical activity—such as 30 minutes a day of brisk walking—significantly contributes to longevity. Even a person with risk factors like high blood pressure, diabetes or even a smoking habit can gain real benefits from incorporating regular physical activity into their daily life.

As many dieters have found, exercise can help you stay on a diet and lose weight. What's more, regular exercise can help lower blood pressure, control blood sugar, improve cholesterol levels and build stronger, denser bones.

The First Step

Before you begin an exercise program, take a fitness test, or substantially increase your level of activity, make sure to answer the following questions. This physical activity readiness questionnaire (PAR-Q) will help determine if you're ready to begin an exercise routine or program.

- Has your doctor ever said that you have a heart condition or that you should participate in physical activity only as recommended by a doctor?
- Do you feel pain in your chest during physical activity?
- In the past month, have you had chest pain when you were not doing physical activity?
- Do you lose your balance from dizziness? Do you ever lose consciousness?
- Do you have a bone or joint problem that could be made worse by a change in your physical activity?
- Is your doctor currently prescribing drugs for your blood pressure or a heart condition?
- Do you know of any reason you should not participate in physical activity?

If you answered yes to one or more questions, if you are over 40 years of age and have recently been inactive, or if you are concerned about your health, consult a physician before taking a fitness test or substantially increasing your physical activity. If you answered no to each question, then it's likely that you can safely begin exercising.

Prior To Exercise

Prior to beginning any exercise program, including the activities depicted in this brochure, individuals should seek medical evaluation and clearance to engage in activity. Not all exercise programs are suitable for everyone, and some programs may result in injury. Activities should be carried out at a pace that is comfortable for the user. Users should discontinue participation in any exercise activity that causes pain or discomfort. In such event, medical consultation should be immediately obtained.

- Drink 20–24 fluid ounces of water or sports beverage for every one pound lost

Overhydration

Overhydration, also called water intoxication, is a condition where the body contains too much water. This can result in behavioral changes, confusion, drowsiness, nausea/vomiting, weight gain, muscle cramps, weakness/paralysis and risk of death.

In general, overhydration is treated by limiting your fluid intake and increasing the salt (sodium) that you consume. If overhydration is suspected, you should see your doctor for appropriate lab tests and treatment. You should not consume more than one liter per hour of fluid.

Part Six
Overcoming Obstacles To Fitness

Chapter 50

Maintaining Fitness Motivation

Motivation And The Power Of Not Giving Up

Have you ever set a goal for yourself, like getting fit, making honor roll, or being picked for a team? Like lots of people, maybe you started out doing great, but then lost some of that drive and had trouble getting motivated again.

You're Not Alone!

Everyone struggles with staying motivated and reaching their goals. Just look at how many people go on diets, lose weight, and then gain it back again!

The reality is that refocusing, changing, or making a new start on something, no matter how small, is a big deal. But it's not impossible. With the right approach, you can definitely do it.

Getting Motivated

So how do you stay motivated and on track with your goal? It all comes down to good planning, realistic expectations, and a stick-to-it attitude. Here's what you need to do:

First, know your goal. Start by writing down your major goal. Your major goal is the ultimate thing you'd like to see happen. For example, "I want to make honor roll," or "I want to get fit enough to make the cross-country team," or even, "I want to play in the Olympics" are all major goals because they're the final thing the goal setter wants to see happen (obviously,

About This Chapter: "Motivation and the Power of Not Giving Up," February 2009, reprinted with permission from www.kidshealth.org. This information was provided by KidsHealth®, one of the largest resources online for medically reviewed health information written for parents, kids, and teens. For more articles like this, visit www .KidsHealth.org or www.TeensHealth.org. Copyright © 1995-2012 The Nemours Foundation. All rights reserved.

some goals take longer and require more work than others). It's OK to dream big. That's how people accomplish stuff. You just have to remember that the bigger the goal, the more work it takes to get there.

No Quick Fix

It often takes several attempts to achieve a goal. For example, the American Lung Association says that the average person who quits smoking tries to stop up to six times before successfully quitting for good.

- I encourage myself every day. I also make plans about eating and exercising. —Kyla, 13
- I remind myself each and every night what my goal is. —Andrew, 16.

Make it specific. It's easier to plan for and master a specific goal than a vague one. Let's say your goal is to get fit. That's pretty vague. Make it specific by defining what you want to achieve (such as muscle tone and definition or endurance), why you want to get fit, and by when. This helps you make a plan to reach your goal.

Make it realistic. People often abandon their goals because their expectations are unreasonable. Maybe they expect to get ripped abs in weeks rather than months, or to quit smoking easily after years of lighting up.

Let's say you want to run a marathon. If you try to run the entire distance of 26.2 miles tomorrow without any training, you're unlikely to succeed. It takes the average person four months of training to run that far! But the bigger risk is that you'll get so bummed out that you'll give up your marathon dreams—and running—altogether.

Part of staying motivated is being realistic about what you can achieve within the timeframe you've planned. Competing on the Olympic ski team is a workable goal if you are 15 and already a star skier. But if you're 18 and only just taking your first lesson, time isn't exactly on your side.

Write it down. Put your specific goal in writing. Then write it down again. And again. Research shows that writing down a goal is part of the mental process of committing to it. Write your goal down every day to keep you focused and remind you how much you want it.

Break it down. Making any change takes self-discipline. You need to pay constant attention so you don't get sidetracked. One way to make this easier is to break a big goal into small steps. For example, let's say you want to run a marathon. If it's February and the marathon is in August, that's a realistic timeframe to prepare. Start by planning to run two miles and work up gradually to the distance you need.

Then set specific daily tasks, like eating five servings of fruit and veggies and running a certain amount a day. Put these on a calendar or planner so you can check them off. Ask a coach to help you set doable mini-goals for additional mile amounts and for tasks to improve your performance, such as exercises to build strength and stamina so you'll stay motivated to run farther.

Reaching frequent, smaller goals is something to celebrate. It gives you the confidence, courage, and motivation to keep running—or doing whatever it is you're aiming to do. So reward yourself!

Staying Motivated

Check in with your goal. Now that you've broken your goal down into a series of mini-goals and daily tasks, check in every day.

It helps to write down your small goals in the same way you wrote down your big goal. That way you can track what you need to do, check off tasks as you complete them, and enjoy knowing that you're moving toward your big goal.

As you accomplish a task, check it off on your list. Tell yourself, "Hey, I've run 10 miles, I'm nearly halfway to my goal!" Reward yourself with something you promised yourself when you set your goal. Feel successful—you are! Now think ahead to accomplishing the rest of your goal: "What do I have to do to reach 26 miles? How am I going to make the time to train?"

Writing down specific steps has another advantage: If you're feeling weak on willpower you can look at your list to help you refocus!

Recommit to your goal if you slip up. If you slip up, don't give up. Forgive yourself and make a plan for getting back on track.

Pat yourself on the back for everything you did right. Don't beat yourself up, no matter how far off track you get. Most people slip up when trying to make a change—it's a natural part of the process.

Writing down daily tasks and mini-goals helps here too. By keeping track of things, you'll quickly recognize when you've slipped up, making it easier to refocus and recommit to your goal. So instead of feeling discouraged, you can know exactly where you got off track and why.

What if you keep slipping up? Ask yourself if you're really committed to your goal. If you are, recommit—and put it in writing. The process of writing everything down may also help you discover when you're not really committed to a goal. For example, perhaps you're more in love with the fantasy of being a star athlete than the reality, and there's something else that you'd rather be or do.

View slip-ups as lessons and reminders of why you're trying to make a change. When you mess up, it's not a fault—it's an opportunity to learn something new about yourself. Say your goal is to fight less with your brother or sister. You may learn that it's better to say, "I can't talk about this right now" and take time to calm down when you feel your temper growing out of control.

Keep a stick-to-it attitude. Visualize yourself achieving your goal: a toned you in your prom dress or a successful you scoring the winning soccer goal. Self-visualization helps you keep what you're trying to accomplish in mind. It helps you believe it's possible. You can also call up your mental picture when willpower and motivation are low.

Positive self-talk also boosts your attitude and motivation. Tell yourself, "I deserve to make the honor roll because I've really been working hard" or "I feel great when I swim—I'm doing well on my exercise plan!"

Share with a friend. Another boost is having supportive people around you. Find a running buddy, a quit smoking buddy, or someone else with a similar goal so you can support each other. Having a goal buddy can make all the difference in times when you don't feel motivated—like getting up for that early-morning run.

If you're not getting support from someone when you really need it, you may need to take a break from that friendship and surround yourself with people who want to help you succeed. For instance, if you've been going to your friend's house to study together every Thursday after school, but now your pal is turning on the TV, IMing friends online, or gabbing on the phone and ignoring your pleas to get down to work, it's time to find another study buddy. You can't stay focused on your goal if your friend doesn't share that goal—or, even worse, is trying to hold you back. Seek out others who are on the same path you are and work with them instead.

Do It For Yourself

The key to making any change is to find the desire within yourself. Don't create a resolution just to please someone else or because others are telling you to change. If you're only doing something because you feel obligated to, you won't be as motivated as if you truly want it for yourself.

Don't Give Up!

Ending an unhealthy behavior or creating a new, exciting one is all about taking responsibility for our lives. Finding the motivation to do it isn't necessarily easy, but it is always possible. You can stay motivated by writing down your goals, sticking to your schedule, and reminding yourself of what led you to set your goal in the first place. Change is exciting—we'd all be very bored without it.

Good luck in reaching your goals!

Chapter 51

You Can Be Active At Any Size

Would you like to be more physically active, but are not sure if you can do it? Good news—if you are a very large person, you can be physically active—and you can have fun and feel good doing it.

There may be special challenges for very large people who are physically active. You may not be able to bend or move in the same way that other people can. It may be hard to find clothes and equipment for exercising. You may feel self-conscious being physically active around other people.

Facing these challenges is hard—but it can be done. The information in this chapter may help you start being more active and healthier, no matter what your size.

Why Should I Be Active?

Being physically active may help you live longer and protect you from type 2 diabetes, heart disease, stroke, and high blood pressure.

If you have any of these health problems, being physically active may help improve your symptoms.

Being Physically Active Can Be A Lot Of Fun

Regular physical activity helps you feel better because it provides these benefits:

- Lowers your stress and boosts your mood

- Increases your strength, movement, balance, and flexibility

- Helps control blood pressure and blood sugar

About This Chapter: Excerpted from "Active at Any Size," National Institute of Diabetes and Digestive and Kidney Diseases (http://win.niddk.nih.gov), 2010.

- Helps build healthy bones, muscles, and joints

- Helps your heart and lungs work better

- Improves your self-esteem

- Boosts energy during the day and may aid in sleep at night

How Do I Get Started?

To start being more active, try these tips:

- **Think about your barriers to being active:** Then try to come up with creative ways to solve them. The following examples may help you overcome barriers.

  - *I don't have enough time:* Be active for a few minutes at a time throughout the day. Sit less. Try to walk more while doing your errands or schedule lunchtime workouts to boost your overall activity. Plan ahead and be creative.

  - *I feel self-conscious when I'm active:* Be active at home while doing household chores and find ways to move more during your day-to-day activities. Try walking with a group of friends with whom you feel comfortable.

  - *I'm worried about my health or injury:* You might feel better if you talk to a health care professional first. Find a fitness provider to guide you or sign up for a class so you feel safe. Remember that activity does not have to be difficult. Gentle activity is good too.

  - *I just don't like exercise:* Good news—you do not have to run or do push-ups to get the benefits of being physically active. Try dancing to the radio, walking outdoors, or being active with friends to spice things up.

  - *I can't stay motivated:* Try to add variety to your activities and ask your friends to help you stay focused on being active. Consider an activity video for extra encouragement. Also, set realistic goals, track your progress, and be sure to celebrate your achievements.

- **Start slowly:** Your body needs time to get used to your new activity.

- **Warm up**: Warm-ups get your body ready for action. Shrug your shoulders, tap your toes, swing your arms, or march in place. Walk more slowly for the first few minutes.

- **Cool down:** Slow down little by little. If you have been walking fast, walk slowly for a few minutes to cool down. Cooling down may protect your heart, relax your muscles, and keep you from getting hurt.

Appreciate Yourself

If you cannot do an activity, do not be hard on yourself. Feel good about what you can do. Be proud of pushing yourself up out of a chair or walking a short distance.

Pat yourself on the back for trying even if you cannot do it the first time. It may be easier the next time.

How Do I Continue To Be Active?

To maintain your active lifestyle, try these suggestions:

- **Pledge to be active:** Making a commitment to yourself to be active may help you stay motivated, stay on track, and reach your goals.

- **Set goals:** Set short-term and long-term goals. A short-term goal may be to walk 5 to 10 minutes, five days a week. It may not seem like a lot, but any activity is better than none. A long-term goal may be to do at least 30 minutes of physical activity at a moderate-intensity level (one that makes you breathe harder but does not overwork or overheat you) on most days of the week. You can break up your physical activity in shorter segments of 10 minutes or more.

- **Set rewards:** Whether your goal was to be active for 15 minutes a day, to walk farther than you did last week, or simply to stay positive, you deserve recognition for your efforts. Some ideas for rewards include purchasing new music to motivate you, new walking shoes, or a new outfit.

- **Get support:** Get a family member or friend to be physically active with you. It may be more fun, and your buddy can cheer you on and help you stick with it.

- **Track progress:** Keep a journal of your physical activity. You may not feel like you are making progress but when you look back at where you started, you may be pleasantly surprised!

- **Have fun!** Try different activities to find the ones you really enjoy.

What Physical Activities Can A Very Large Person Do?

Most very large people can do some or all of the physical activities in this chapter. You do not need special skills or a lot of equipment. Here are example of what you can do:

- **Weight-bearing activities,** like walking and climbing stairs, which involve lifting or pushing your own body weight.

- **Nonweight-bearing activities,** like swimming and water workouts, which put less stress on your joints because you do not have to lift or push your own weight. If your feet or joints hurt when you stand, nonweight-bearing activities may be best for you.

- **Lifestyle activities,** like gardening or washing the car, which are great ways to get moving. Lifestyle activities do not have to be planned out ahead of time.

Remember that physical activity does not have to be hard or boring to be good for you. Anything that gets you moving around-even for only a few minutes a day-is a healthy start to getting more fit.

Walking (Weight Bearing)

Walking may help you improve your fitness, increase the number of calories your body uses, and increase your energy levels.

Tips For Walking

- **Try to walk 5 minutes a day for the first week.** Walk 8 minutes the next week. Stay at 8-minute walks until you feel comfortable. Then increase your walks to 11 minutes. Slowly lengthen each walk, or try walking faster.

- **Gradually increase your walks** to give your heart and lungs—as well as your leg muscles—a good workout.

- **Wear comfortable walking shoes** with a lot of support. If you walk frequently, you may need to buy new shoes often. You may wish to speak with a podiatrist about when you need to purchase new walking shoes.

- **Wear garments that prevent inner-thigh chafing,** such as tights or spandex shorts.

- **Make walking fun.** Walk with a friend or pet. Walk in places you enjoy, like a park or shopping mall.

Dancing (Weight Bearing Or Nonweight Bearing)

Dancing may help tone your muscles, improve your flexibility, make your heart stronger, and make your lungs work better. You can dance in a health club, in a nightclub, or at home. To dance at home, just move your body to some lively music.

Do I need to see my health care provider before I start being physically active?

You should talk to your health care provider if you have a chronic disease or have risk factors for a chronic disease, such as asthma or diabetes, or have high blood pressure, high cholesterol, or a personal or family history of heart disease. You should also see a health care provider if you are pregnant or are a smoker. If you are unsure of your health status or have any concerns that exercise might be unsafe for you, ask your health care provider.

Chances are your health care provider will be pleased with your decision to start an activity program. It is unlikely that you will need a complete medical exam before you go out for a short walk.

Dancing on your feet is a weight-bearing activity. Dancing while seated is a nonweight-bearing activity. Sometimes called chair dancing, this activity lets you move your arms and legs to music while taking the weight off your feet. This may be a good choice if you cannot stand on your feet for a long time.

Water Workouts (Nonweight Bearing)

Exercising in water helps flexibility. You can bend and move your body in water in ways you cannot on land. It also reduces risk of injury. Water makes your body float. This keeps your joints from being pounded or jarred and helps prevent sore muscles and injury. Exercising in water also keeps you refreshed. You can keep cool in water—even when you are working hard.

You do not need to know how to swim to work out in water—you can do shallow-water or deep-water exercises without swimming.

For shallow-water workouts, the water level should be between your waist and your chest. If the water is too shallow, it will be hard to move your arms underwater. If the water is deeper than chest-height, it will be hard to keep your feet on the pool bottom.

For deep-water workouts, most of your body is underwater. This means that your whole body will get a good workout. For safety and comfort, wear a foam belt or life jacket.

Many swim centers offer classes in water workouts. Check with the pools in your area to find the best water workout for you.

Weight Training (Weight Bearing Or Nonweight Bearing)

Weight training may help you build strong muscles and bones. You can weight train at home or at a fitness center. It also can help you increase the number of calories your body uses.

You do not need benches or bars to begin weight training at home. You can use a pair of hand weights or even two soup cans. To make sure you are using the correct posture, and that your movements are slow and controlled, you may want to schedule a session with a personal trainer. Ask your health care provider for a referral to a personal trainer. You may need to check with your health insurer about whether this service is covered by your plan.

If you decide to buy a home gym, check its weight rating (the number of pounds it can support) to make sure it is safe for your size. If you want to join a fitness center where you can use weights, shop around for one where you feel at ease.

Weight Training Rule Of Thumb: If you cannot lift a weight six times in a row, the weight you are lifting is too heavy. If you can easily lift a weight 15 times in a row, your weight is too light.

Bicycling (Nonweight Bearing)

You can bicycle indoors on a stationary bike or outdoors on a road bike. Biking does not stress any one part of the body—your weight is spread among your arms, back, and hips.

You may want to use a recumbent bike. On this type of bike, you sit low to the ground with your legs reaching forward to the pedals. This may feel better than sitting upright. The seat on a recumbent bike is also wider than the seat on an upright bike.

For biking outdoors, you may want to try a mountain bike. These bikes have wider tires and are heavy. You can also buy a larger seat to put on your bike. Make sure the bike you buy has a weight rating at least as high as your own weight.

Yoga (Weight Bearing Or Nonweight Bearing)

Yoga may help you be more flexible, feel more relaxed, and improve posture. Yoga may also help you breathe deeply, relax, and get rid of stress. Your local fitness center may offer yoga, tai chi, or other mind/body classes. You may want to start with "gentle" classes, like those aimed at seniors.

Lifestyle Activities

Lifestyle physical activities do not have to be planned. You can make small changes to make your day more physically active and improve your health. Here are some examples:

- If possible, take two- to three-minute walking breaks a few times a day.
- Put away the TV remote control—get up to change the channel.
- March in place during TV commercials.
- Stand or walk, rather than sit, while talking on the phone.
- Play with your family.

Even a shopping trip can be exercise, since it is a chance to walk and carry your bags. In addition, doing chores like lawn mowing, raking leaves, gardening, and housework can count as activity.

Tips For Safe Physical Activity

Stop your activity right away if you experience these symptoms:

- Have pain, tightness, or pressure in your chest or neck, shoulder, or arm
- Feel dizzy or sick
- Break out in a cold sweat
- Have muscle cramps
- Are extremely short of breath
- Feel pain in your joints, feet, ankles, or legs. You could hurt yourself if you ignore the pain

Ask your health care provider what to do if you have any of these symptoms.

Questions To Ask When Choosing A Fitness Center

- Can the treadmills or benches support people who are large?
- Does the fitness staff know how to work with people of larger sizes?
- Can I take time to see how I like the center before I sign up?
- Is the aim of signing up to have fun and get healthy?
- What are the hours? What time of day is it crowded?

Slow down if you feel out of breath. The "Talk Test" is an easy way to monitor your physical activity intensity:

- You should be able to talk during your activity without gasping for breath.

- When talking becomes difficult, your activity may be too hard.

- If talking becomes difficult for you while exercising, slow down until you are able to talk comfortably again.

Wear Suitable Clothes

- Wear lightweight, loose-fitting tops so you can move easily.

- Wear clothes made of fabrics that absorb sweat and remove it from your skin.

- Never wear rubber or plastic suits. Plastic suits could hold the sweat on your skin and make your body overheat.

- Women should wear a good support bra.

- Wear supportive athletic shoes for weight-bearing activities.

- Wear a knit hat to keep you warm when you are physically active outdoors in cold weather. Wear a tightly woven, wide-brimmed hat in hot weather to help keep you cool and protect you from the sun.

- Wear sunscreen when you are physically active outdoors.

- Wear garments that prevent inner-thigh chafing, such as tights or spandex shorts.

Drink Fluids When You Are Thirsty.

Drink fluids regularly while you are being physically active. Water or other fluids will help keep you hydrated when you are sweating.

Applaud Yourself

If you can do only a few or none of the activities mentioned in this chapter activities, it is OK. Appreciate what you can do, even if you think it is a small amount. Doing any movement—even for a short time—can make you healthier. Remember, each activity you do is a step toward a more active lifestyle.

Healthy, fit bodies come in all sizes. Whatever your size or shape, get physically active now and keep moving for a healthier you.

Chapter 52

Sports Injuries

Childhood Sports Injuries: A Common And Serious Problem

More than 38 million children and adolescents participate in organized sports in the United States each year. Still more participate in informal recreational activities. Although sports participation provides numerous physical and social benefits, it also has a downside: the risk of sports-related injuries. In fact, according to a 2002 report by the Centers for Disease Control, nearly 1.9 million children under 15 were treated in emergency departments the year before for sports-related injuries.

These injuries are by far the most common cause of musculoskeletal injuries in children treated in emergency departments. They are also the single most common cause of injury-related primary care office visits.

The Most Common Sports-Related Injuries In Kids

Although sports injuries can range from scrapes and bruises to serious brain and spinal cord injuries, most fall somewhere between the two extremes. Here are some of the more common types of injuries.

About This Chapter: Excerpted and adapted from "Childhood Sports Injuries and Their Prevention," National Institute of Arthritis and Musculoskeletal and Skin Disease (http://www.niams.nih.gov), July 2009.

Sprains And Strains

A sprain is an injury to a ligament, one of the bands of tough, fibrous tissue that connects two or more bones at a joint and prevents excessive movement of the joint. An ankle sprain is the most common athletic injury.

A strain is an injury to either a muscle or a tendon. A muscle is a tissue composed of bundles of specialized cells that, when stimulated by nerve messages, contract and produce movement. A tendon is a tough, fibrous cord of tissue that connects muscle to bone. Muscles in any part of the body can be injured.

Growth Plate Injuries

In some sports accidents and injuries, the growth plate may be injured. The growth plate is the area of developing tissues at the end of the long bones in growing children and adolescents. When growth is complete, sometime during adolescence, the growth plate is replaced by solid bone. The long bones in the body include these:

- The long bones of the hand and fingers (metacarpals and phalanges)
- Both bones of the forearm (radius and ulna)
- The bone of the upper leg (femur)
- The lower leg bones (tibia and fibula)
- The foot bones (metatarsals and phalanges)

If any of these areas become injured, it's important to seek professional help from an orthopaedic surgeon, a doctor who specializes in bone injuries.

Repetitive Motion Injuries

Painful injuries such as stress fractures (a hairline fracture of the bone that has been subjected to repeated stress) and tendinitis (inflammation of a tendon) can occur from overuse of muscles and tendons. Some of these injuries don't always show up on x-rays, but they do cause pain and discomfort. The injured area usually responds to rest, ice, compression, and elevation (RICE). Other treatments can include crutches, cast immobilization, and physical therapy.

Heat-Related Illnesses

Heat-related illnesses include the following:

- Dehydration (deficit in body fluids)

- Heat exhaustion (nausea, dizziness, weakness, headache, pale and moist skin, heavy perspiration, normal or low body temperature, weak pulse, dilated pupils, disorientation, and fainting spells)

- Heat stroke (headache, dizziness, confusion, and hot dry skin, possibly leading to vascular collapse, coma, and death).

Heat injuries are always dangerous and can be fatal. Heat-related injuries are a particular problem for children because children perspire less than adults and require a higher core body temperature to trigger sweating. Playing rigorous sports in the heat requires close monitoring of both body and weather conditions. Fortunately, heat-related illnesses can be prevented.

Preventing And Treating Injuries

Injuries can happen to anyone who plays sports, but there are some things that can help prevent and treat injuries.

Prevention

- Enroll in organized sports through schools, community clubs, and recreation areas that are properly maintained. Any organized team activity should demonstrate a commitment to injury prevention. Coaches should be trained in first aid and CPR, and should have a plan for responding to emergencies. Coaches should be well versed in the proper use of equipment, and should enforce rules on equipment use.

- Organized sports programs may have adults on staff who are Certified Athletic Trainers. These individuals are trained to prevent, recognize, and provide immediate care for athletic injuries.

- Make sure you have—and consistently use—proper gear for a particular sport. This may reduce the chances of being injured.

- Make warm-ups and cool-downs part of your routine before and after sports participation. Warm-up exercises, such as stretching and light jogging, can help minimize the chance of muscle strain or other soft tissue injury during sports. Warm-up exercises make the body's tissues warmer and more flexible. Cool-down exercises loosen muscles that have tightened during exercise.

- Make sure you have access to water or a sports drink while playing. Drink frequently and stay properly hydrated. Remember to include sunscreen and a hat (when possible) to reduce the chance of sunburn, which is a type of injury to the skin. Sun protection may also decrease the chances of malignant melanoma—a potentially deadly skin cancer—or other skin cancers that can occur later in life.

- Learn and follow safety rules and suggestions for your particular sport. You'll find some more sport-specific safety suggestions below.

Treatment

Treatment for sports-related injuries will vary by injury. But if you suffer a soft tissue injury (such as a sprain or strain) or a bone injury, the best immediate treatment is easy to remember: RICE (rest, ice, compression, elevation) the injury. Get professional treatment if any injury is severe. A severe injury means having an obvious fracture or dislocation of a joint, prolonged swelling, or prolonged or severe pain.

Keep Kids Exercising

It's important to continue some type of regular exercise and sports involvement after the injury heals. Exercise may reduce chances of obesity, which is becoming more common in children. It may also reduce risk of diabetes, a disease that can be associated with a lack of exercise and poor eating habits. Exercise also helps build social skills and provides a general sense of well-being. Sports participation is an important part of learning how to build team skills.

You should be mindful of the risks associated with different sports and take important measures to reduce the chance of injury. For sport-specific suggestions, see the following information.

Sport-Specific Safety Information

Here are some winning ways to help prevent an injury from occurring.

Basketball

- **Common Injuries And Locations:** Sprains; strains; bruises; fractures; scrapes; dislocations; cuts; injuries to teeth, ankles and knees. (Injury rates are higher in girls, especially for the anterior cruciate ligament (ACL), the wide ligament that limits rotation and forward movement of the shin bone.)

- **Safest Playing With:** Eye protection, elbow and knee pads, mouth guard, athletic supporters for males, proper shoes, water. If playing outdoors, wear sunscreen and, when possible, a hat.

- **Injury Prevention:** Strength training (particularly knees and shoulders), aerobics (exercises that develop the strength and endurance of heart and lungs), warm-up exercises, proper coaching, and use of safety equipment.

Track And Field

- **Common Injuries:** Strains, sprains, scrapes from falls.
- **Safest Playing With:** Proper shoes, athletic supporters for males, sunscreen, water.
- **Injury Prevention:** Proper conditioning and coaching.

Football

- **Common Injuries And Locations:** Bruises; sprains; strains; pulled muscles; tears to soft tissues such as ligaments; broken bones; internal injures (bruised or damaged organs); concussions; back injuries; sunburn. Knees and ankles are the most common injury sites.
- **Safest Playing With:** Helmet; mouth guard; shoulder pads; athletic supporters for males; chest/rib pads; forearm, elbow, and thigh pads; shin guards; proper shoes; sunscreen; water.
- **Injury Prevention:** Proper use of safety equipment, warm-up exercises, proper coaching techniques and conditioning.

Baseball And Softball

- **Common Injuries:** Soft tissue strains; impact injuries that include fractures caused by sliding and being hit by a ball; sunburn.
- **Safest Playing With:** Batting helmet; shin guards; elbow guards; athletic supporters for males; mouth guard; sunscreen; cleats; hat; detachable, "breakaway bases" rather than traditional, stationary ones.
- **Injury Prevention:** Proper conditioning and warm-ups.

Soccer

- **Common Injuries:** Bruises, cuts and scrapes, headaches, sunburn.
- **Safest Playing With:** Shin guards, athletic supporters for males, cleats, sunscreen, water.
- **Injury Prevention:** Aerobic conditioning and warm-ups, and proper training in "heading" (that is, using the head to strike or make a play with the ball).

Gymnastics

- **Common Injuries:** Sprains and strains of soft tissues.

- **Safest Playing With:** Athletic supporters for males, safety harness, joint supports (such as neoprene wraps), water.

- **Injury Prevention:** Proper conditioning and warm-ups.

Treat Injuries With "RICE"

Rest: Reduce or stop using the injured area for at least 48 hours. If you have a leg injury, you may need to stay off of it completely.

Ice: Put an ice pack on the injured area for 20 minutes at a time, four to eight times per day. Use a cold pack, ice bag, or a plastic bag filled with crushed ice that has been wrapped in a towel.

Compression: Ask your doctor about elastics wraps, air casts, special boots, or splints that can be used to compress an injured ankle, knee, or wrist to reduce swelling.

Elevation: Keep the injured area elevated above the level of the heart to help decrease swelling. Use a pillow to help elevate an injured limb.

Play It Safe In The Heat

- Schedule regular fluid breaks during practice and games. Kids need to drink 8 ounces of fluid—preferably water—every 20 minutes, and more after playing.

- Wear light-colored, "breathable" clothing.

- Make player substitutions more frequently in the heat.

- Use misting sprays on the body to keep cool.

- Know the signs of heat-related problems, including confusion; dilated pupils; dizziness; fainting; headache; heavy perspiration; nausea; pale and moist or hot, dry skin; weak pulse; and weakness. If you experience any combination of these symptoms or don't feel quite right, seek medical attention immediately.

This list adapted with permission from *Patient Care* magazine, copyrighted by Medical Economics.

Safety Tips For All Sports

- Be in proper physical condition to play the sport.

- Follow the rules of the sport.

- Wear appropriate protective gear (for example, shin guards for soccer, a hard-shell helmet when facing a baseball or softball pitcher, a helmet and body padding for ice hockey).

- Know how to use athletic equipment.

- Always warm up before playing.

- Avoid playing when very tired or in pain.

- Get a preseason physical examination.

- Make sure adequate water or other liquids are available to maintain proper hydration.

This list adapted from *Play It Safe, a Guide to Safety for Young Athletes*, with permission of the American Academy of Orthopaedic Surgeons.

Chapter 53

Exercising While Recovering From An Injury

A strained muscle, sprained ankle, or foot injury can make even the most motivated exerciser feel discouraged when it comes to working out.

But being injured doesn't necessarily mean you can't exercise, says Colleen Greene, wellness coordinator with MFit, the University of Michigan Health System's health promotion division. By speaking with an expert and finding a plan that will work as you heal, you can still hit the gym while recovering.

"Exercise can definitely be beneficial for a person dealing with an injury. Depending on its type, the injured area should be moved and not left in place for a long period of time," explains Greene. "Some people think they should just rest and not move at all with an injury. Doing that can actually be worse because—depending on the amount of time one does not move the appendage—the muscle might begin to atrophy."

Greene notes that the general rule of thumb when initially handling an injury is to follow RICE—rest, ice, compression, and elevation. Once you have done this, consult a doctor to look at the injury as soon as possible. You may be referred to a physical therapist or specialist trainer if the injury is severe enough. These professionals can provide guidance for your recovery, as well as give you tips on how to maintain strength while recovering.

Greene also notes that there are "dos and don'ts" when it comes to specific injuries. Because each condition is unique, there are certain things a person can do and other activities the injured person should avoid while healing. She offers these tips on three common injuries:

General Advice For Any Injury: See a physician or physical therapist to learn what exercises are possible with your type of injury. Focus on the goal of maintaining strength, not gaining it, while you are recovering. And always be wary of pain as you explore different workouts.

"Pain is always the indicator; discomfort is OK, but pain tells you when you should stop what you are doing and do something else," Greene says. "You always want to keep in mind that you should be doing something that doesn't re-injure or further injure yourself."

Sprained Ankle: When seeking out cardiovascular exercises, Greene suggests sticking with low-impact workouts, such as swimming or riding a stationary bike. She notes that running or aerobics are generally activities that are too high in impact. A person with a sprained ankle can also do upper-body or core impact exercises for strength training.

Plantar Fasciitis: Plantar fasciitis is an overuse injury normally caused by a lack of cross training. For example, a person may develop plantar fasciitis by only running when training for a marathon, but not preparing through other exercises, such as swimming or biking. Greene notes that people dealing with this type of injury need to focus on resting in order to heal, but it is possible to explore low-impact core and upper-body exercises while recovering.

"There are not a lot of ways other than physical therapy to recover from plantar fasciitis except for resting," she says. "You want to do things that are low impact without a lot of pressure on the area."

Grab an ice pack, get some rest and allow your injury to fully recover before trying to get stronger.

Strained And Pulled Muscle: "The first thing a person with a pulled or strained muscle should know is that they, like everyone, should warm up thoroughly before doing anything," Greene notes.

She also says that people with this type of injury should stay in a pain-free range by focusing on conditioning the side of the body opposite of the strained or torn muscle. If you have pulled a hamstring, for example, then aim to work on your upper-body.

Greene also notes that there are preventative measures that a person can take to avoid pulling or training a muscle. First, Greene recommends a good warm-up for five to 10 minutes. Second, be sure to cool down at the end of your workout. And don't forget to stretch.

"We find that as people age, they can actually pull muscles by doing everyday things such as bending over to grab a bag of groceries or leaning over to put something on a shelf," she explains. "So the preventative measures that can be taken to avoid pulling or tearing a muscle with exercise are also measures that should be taken to avoid tearing or pulling a muscle in everyday life, not just on a basketball court."

Overall, Greene believes the most important thing injured exercisers can do when hitting the gym is to pay attention to their body. She also advises to stop immediately if a workout becomes painful.

"One of the basic exercise myths is 'no pain, no gain.' We used to think that a long time ago," says Greene. "If you are actually in pain, you should stop immediately. Now we say, 'no discomfort, no gain.' There is a big difference."

Chapter 54

Exercise Suggestions For People With Asthma

Exercise And Asthma

Many people with asthma believe exercise is not an option for them, that it will do more harm than good. The truth is that most asthmatics would likely benefit from some form of regular physical activity.

The ABCs Of Asthma

Twelve percent to 15 percent of the population are considered asthmatics and suffer recurrent attacks of breathlessness. The severity of an asthma attack can vary greatly, from slight breathlessness to respiratory failure. Common symptoms include wheezing, a dry cough, and tightness in the chest.

Attacks may be brought on by an allergic response, a respiratory infection, tobacco smoke, air pollutants, anxiety, or stress. Exercise induced asthma (EIA) is usually brought on by vigorous aerobic activity.

Exercising With Asthma

Despite the fact that asthma may be brought on by aerobic activity, exercise may still be a desirable option for many asthmatics. Research indicates that as tolerance for physical exertion is built up over time, it is less likely that an asthmatic will experience an attack during exercise. And, in addition to reducing the risk of developing many other diseases, appropriate exercise can help asthmatics reduce stress, sleep better, and feel more energized.

About This Chapter: This chapter begins with "Exercise and Asthma," American Council on Exercise (ACE) Fit Facts®. Copyright © 2009 American Council on Exercise. All rights reserved. Reprinted by permission. Fit Facts is a registered trademark of the American Council on Exercise. Additional information from A.D.A.M, Inc. about exercise-induced asthma is cited separately within the chapter.

It might surprise you to know that even world-class athletes, such as Olympic gold medalist Jackie Joyner-Kersee, continue to compete after being diagnosed with asthma.

Have a thorough medical evaluation and obtain your doctor's permission before beginning any type of exercise program. This is an absolutely essential first step. Your physician may prescribe medications that might further aid in controlling your condition. You will need specific instructions on when to take the medication before exercising and how long the effects will last.

Once you have received clearance from your doctor to begin an exercise program, consider the following guidelines:

Take extra time to warm up before exercising. A prolonged period of low-level aerobic activity will help prepare your body for higher-intensity exercise.

Exercise toward the lower end of your target heart rate. Exercises such as walking or swimming are great for asthmatics because they are low intensity and may be done for longer periods of time. Those who wish to participate in higher-intensity exercise, such as running or fast-paced sports, should slowly increase intensity over time.

Rest when necessary and listen to what your body is telling you. Strength-training exercises are unlikely to cause an asthma attack if you rest between sets.

Avoid exercising in polluted environments, or in cold or dry air.

Don't rush through your cool down; extending it can help prevent the asthma attacks that occur immediately following an exercise session. A warm bath or shower may also help.

Keep Your Options Open

Asthma does not necessarily mean you have to live an inactive life. Regular physical activity is one of the best things you can do for both your health and your overall well-being. As long as you and your physician are comfortable with your level of activity, nothing should keep you from doing the activities that keep you happy and healthy.

These exercises are listed in order from most to least likely to induce an asthma attack:

- Outdoor running
- Treadmill running
- Cycling
- Walking
- Pool swimming

Exercise-Induced Asthma

© 2012 A.D.A.M., Inc. Reprinted with permission.

Sometimes exercise triggers asthma symptoms. This is called exercise-induced asthma (EIA).

The symptoms of EIA are coughing, wheezing, a feeling of tightness in your chest, or shortness of breath. Most times, these symptoms start soon after you stop exercising. But, some people may have symptoms after they start exercising.

Having asthma symptoms when you exercise does not mean you cannot or should not exercise. The tips below may keep you from getting EIA.

Be Careful Where And When You Exercise

Cold or dry air may trigger your asthma symptoms. If you do exercise in cold or dry air:

- Breathe through your nose.
- Wear a scarf or mask over your mouth.

Do not exercise when the air is dirty or polluted. Do not exercise near fields or lawns that have just been mowed. Warm up before you exercise, and cool down after you exercise.

- To warm up, walk or do your exercise activity slowly before you speed up.
- The longer you warm up, the better.
- To cool down, walk or do your exercise activity slowly for several minutes.

Some kinds of exercise may trigger your asthma less than others.

- Swimming is a good sport for people with EIA. The warm, moist air helps keep asthma symptoms away.
- Football, baseball, and other sports with periods when you do not move fast are less likely to trigger your asthma symptoms.

Activities that keep you moving fast all the time are more likely to trigger asthma symptoms. Some of these are running, basketball, and soccer.

Use Your Asthma Drugs Before Exercise

Take your short-acting inhaled beta-agonists before you exercise. These are called quick-relief drugs.

- Take them 10 to 15 minutes before exercise.

- They can help for up to four hours.

Long-acting inhaled beta-agonists may also help.

- Use them at least 30 minutes before exercise.

- They can help for up to 12 hours. Children can take this medicine before school, and it will help for the whole day.

- But, using this medicine every day before exercise will make it less effective over time.

Inhaled cromolyn can also be used before exercise. But, most times, it is not as effective as other medicines.

References

National Asthma Education and Prevention Program Expert Panel Report 3: *Guidelines for the Diagnosis and Management of Asthma*. Rockville, MD. National Heart, Lung, and Blood Institute, US Dept of Health and Human Services; 2007. NIH publications 08-4051.

Szefler SJ. Advances in pediatric asthma in 2009: gaining control of childhood asthma. *J Allergy Clin Immunol.* 2010 Jan;125(1):69-78.

Chapter 55

Exercise Suggestions For People With Diabetes

How can I take care of my diabetes?

Diabetes means your blood glucose, also called blood sugar, is too high. Your body uses glucose for energy. But having too much glucose in your blood can hurt you.

When you take care of your diabetes, you'll feel better. You'll reduce your risk for problems with your kidneys, eyes, nerves, feet and legs, and teeth. You'll also lower your risk for a heart attack or a stroke. You can take care of your diabetes by being physically active, following a healthy meal plan, and taking medicines, if prescribed by your doctor.

What can a physically active lifestyle do for me?

- Lower your blood glucose and your blood pressure
- Lower your bad cholesterol and raise your good cholesterol
- Improve your body's ability to use insulin
- Lower your risk for heart disease and stroke
- Keep your heart and bones strong
- Keep your joints flexible
- Lower your risk of falling

About This Chapter: From "What I Need to Know about Physical Activity and Diabetes," National Institute of Diabetes and Digestive and Kidney Diseases (http://www.niddk.nih.gov), March 2008.

- Help you lose weight

- Reduce your body fat

- Give you more energy

- Reduce your stress levels

Physical activity also plays an important part in preventing type 2 diabetes. A major government study, the Diabetes Prevention Program (DPP), showed that modest weight loss of 5 to 7 percent—for example, 10 to 15 pounds for a 200-pound person—can delay and possibly prevent type 2 diabetes. People in the study used diet and exercise to lose weight.

What kinds of physical activity can help me?

Four kinds of activity can help. You can be extra active every day, do aerobic exercise, do strength training, and stretch.

Be Extra Active Every Day

Being extra active can increase the number of calories you burn. Try these ways to be extra active, or think of other things you can do.

- Walk around while you talk on the phone.

- Play outside

- Take the dog for a walk.

- Get up to change the TV channel instead of using the remote control.

- Work in the garden or rake leaves.

- Clean the house.

- Wash the car.

- Stretch out your chores. For example, make two trips to take the laundry downstairs instead of one.

- Park at the far end of the shopping center parking lot and walk to the store.

- At the grocery store, walk down every aisle.

- Take the stairs instead of the elevator.

- Other things I can do: _____

Do Aerobic Exercise

Aerobic exercise is activity that requires the use of large muscles and makes your heart beat faster. You will also breathe harder during aerobic exercise. Doing aerobic exercise for 30 minutes a day at least five days a week provides many benefits. You can even split up those 30 minutes into several parts. For example, you can take three brisk 10-minute walks, one after each meal.

If you haven't exercised lately, see your doctor first to make sure it's OK for you to increase your level of physical activity. Talk with your doctor about how to warm up and stretch before you exercise and how to cool down after you exercise. Then start slowly with five to ten minutes a day. Add a little more time each week, aiming for at least 150 minutes per week. Here are some things you can try:

- Walking briskly
- Hiking
- Climbing stairs
- Swimming or taking a water-aerobics class
- Dancing
- Riding a bicycle outdoors or a stationary bicycle indoors
- Taking an aerobics class
- Playing basketball, volleyball, or other sports
- In-line skating, ice skating, or skate boarding
- Playing tennis
- Cross-country skiing

Do Strength Training

Doing exercises with hand weights, elastic bands, or weight machines three times a week builds muscle. When you have more muscle and less fat, you'll burn more calories because muscle burns more calories than fat, even between exercise sessions. Strength training can help make daily chores easier, improving your balance and coordination, as well as your bones' health. You can do strength training at home, at a fitness center, or in a class. Your health care team can tell you more about strength training and what kind is best for you.

Stretch

Stretching increases your flexibility, lowers stress, and helps prevent muscle soreness after other types of exercise. Your health care team can tell you what kind of stretching is best for you.

Can I exercise any time I want?

Your health care team can help you decide the best time of day for you to exercise. Together, you and your team will consider your daily schedule, your meal plan, and your diabetes medicines.

If you have type 1 diabetes, avoid strenuous exercise when you have ketones in your blood or urine. Ketones are chemicals your body might make when your blood glucose level is too high and your insulin level is too low. Too many ketones can make you sick. If you exercise when you have ketones in your blood or urine, your blood glucose level may go even higher.

If you have type 2 diabetes and your blood glucose is high but you don't have ketones, light or moderate exercise will probably lower your blood glucose. Ask your health care team whether you should exercise when your blood glucose is high.

Are there any types of physical activity I shouldn't do?

If you have diabetes complications, some kinds of exercise can make your problems worse. For example, activities that increase the pressure in the blood vessels of your eyes, such as lifting heavy weights, can make diabetic eye problems worse. If nerve damage from diabetes has made your feet numb, your doctor may suggest that you try swimming instead of walking for aerobic exercise.

When you have numb feet, you might not feel pain in your feet. Sores or blisters might get worse because you don't notice them. Without proper care, minor foot problems can turn into serious conditions, sometimes leading to amputation. Make sure you exercise in cotton socks and comfortable, well-fitting shoes designed for the activity you are doing. After you exercise, check your feet for cuts, sores, bumps, or redness. Call your doctor if any foot problems develop.

Can physical activity cause low blood glucose?

Physical activity can cause low blood glucose, also called hypoglycemia, in people who take insulin or certain types of diabetes medicines. Ask your health care team whether your diabetes medicines can cause low blood glucose.

Low blood glucose can happen while you exercise, right afterward, or even up to a day later. It can make you feel shaky, weak, confused, grumpy, hungry, or tired. You may sweat a lot or get a headache. If your blood glucose drops too low, you could pass out or have a seizure.

However, you should still be physically active. These steps can help you be prepared for low blood glucose:

Before Exercise

- Ask your health care team whether you should check your blood glucose level before exercising.
- If you take diabetes medicines that can cause low blood glucose, ask your health care team whether you should change the amount you take before you exercise or have a snack if your blood glucose level is below 100.

During Exercise

- Wear your medical identification (ID) bracelet or necklace or carry your ID in your pocket.
- Always carry food or glucose tablets so you'll be ready to treat low blood glucose.
- If you'll be exercising for more than an hour, check your blood glucose at regular intervals. You may need snacks before you finish.

After Exercise

- Check to see how exercise affected your blood glucose level.

Treating Low Blood Glucose

If your blood glucose is below 70, have one of the following right away:

- 3 or 4 glucose tablets
- 1 serving of glucose gel—the amount equal to 15 grams of carbohydrate
- 1/2 cup (4 ounces) of any fruit juice
- 1/2 cup (4 ounces) of a regular—not diet—soft drink
- 1 cup (8 ounces) of milk
- 5 or 6 pieces of hard candy
- 1 tablespoon of sugar or honey

After 15 minutes, check your blood glucose again. If it's still too low, have another serving. Repeat until your blood glucose is 70 or higher. If it will be an hour or more before your next meal, have a snack as well.

What should I do before I start a physical activity program?

Check with your doctor. Always talk with your doctor before you start a new physical activity program. Ask about your medicines—prescription and over-the counter—and whether you should change the amount you take before you exercise. If you have heart disease, kidney disease, eye problems, or foot problems, ask which types of physical activity are safe for you.

Decide exactly what you'll do and set some goals. Choose the type of physical activity you want to do. Be sure you have the clothes and items you'll need to get ready. Select the days and times you'll add activity and the length of each session. Develop a plan for warming up, stretching, and cooling down for each session. Be sure to have a backup plan if the weather is bad (such as where you'll walk). Know how you will measure of your progress.

Find an exercise buddy. Many people find they are more likely to do something active if a friend joins them. If you and a friend plan to walk together, for example, you may be more likely to do it.

Keep track of your physical activity. Write down when you exercise and for how long in your blood glucose record book. You'll be able to track your progress and see how physical activity affects your blood glucose.

Decide how you'll reward yourself. Do something nice for yourself when you reach your activity goals. For example, treat yourself to a movie or buy a new plant for the garden.

What can I do to make sure I stay active?

One of the keys to staying on track is finding some activities you like to do. If you keep finding excuses not to exercise, think about why. Are your goals realistic? Do you need a change in activity? Would another time be more convenient? Keep trying until you find a routine that works for you. Once you make physical activity a habit, you'll wonder how you lived without it.

Chapter 56

Exercise Suggestions For People With Physical Disabilities

No Limits—Exercising With A Disability

You've heard that everyone should be exercising, but what if you have a disability? It's hard enough taking care of the basics if you're in a wheelchair or have other physical disabilities, much less exercise. However, exercise is even more important for people with disabilities. It keeps your body strength, gives you energy, improves stress, and can help reduce fatigue. The key is to find the right kind of exercise for your situation.

Wheelchair Users

Generally, wheelchair users can focus on resistance exercises to improve your upper body strength and help reduce your chances of injury. You should always talk to your doctor or physical therapist to get clearance and guidance for your best options. One place to start is with videos (check out Collage Video [http://www.collagevideo.com] for ideas) you can do at home or workouts, such as this Seated Strength Workout (http://exercise.about.com/cs/exerciseworkouts/l/blobeseexercise.htm) or this Seated Upper Body Workout (http://exercise.about.com/library/blseatedupperbody.htm).

If you're interested in doing more, you might want to think about investing in some specialized exercise equipment. There are many new strength training machines available for people in wheelchairs, as well as hand-cyclers and other cardio equipment. But, don't let a lack of special equipment keep you from your work out. If you have upper body mobility, try lifting

About This Chapter: This chapter begins with "No Limits—Exercising With A Disability," © 2012 About.com. Used with permission of About, Inc. which can be found online at www.About.com. All rights reserved. Text under the heading "Sports and Recreation for Teens with Illnesses or Disabilities," is from "Sports and Recreation: Illness and Disability," produced by the Office on Women's Health (www.girlshealth.gov), February 2011.

your arms straight out in front of you, hold for a few seconds then lower. Next, lift your arms out to the sides (stopping at shoulder level), hold, then lower. Do both of these exercise 15 to 20 times and, as you get stronger, hold light hand weights. More specific upper body activities include shoulder shrugs, overhead presses, and bicep curls.

If you're competitive, another option is to try organized sports. Wheelchair Sports (http://www.wsusa.org) can help you find events near you that include basketball, archery, fencing, and more. If you need help with training for a specific sport or event, the National Center on Physical Activity and Disability (NCPAD; http://www.ncpad.org/) can help you find fitness programs in your area.

Stretching and flexibility is important too for reducing the chance of injury. Specifically, you should be stretching all the major muscles in your upper body, including your shoulders, arms, back, and neck. Exercises for Wheelchair Users (http://www.amsvans.com/Exercises_for_Wheelchair_Users.article) offers examples of exercises and stretches you can do for your upper body and includes tips on proper form.

If you have a disability, you have to work much harder and be much more creative about exercise. Talking to your doctor, physical therapist, or other experts can help you find activities to keep your body strong and active.

Sight/Hearing Impaired

People who are sight or hearing impaired have plenty of obstacles to overcome in daily life, and that goes double when you add the element of exercise. However, with the advent of blind athletes like Marla Runyon, who ran in the 2000 Olympic games, more and more people are getting involved in sports and exercise.

The specific concerns for the sight- and hearing-impaired involve exercising safely. Like any new exerciser, your first concern should be starting slowly with cardio exercise and a weight training routine and making sure you are using proper form. One option is to join a health club and check out their personal training options. A trainer can help guide you through both the gym as well as the equipment available to you. He or she can show you how to correctly do the exercises, how to use the cardio machines safely and put you on a routine that will work for you. If you like the outdoors, consider getting involved in sports. The Association of Blind Athletes (http://www.usaba.org) and Deaf Sports Federation (http://www.usadsf.org) are good resources for the sight or hearing impaired. They offer information about organizations you can join and specific ways to work out safely and effectively. Guiding Eyes (http://www.guiding-eyes.org) is another option, if you're wondering whether a guide dog is right for you.

Living with a disability can be challenging and exercise can feel like just another burden to add to the mix. However, with a little guidance, you can be on your way to healthier and less stressful life.

Other Organizations That Offer Activities And Sports

- Adaptive Adventures (http://adaptiveadventures.org) has links to youth programs and camps around the country.
- BlazeSports (www.blazesports.org) provides training and competition for people with physical disabilities.
- Deaflympics (www.deaflympics.com)
- Disabled Sports USA (www.dsusa.org)
- Let's Move (www.letsmove.gov) offers fun tips and tools from the government.
- National Center on Physical Activity and Disability (http://www.ncpad.org)
- National Sports Center for the Disabled (www.nscd.org)
- National Wheelchair Basketball Association www.nwba.org) (Check out the Youth Sports Corner)
- The Amputee Coalition of America (www.amputee-coalition.org)
- USA Deaf Sports Federation (www.usdeafsports.org)
- U.S. Paralympics Team (www.usparalympics.org)
- United States Association of Blind Athletes (www.usaba.org)
- United States Handcycling Federation (www.ushf.org)
- Wheelchair and Ambulatory Sports USA (www.wsusa.org)

Source: Office on Women's Health, 2011; websites verified in June 2012.

Sports And Recreation For Teens With Illnesses Or Disabilities

Physical activity comes in many forms. Types of exercise include swimming laps, taking a walk, playing wheelchair basketball, or walking up the stairs. Here are some important physical activity tips:

- Before you start any physical activity program, talk to your doctor to make sure that it is okay. Your doctor will help you be active in the safest way possible.

- Make sure you stop being physically active or playing a sport if you feel pain, feel sick, feel dizzy, or are short of breath.

- Make sure to drink plenty of water before, during, and after you are physically active.

How To Find Activities And Sports

Your community probably has many places where you can take part in activities you love and even try new ones. To start, call your city's recreation department, your own school, health clubs, YMCA, YWCA, the local Girls Scout or Boy Scout council, and nearby colleges. They might have pools, sports teams, exercise rooms, and more. You can also call the local Chamber of Commerce to find out where else you can find programs in your area.

Another place to try calling is your nearby Center for Independent Living http://www .ilru.org/html/publications/directory/index.html). CILs are agencies staffed mainly by people with disabilities. They know all about resources in your community for people with disabilities.

Questions To Ask About Fitness Or Exercise Programs

- Where are you located?

- What sports teams, games, programs, or exercise equipment do you offer?

- How much does it cost?

- How can I apply for financial help if I need it?

- What are the times and dates of your programs?

- How do you register?

- Are your facilities and programs accessible to people with disabilities?

- Do you have any adaptive equipment or tools that people with disabilities can use?

- Do you have anyone on the staff who can help people with disabilities use your facilities? (These people are sometimes called "inclusion aides.")

- Do you have any programs that are just for people with disabilities?

- Can teenagers use the facility?

Tips For Playing Sports Differently To Meet Your Needs

- **Soccer:** Walk instead of run if you need to, or hold the ball in your lap if you use a wheelchair.

- **Volleyball:** Use a larger ball that is softer or brightly colored, or allow the ball to bounce on the ground before hitting it.

- **Bowling:** Use two hands instead of one, or use a ramp.

- **Tennis:** Use a racquet with a large head, or don't use a net.

For many sports, you could try using an inclusion aide. An inclusion aide is a person who helps people with disabilities participate in sports and other activities. For example, if you are interested in horseback riding but have an illness or disability that makes this hard for you to do alone, an inclusion aide would assist you.

Some Specific Fitness Options

People of all levels of ability can find sports and activities that suit them. Find out if one of these is right for you:

- Interested in dance? Check out AXIS Dance Company's program for girls with and without disabilities (http://www.axisdance.org).

- Do you love horses? Visit the North American Riding for the Handicapped Association (http://www.narha.org), which serves horseback riders with disabilities across the United States and Canada.

- Has it always been your dream to skate? If so, visit the Skating Athletes Bold at Heart website (http://www.sabahinc.org). The association teaches people who are physically, emotionally, or mentally challenged how to ice skate.

- Could you be a future Olympian? If the answer is yes, the Special Olympics can offer you an amazing experience (http://www.specialolympics.org).

- Fitness can be relaxing. Yoga for the Special Child (http://www.specialyoga.com) offers yoga for kids who have special needs such as Down syndrome, cerebral palsy, autism, attention deficit hyperactivity disorder, and learning disabilities, and other conditions.

- Want to go on hiking trails in a wheelchair? Call a national park or state park and ask if they have any paved hiking trails (http://home.nps.gov/findapark/index.htm).

Chapter 57

Compulsive Exercise: When Exercise Turns Unhealthy

Melissa has been a track fanatic since she was 12 years old. She has run the mile in meets in junior high and high school, constantly improving her times and winning several medals. Best of all, Melissa truly loves her sport.

Recently, however, Melissa's parents have noticed a change in their daughter. She used to return tired but happy from practice and relax with her family, but now she's hardly home for 15 minutes before she heads out for another run on her own. On many days, she gets up to run before school. When she's unable to squeeze in extra runs, she becomes irritable and anxious. And she no longer talks about how much fun track is, just how many miles she has to run today and how many more she should run tomorrow.

Melissa is living proof that even though exercise has many positive benefits, too much can be harmful. Teens who exercise compulsively are at risk for both physical and psychological problems.

About Compulsive Exercise

Compulsive exercise (also called obligatory exercise and anorexia athletica) is best defined by an exercise addict's frame of mind: He or she no longer chooses to exercise but feels compelled to do so and struggles with guilt and anxiety if he or she doesn't work out. Injury, illness, an outing with friends, bad weather—none of these will deter those who compulsively exercise. In a sense, exercising takes over a compulsive exerciser's life because he or she plans life around it.

About This Chapter: "Compulsive Exercise," October 2010, reprinted with permission from www.kidshealth .org. This information was provided by KidsHealth®, one of the largest resources online for medically reviewed health information written for parents, kids, and teens. For more articles like this, visit www.KidsHealth.org or www.TeensHealth.org. Copyright © 1995-2012 The Nemours Foundation. All rights reserved. Although this chapter addresses parents, teens will still find it informative.

Of course, it's nearly impossible to draw a clear line dividing a healthy amount of exercise from too much. The government's 2005 dietary guidelines, published by the U.S. Department of Agriculture (USDA) and the U.S. Department of Health and Human Services (HHS), recommend at least 60 minutes of physical activity for kids and teens on most—if not all—days of the week.

Experts say that repeatedly exercising beyond the requirements for good health is an indicator of compulsive behavior, but because different amounts of exercise are appropriate for different people, this definition covers a range of activity levels. However, several workouts a day, every day, is overdoing it for almost anyone.

Much like with eating disorders, many people who engage in compulsive exercise do so to feel more in control of their lives, and the majority of them are female. They often define their self-worth through their athletic performance and try to deal with emotions like anger or depression by pushing their bodies to the limit. In sticking to a rigorous workout schedule, they seek a sense of power to help them cope with low self-esteem.

Although compulsive exercising doesn't have to accompany an eating disorder, the two often go hand in hand. In anorexia nervosa, the excessive workouts usually begin as a means to control weight and become more and more extreme. As the rate of activity increases, the amount the person eats might decrease. Someone with bulimia also may use exercise as a way to compensate for binge eating.

Compulsive exercise behavior can grow out of student athletes' demanding practice schedules and their quest to excel. Pressure, both external (from coaches, peers, or parents) and internal, can drive an athlete to go too far to be the best. He or she ends up believing that just one more workout will make the difference between first and second place . . . then keeps adding more workouts.

Eventually, compulsive exercising can breed other compulsive behavior, from strict dieting to obsessive thoughts about perceived flaws. Exercise addicts may keep detailed journals about their exercise schedules and obsess about improving themselves. Unfortunately, these behaviors often compound each other, trapping the person in a downward spiral of negative thinking and low self-esteem.

Why Is Exercising Too Much A Bad Thing?

We all know that regular exercise is an important part of a healthy lifestyle. But few people realize that too much can cause physical and psychological harm:

- Excessive exercise can damage tendons, ligaments, bones, cartilage, and joints, and when minor injuries aren't allowed to heal, they often result in long-term damage. Instead of building muscle, too much exercise actually destroys muscle mass, especially if the body isn't getting enough nutrition, forcing it to break down muscle for energy.

- Girls who exercise compulsively may disrupt the balance of hormones in their bodies. This can change their menstrual cycles (some girls lose their periods altogether, a condition known as amenorrhea) and increase the risk of premature bone loss (osteoporosis). And of course, working their bodies so hard leads to exhaustion and constant fatigue.

- An even more serious risk is the stress that excessive exercise can place on the heart, particularly when someone is also engaging in unhealthy weight loss behaviors such as restricting intake, vomiting, and using diet pills or supplements. In extreme cases, the combination of anorexia and compulsive exercise can be fatal.

- Psychologically, exercise addicts are often plagued by anxiety and depression. They may have a negative image of themselves and feel worthless. Their social and academic lives may suffer as they withdraw from friends and family to fixate on exercise. Even if they want to succeed in school or in relationships, working out always comes first, so they end up skipping homework or missing out on time spent with friends.

Warning Signs

Someone may be exercising compulsively if he or she:

- won't skip a workout, even if tired, sick, or injured
- doesn't enjoy exercise sessions, but feels obligated to do them
- seems anxious or guilty when missing even one workout
- does miss one workout and exercises twice as long the next time
- is constantly preoccupied with his or her weight and exercise routine
- doesn't like to sit still or relax because of worry that not enough calories are being burnt
- has lost a significant amount of weight
- exercises more after eating more
- skips seeing friends, gives up activities, and abandons responsibilities to make more time for exercise
- seems to base self-worth on the number of workouts completed and the effort put into training

- is never satisfied with his or her own physical achievements

It's important, too, to recognize the types of athletes who are more prone to compulsive exercise because their sports place a particular emphasis on being thin. Ice skaters, gymnasts, wrestlers, and dancers can feel even more pressure than most athletes to keep their weight down and their body toned. Runners also frequently fall into a cycle of obsessive workouts.

Getting Professional Help

If you recognize two or more warning signs of compulsive exercise in your child, call your doctor to discuss your concerns. After evaluating your child, the doctor may recommend medical treatment and/or other therapy.

Because compulsive exercise is so often linked to an eating disorder, a community agency that focuses on treating these disorders might be able to offer advice or referrals. Extreme cases may require hospitalization to get a child's weight back up to a safe range.

Treating a compulsion to exercise is never a quick-fix process—it may take several months or even years. But with time and effort, kids can get back on the road to good health. Therapy can help improve self-esteem and body image, as well as teach them how to deal with emotions. Sessions with a nutritionist can help develop healthy eating habits. Once they know what to watch out for, kids will be better equipped to steer clear of unsafe exercise and eating patterns.

Ways To Help At Home

Parents can do a lot to help a child overcome a compulsion to exercise:

- Involve kids in preparing nutritious meals.

- Combine activity and fun by going for a hike or a bike ride together as a family.

- Be a good body-image role model. In other words, don't fixate on your own physical flaws, as that just teaches kids that it's normal to dislike what they see in the mirror.

- Never criticize another family member's weight or body shape, even if you're just kidding around. Such remarks might seem harmless, but they can leave a lasting impression on kids or teens struggling to define and accept themselves.

- Examine whether you're putting too much pressure on your kids to excel, particularly in a sport (because some teens turn to exercise to cope with pressure). Take a look at where kids might be feeling too much pressure. Help them put it in perspective and find other ways to cope.

Most important, just be there with constant support. Point out all of your child's great qualities that have nothing to do with working out—small daily doses of encouragement and praise can help improve self-esteem.

If you teach kids to be proud of the challenges they've faced and not just the first-place ribbons they've won, they will likely be much happier and healthier kids now and in the long run.

Chapter 58

Female Athlete Triad: Three Symptoms That Mean Trouble

Female Athlete Triad

The female athlete triad is a syndrome that consists of three related conditions:

- Disordered eating habits

- Irregular or absent menstrual periods

- Osteopenia (thinning of the bones)

This syndrome occurs most commonly in sports where a lean physique is thought to provide a competitive advantage, such as cross-country running, gymnastics, figure skating, and dance. However, any female athlete with unhealthy eating habits is at risk for female athlete triad.

How It Occurs

All athletes need a constant source of energy to perform at their best. This energy is provided by the calories found in the food they eat. When an athlete is training very hard (burning energy) and not eating enough calories, the body does not have enough energy to support normal body functions like the menstrual cycle. When menstrual cycles are disrupted, estrogen levels fall. Estrogen plays a key role in building bone density. Without sufficient estrogen, the body cannot absorb calcium from food. This causes the bones to become thin and susceptible to fractures.

About This Chapter: "Female Athletic Triad," reprinted with permission from Ann & Robert H. Lurie Children's Hospital of Chicago (www.luriechildrens.org). © 2012. All rights reserved. Although this chapter addresses parents, teens will still find it informative.

Signs And Symptoms

Your child may exhibit changes in her eating behaviors, such as restricting food intake, fasting, or eliminating entire food groups, such as dairy products or meat. She may also try to lose weight by inducing vomiting or using laxatives, water pills, or diet pills. She may insist on exercising beyond what is required by her team. She may lose weight, develop irregular menstrual cycles, or still not have had her first menstrual period well beyond the age when most of her peers have started having periods. She may complain of feeling cold, lightheaded, or fatigued. She may have noticed a decrease in her athletic performance or inability to complete her usual workouts. She may have developed one or more stress fractures.

Diagnosis

Your doctor will gather information about your child's eating habits, menstrual cycles, and attitude about her weight and body image. He/she will also take a family history and measure your child height and weight to determine if her body mass index (BMI) is abnormally low (less than the 5th percentile for her age). Blood tests may be ordered to look for other causes of menstrual cycle dysfunction. If there is a history of stress fractures, your doctor may recommend a bone density test that assesses the level of calcium in your child's bones.

Treatment

The most effective treatment for the female athlete triad involves a team approach where your child and family will have regular meetings with your doctor, a nutritionist, and a clinical psychologist. Your doctor will monitor the medical status of your child. A nutritionist creates a plan with your child for healthy eating behaviors and a diet with an appropriate amount of calories to maintain normal body functions as well as exercise. A psychologist is helpful for athletes who are struggling with stressful circumstances in their lives or are feeling pressure to succeed, both of which may cause athletes to adopt disordered eating patterns in an attempt to relieve stress and maintain control. Your family can continue to offer a supportive environment for your child, encouraging her to use healthy eating behaviors and safe training practices to achieve her athletic goals.

Returning To Activity And Sports

The goal is to return your child to her sport as quickly and safely as possible.

In mild cases, your child may be able to continue practicing and competing during treatment. Exercise duration and frequency, along with calorie intake should be closely monitored.

In more serious cases, your child may not be returned to sport until she has demonstrated that she can sustain healthy eating behaviors and consistently take in an adequate number of calories to maintain normal menstrual function.

Potential Long-Term Effects Of The Female Athlete Triad

If left untreated, female athlete triad can have detrimental effects on the athlete's health. Serious medical complications may occur. Osteopenia can lead to recurrent stress fractures that may cause chronic pain if they do not heal properly. Persistent low weight and absent menstrual cycles may lead to problems with fertility later in life. Eating habits such as induced vomiting, use of laxatives, diet pills or water pills may lead to alterations in the body's chemistry that are life threatening and require hospitalization to safely correct.

Preventing The Female Athlete Triad

Educating athletes, parents, and coaches about the signs, symptoms, and negative health consequences of the female athlete triad is the most important step in prevention. Taking your child to her doctor for regular check-ups and sports physicals is important so the doctor can discuss issues relating to diet, exercise, stress, and menstrual cycles. Loss of a previously normal menstrual cycle should not be considered a normal response to exercise. Any female athlete with irregular menstrual cycles should be evaluated by a physician. Parents and coaches should be reminded to emphasize that success in sports depends on talent, proper training, and a healthy diet with adequate calories, not on attaining a specific body weight, size, or shape.

Chapter 59

Steroids And Other Performance Enhancers Are Risky

Anabolic Steroids

The Brain's Response To Anabolic Steroids

Anabolic steroids are artificial versions of a hormone that's in all of us—testosterone. (That's right, testosterone is in girls as well as guys.) Testosterone not only brings out male sexual traits, it also causes muscles to grow.

Some people take anabolic steroid pills or injections to try to build muscle faster. ("Anabolic" means growing or building.) But these steroids also have other effects. They can cause changes in the brain and body that increase risks for illness and they may affect moods.

Scientists are still learning about how anabolic steroids affect the brain, and in turn, behavior. Research has shown that anabolic steroids may trigger aggressive behavior in some people. This means that someone who abuses anabolic steroids may act mean to people they're normally nice to, like friends and family, and they may even start fights. Some outbursts can be so severe they have become known in the media as "roid rages." And when a steroid abuser stops using the drugs, they can become depressed, even suicidal. Researchers think that some of the changes in behavior may be caused by hormonal changes that are caused by steroids, but there is still a lot that is not known.

About This Chapter: This chapter begins with excerpts from "Mind Over Matter: Anabolic Steroids," National Institute on Drug Abuse (www.nida.nih.gov), 2009. It continues with "Warning on Body Building Products Marketed as Containing Steroids or Steroid-Like Substances," U.S. Food and Drug Administration (www.fda.gov), 2011.

Do anabolic steroids really make the body stronger?

You may have heard that some athletes use anabolic steroids to gain size and strength. Maybe you've even seen an anabolic steroid user develop bigger muscles over time.

But while anabolic steroids can make some people look stronger on the outside, they may create weaknesses on the inside. For example, anabolic steroids are bad for the heart—they can increase fat deposits in blood vessels, which can cause heart attacks and strokes. They may also damage the liver. Steroids can halt bone growth—which means that a teenage steroid user may not grow to his/her full adult height.

Source: National Institute on Drug Abuse, 2009.

Anabolic Steroids Can Confuse The Brain And Body

Your body's testosterone production is controlled by a group of nerve cells at the base of the brain, called the hypothalamus. The hypothalamus also does a lot of other things. It helps control appetite, blood pressure, moods, and reproductive ability.

Anabolic steroids can change the messages the hypothalamus sends to the body. This can disrupt normal hormone function.

In guys, anabolic steroids can interfere with the normal production of testosterone. They can also act directly on the testes and cause them to shrink. This can result in a lower sperm count. They can also cause an irreversible loss of scalp hair.

In girls, anabolic steroids can cause a loss of the monthly period by acting on both the hypothalamus and reproductive organs. They can also cause loss of scalp hair, growth of body and facial hair, and deepening of the voice. These changes can also be irreversible.

Anabolic Steroids In Medicine

Doctors never prescribe anabolic steroids for building muscle in young, healthy people. (Try push-ups instead!) But doctors sometimes prescribe anabolic steroids to treat some types of anemia or disorders in men that prevent the normal production of testosterone.

You may have heard that doctors sometimes prescribe steroids to reduce swelling. This is true, but these aren't anabolic steroids. They're corticosteroids. Since corticosteroids don't build muscles the way that anabolic steroids do, people don't abuse them.

Warning On Body Building Products Marketed As Containing Steroids Or Steroid-Like Substances

The U.S. Food and Drug Administration (FDA) issued a public health advisory warning consumers to stop using any body building products that are represented to contain steroids or steroid-like substances. Many of these products are marketed as dietary supplements. Although these products are marketed as dietary supplements, they are NOT dietary supplements, but instead are unapproved and misbranded drugs.

What types of products are affected by this public health advisory?

FDA is warning consumers about products that are being marketed for body building and that claim to contain steroids or steroid-like substances. These products are sold online and in retail stores and are promoted as hormone products and/or as alternatives to anabolic steroids for increasing muscle mass and strength. Many of these products are labeled as dietary supplements and make claims about the ability of the active ingredients to enhance or diminish androgen, estrogen, or progestin-like effects in the body. Consumers should be aware that these products are potentially harmful and that FDA has not approved them nor reviewed their safety before marketing.

What are some examples of these types of products?

These body building products are often marketed as being anabolic (promoting muscle building) and/or being similar to anabolic steroids (such as testosterone). A few examples of the body building products about which FDA has safety concerns are:

- TREN-Xtreme: 19-Norandrosta-4,9-diene-3,17 dione, marketed as "similar to Trenbolone"

- MASS Xtreme: 17α-methyl-etioallocholan-2-ene-17b-ol, marketed as "similar to Methyl Testosterone"

- ESTRO Xtreme: 4-hydroxyandrostenedione (4-OHA)

- AH-89-Xtreme: 5α-androstano[3,2-c]pyrazole-3-one-17β-ol-THP-ether, marketed as "similar to Stanozolol"

- HMG Xtreme: 2α,3α-epithio-17α-methyl-17β-hydroxy-5α-etioallocholane

- MMA-3 Xtreme: Androsta-1,4-dien-3,17-dione, marketed as "similar to Boldenone (Equipoise)"

- VNS-9 Xtreme: 17α-methyl-4-chloro-androsta-1,4-diene-3β,17β-diol, marketed as "similar to Turinabol"

- TT-40-Xtreme: 1-androsterone, marketed as "very similar to 1-Testosterone" and "converts to 1-Testosterone"

What are the health risks of these types of products?

Adverse event reports received by FDA for body building products that are labeled to contain steroids or steroid alternatives involve men (ages 22–55) and include cases of serious liver injury, stroke, kidney failure, and pulmonary embolism (blockage of an artery in the lung). Acute liver injury is known to be a possible harmful effect of using anabolic steroid-containing products. In addition, anabolic steroids may cause other serious long-term adverse health consequences in men, women, and children. These include shrinkage of the testes and male infertility, masculinization of women, breast enlargement in males, short stature in children, adverse effects on blood lipid levels, and increased risk of heart attack and stroke.

Why does FDA say these products are illegally marketed?

These products are NOT dietary supplements because they contain synthetic steroid or steroid-like active ingredients. These products are unapproved new drugs because they are not generally recognized as safe and effective. In fact, they are potentially harmful. In addition, the products are misbranded because the labeling is misleading and does not provide adequate directions for use.

What action is FDA taking?

FDA has issued a public health advisory to highlight the risks of products that are marketed for body building and that contain or claim to contain steroids or steroid-like substances. The agency has executed a search warrant and issued a warning letter to American Cellular Laboratories Inc., which markets a number of these products, because the products are unapproved new drugs and are misbranded. FDA is gathering and reviewing additional data about other products that are marketed for body building and that claim to contain steroids or steroid-like substances.

What should consumers do if they have been using these products?

Due to the potential serious health risks, FDA recommends that consumers immediately stop using these products. Consumers should also consult their health care professional if they are experiencing symptoms possibly associated with these products, particularly nausea, weakness or fatigue, fever, abdominal pain, chest pain, shortness of breath, yellowing of the skin or whites of the eyes, or brown/discolored urine. FDA also recommends that consumers talk with their health care professional about body building supplements they are taking, particularly if they are uncertain about the product's ingredients.

These products are often promoted to athletes to improve sports performance and to aid in recovery from training and sporting events. FDA cautions that athletes taking these products may test positive for performance-enhancing drugs.

Part Seven
If You Need More Information

Chapter 60

The President's Challenge

The President's Challenge is the premier program of the President's Council on Fitness, Sports, and Nutrition administered through a co-sponsorship agreement with the Amateur Athletic Union. The President's Challenge helps people of all ages and abilities increase their physical activity and improve their fitness through research-based information, easy-to-use tools, and friendly motivation.

Since our founding as a fitness test for youth in the 1960s, we've grown to include these challenges:

- The Physical Fitness Test measures the physical fitness of kids and teens.

- The Adult Fitness Test measures an adult's aerobic fitness, muscular strength, flexibility, and other aspects of health-related fitness.

- The Presidential Active Lifestyle Award (PALA) challenge is for people who want to make physical activity and healthy eating part of their everyday lives.

- The Presidential Champions challenge is for people who want to be more active more often.

Over the years, we've recognized the fitness achievements of more than 50 million kids and teens, bestowed more than one million PALA and Presidential Champions awards, and helped countless people live more active, healthier lives.

About This Chapter: This chapter includes "About," "Who Can Participate," and "Choose A Challenge: Physical Fitness Test," reprinted with permission from www.presidentschallenge.org. © 2012 The President's Challenge.

Individuals

The President's Challenge isn't just for schoolkids anymore. It's for anyone who wants to track their physical activities and improve their fitness, while eating better. Maybe you want to lose a few pounds or gain muscle mass? We can help you do that. (And our BMI calculator will help put your weight in perspective.)

The bottom line is this: Couch potato or triathlete—the President's Challenge is an equal-opportunity program.

Physical Activity Is Your Friend

Think about your current level of physical activity for a minute. Which one of these challenges is right for you?

- The Presidential Active Lifestyle Award (PALA) challenge is for people who want to make physical activity and eating well part of their everyday lives. If you want to set yourself on the path to better health, try this entry-level challenge.

- The Presidential Champions challenge is for people who want to be more active more often. Try this program if you want to step your current fitness plan up a notch or two.

Sign Up Today

Go ahead—pick a program. No matter which you choose, you'll get encouragement and tips to stay active and eat well, and you can even earn awards from the President's Challenge (www.presidentschallenge.org). We want you to be active—why not create an account today?

Physical Fitness Test

Today more than ever, our students need help leading active, healthy lives. That's where educators come in. They're on the front lines of fitness, working to teach our kids the fundamentals of healthy living.

The President's Challenge wants to help. We've created the Physical Fitness Test as a tool to help educators bring out the best in their students.

Awards For Everyone

The Physical Fitness Test recognizes students for their level of physical fitness in five activities:

- Curl-ups (or partial curl-ups)

- Shuttle run

- Endurance run/walk

- Pull-ups (or right angle push-ups or flexed-arm hang)

- V-sit reach (or sit and reach)

We know that just completing all five activities is an accomplishment. To celebrate this fitness feat, we offer three awards for students, based on their scores.

Fitness File Makes Testing Easy

Educators who create an account with us gain access to the Physical Fitness Test's free official software, Fitness File.

Fitness File is one handy tool, allowing instructors to enter students' scores, keep track of tests, and generate reports of student scores and other data. With less time spent on the computer, educators can spend more time where they're needed—in the gym helping kids get fit.

Chapter 61

Resources For More Information About Fitness

Action for Healthy Kids

600 West Van Buren Street, Suite 720
Chicago, IL 60607
Toll-Free: 800-416-5136
Fax: 312-212-0098
Website:
http://www.actionforhealthykids.org

Aerobics and Fitness Association of America

15250 Ventura Boulevard, Suite 200
Sherman Oaks, CA 91403
Toll-Free: 877-YOUR-BODY
(877-968-7263)
Website: http://www.afaa.com

Amateur Athletic Union

National Headquarters
P.O. Box 22409
Lake Buena Vista, FL 32830
Toll-Free: 800-AAU-4USA
(800-228-4872)
Phone: 407-934-7200
Fax: 407-934-7242
Website: http://www.aausports.org

Amateur Endurance

Endurance Media, Inc.
P.O. Box 9799
San Diego, CA 92169
Website:
http://www.amateurendurance.com
E-mail: service@amateurendurance.com

About This Chapter: Information in this chapter was compiled from many sources deemed reliable. Inclusion does not constitute endorsement and there is no implication associated with omission. All contact information was verified in 2012.

American Alliance for Health, Physical Education, Recreation, and Dance

1900 Association Drive
Reston, VA 20191-1598
Toll-Free: 800-213-7193
Phone: 703-476-3400
Fax: 703-476-9527
Website: http://www.aahperd.org

American Athletic Institute

Website:
http://www.americanathleticinstitute.org

American College of Sports Medicine

401 West Michigan Street
Indianapolis, IN 46202-3233
Phone: 317-637-9200
Fax: 317-634-7817
Website: http://www.acsm.org

American Council on Exercise

4851 Paramount Drive
San Diego, CA 92123
Toll-Free: 888-825-3636
Phone: 858-279-8227
Fax: 858-576-6564
Website: http://www.acefitness.org
E-mail: support@acefitness.org

American Diabetes Association

Center for Information
1701 North Beauregard Street
Alexandria, VA 22311
Toll-Free: 800-DIABETES (342-2383)
Phone: 703-549-1500
Fax: 703-739-9346
Website: http://www.diabetes.org
E-mail: AskADA@diabetes.org

American Heart Association

7272 Greenville Avenue
Dallas, TX 75231-4596
Toll-Free: 800-AHA-USA1
(800-242-8721)
Website: www.americanheart.org

American Lung Association

National Headquarters
1301 Pennsylvania Avenue NW, Suite 800
Washington, DC 20004
Toll-Free: 800-LUNGUSA (800-586-4872)
Toll-Free: 800-548-8252 (Helpline)
Phone: 202-785-3355
Fax: 202-452-1805
Website: http://www.lung.org
E-mail: info@lung.org

Ann and Robert H. Lurie Children's Hospital of Chicago

225 East Chicago Avenue
Chicago, IL 60611
Toll-Free: 800-KIDS-DOC
(800-543-7362)
Website: http://www.luriechildrens.org

Bone Builders

University of Arizona
4341 East Broadway
Phoenix, AZ 85040
Phone: 602-827-8200, ext. 316
Website: http://www.bonebuilders.org
E-mail: bones@ag.arizona.edu

Canadian Society for Exercise Physiology

1800 Louisa Street, Suite 370
Ottawa, Ontario CANADA K1R 6Y6
Website: http://www.csep.ca
E-mail: info@csep.ca

Centers for Disease Control and Prevention (CDC)

Division of Nutrition, Physical Activity,
and Obesity
1600 Clifton Road
Atlanta, GA 30333
Toll-Free: 800-CDC-INFO
(800-232-4636)
Toll-Free TTY: 888-232-6348
Website: http://www.cdc.gov/nccdphp/
dnpao/index.html
Email: cdcinfo@cdc.gov

Consumer Product Safety Commission

4330 East West Highway
Bethesda, MD 20814
Toll-Free: 800-638-2772
Phone: 301-504-7923
TTY: 301-595-7054
Website: http://www.cpsc.gov

Disabled Sports USA

451 Hungerford Drive
Suite 100
Rockville, MD 20850
Phone: 301-217-0960
Fax: 301-217-0968
Website: http://www.dsusa.org
Email: information@dsusa.org

Go Ask Alice, Columbia University Health Education Program

Website: http://goaskalice.columbia.edu

HealthyWomen

157 Broad Street, Suite 106
Red Bank, NJ 07701
Toll-Free: 877-986-9472
Fax: 732-530-3347
Website: http://www.healthywomen.org
E-mail: info@healthywomen.org

IDEA Health & Fitness Association

10455 Pacific Center Court
San Diego, CA 92121
Toll-Free: 800-999-4332, ext. 7
Phone: 858-535-8979, ext. 7
Fax: 858-535-8234
Website: http://www.ideafit.com
E-mail: contact@ideafit.com

iEmily

Website: http://www.iemily.com
E-mail: iemilyinfo@yahoo.com

International Fitness Association

12472 Lake Underhill Road, #341
Orlando, FL 32828-7144
Toll-Free: 800-227-1976
Phone: 407-579-8610
Website: http://www.ifafitness.com

Kidshealth.org

Nemours Foundation
10140 Centurion Parkway
Jacksonville, FL 32256
Phone: 904-697-4100
Fax: 904-697-4220
Website: http://www.kidshealth.org

LiveStrong

Website: http://www.livestrong.com

National Alliance for Youth Sports

National Headquarters
2050 Vista Parkway
West Palm Beach, FL 33411
Toll-Free: 800-688-KIDS
(800-729-2057)
Phone: 561-684-1141
Fax: 561-684-2546
Website: http://www.nays.org
E-mail: nays@nays.org

National Association for Health and Fitness

c/o Be Active New York State
65 Niagara Square, Room 607
Buffalo, NY 14202
Phone: 716-851-4052
Fax: 716-851-4309
Website: http://www.physicalfitness.org
E-mail: wellness@city-buffalo.org

National Center on Physical Activity and Disability

University of Illinois at Chicago
Department of Disability and Human
Development
1640 West Roosevelt Road
Chicago, IL 60608-6904
Toll-Free: 800-900-8086
Toll-Free TTY: 800-900-8086
Fax: 312-355-4058
Website: http://www.ncpad.org
E-mail: ncpad@uic.edu

National Coalition for Promoting Physical Activity

1100 H Street, NW, Suite 510
Washington, DC 20005
Phone: 202-454-7521
Fax: 202-454-7598
Website: http://www.ncppa.org
Email: info@ncppa.org

National Collegiate Athletic Association

Website: http://www.ncaa.org

National Heart, Lung, and Blood Institute

NHLBI Health Information Center
P.O. Box 30105
Bethesda, MD 20824-0105
Phone: 301-592-8573
TTY: 240-629-3255
Fax: 240-629-3246
Website: http://www.nhlbi.nih.gov
E-mail: nhlbiinfo@rover.nhlbi.nih.gov

National Institute of Arthritis and Musculoskeletal and Skin Diseases

Information Clearinghouse
National Institutes of Health
1 AMS Circle
Bethesda, MD 20892-3675
Toll-Free: 877-22-NIAMS
(877-226-4267)
Phone: 301-495-4484
TTY: 301-565-2966
Fax: 301-718-6366
Website: http://www.niams.nih.gov
E-mail: NIAMSinfo@mail.nih.gov

National Institute of Diabetes and Digestive and Kidney Diseases

Office of Communications and
Public Liaison
Building 31, Room 9A06
31 Center Drive, MSC 2560
Bethesda, MD 20892-2560
Phone: 301-496-3583
Website: http://www.niddk.nih.gov

National Osteoporosis Foundation

1150 17th Street, NW, Suite 850
Washington, DC 20036
Toll-Free: 800-231-4222
Phone: 202-223-2226
Fax: 202-223-2237
Website: http://www.nof.org

National Recreation and Park Association

22377 Belmont Ridge Road
Ashburn, VA 20148-4501
Toll-Free: 800-626-NRPA
(800-626-6772)
Website: http://www.nrpa.org
E-mail: customerservice@nrpa.or

National Strength and Conditioning Association

1885 Bob Johnson Drive
Colorado Springs, CO 80906
Toll-Free: 800-815-6826
Phone: 719-632-6722
Fax: 719-632-6367
Website: http://www.nsca-lift.org
E-mail: nsca@nsca-lift.org

National Women's Health Information Center

U.S. Department of Health and Human Services
8270 Willow Oaks Corporate Drive
Fairfax, VA 22031
Toll-Free: 800-994-9662
Toll-Free TTD: 888-220-5446
Phone: 202-690-7650
Fax: 202-205-2631
Website: http://www.womenshealth.gov

PE Central

P.O. Box 10262
1995 South Main Street, Suite 902
Blacksburg, VA 24062
Phone: 540-953-1043
Fax: 540-301-0112
Website: http://www.pecentral.org
E-mail: pec@pecentral.org

President's Challenge

501 North Morton Street, Suite 203
Bloomington, IN 47404
Toll-Free: 800-258-8146
Fax: 812-855-8999
Website:
http://www.presidentschallenge.org
E-mail: preschal@indiana.edu

President's Council on Fitness, Sports, and Nutrition

1101 Wootton Parkway, Suite 560
Rockville, MD 20852
Phone: 240-276-9567
Fax: 240-276-9860
Website: http://www.fitness.gov
Email: fitness@hhs.gov

Right to Play International

65 Queen Street West
Thomson Building, Suite 1900
Box 64
Toronto, Ontario M5H2M5
Phone: +1 416 498 1922
Fax: +1 416 498 1942
Website: http://www.righttoplay.com
E-mail: info@righttoplay.com

Safe Kids Canada

555 University Avenue
Toronto, Ontario M5G 1X8
Website: http://www.safekidscanada.ca

Safe Kids USA

1301 Pennsylvania Avenue NW
Suite 1000
Washington, DC 20004-1707
Phone: 202-662-0600
Fax: 202-393-2072
Website: http://www.safekids.org

Shape Up America

P.O. Box 149
506 Brackett Creek Road
Clyde Park, MT 59018-0149
Phone: 406-686-4844
Website: http://www.shapeup.org

Weight-Control Information Network

1 WIN Way
Bethesda, MD 20892-3665
Toll-Free: 877-946-4627
Fax: 202-828-1028
Website: http://win.niddk.nih.gov
E-mail: win@info.niddk.nih.gov

Women's Sports Foundation

Eisenhower Park
1899 Hempstead Turnpike
Suite 400
East Meadow, NY 11554
Toll-Free: 800-227-3988
Phone: 516-542-4700
Fax: 516-542-4716
Website:
http://www.womenssportsfoundation.org
E-mail:
Info@WomensSportsFoundation.org

Chapter 62

Resources For More Information About Specific Sports And Activities

Amateur Athletic Union Basketball

P.O. Box 22409
Lake Buena Vista, FL 32830
Toll-Free: 800-AAU-4USA
(800-228-4872)
Phone: 407-934-7200
Fax: 407-934-7242
Boys website: http://aauboysbasketball.org
Girls website: http://aaugirlsbasketball.org

Amateur Softball Association of America

2801 NE 50th Street
Oklahoma City, OK 73111
Phone: 405-424-5266
Website: http://www.asasoftball.com

American Hiking Society

1422 Fenwick Lane
Silver Spring, MD 20910
Toll-Free: 800-972-8608
Phone: 301-565-6704
Fax: 301-565-6714
Website: http://www.americanhiking.org
E-mail: info@americanhiking.org

American Running Association

4405 East-West Highway, Suite 405
Bethesda, MD 20814
Phone: 800-776-2732 (ext. 13 or 12)
Fax: 301-913-9520
Website: http://www.americanrunning.org

About This Chapter: Information in this chapter was compiled from many sources deemed reliable. Inclusion does not constitute endorsement and there is no implication associated with omission. All contact information was verified in 2012.

American Whitewater

P.O. Box 1540
Cullowhee, NC 28723
Toll-Free: 866-BOAT-4-AW
(866-262-8429)
Website:
http://www.americanwhitewater.org
E-mail: info@americanwhitewater.org

American Youth Soccer Association

19750 South Vermont Avenue
Suite 200
Torrance, CA 90502
Toll-Free: 800-USA-AYSO
(800-872-2976)
Fax: 310-525-1155
Website: http://www.ayso.org

Aquatic Exercise Association

P.O. Box 1609
Nokomis, FL 34274-1609
Toll-Free: 888-232-9283
Website: http://www.aeawave.com

Bicycle Helmet Safety Institute

4611 Seventh Street South
Arlington, VA 22204-1419
Phone: 703-486-0100
Website: http://www.bhsi.org
E-mail: info@helmets.org

College and Junior Tennis

Port Washington Tennis Academy
100 Harbor Road
Port Washington, NY 11050
Phone: 516-883-6601
Fax: 516-883-5241
Website: http://www.clgandjrtennis.com
E-mail: info@collegeandjuniortennis.com

Dance USA

1111 16th Street NW
Suite 300
Washington, DC 20036
Phone: 202-833-1717
Fax: 202-833-2686
Website: http://www.danceusa.org

Inline Skating Resource Center

Website: http://www.iisa.org
E-mail: contact@iisa.org

International Skateboarding Federation

Website:
http://www.international
skateboardingfederation.org
E-mail: president@
internationalskateboardingfederation.org

Little League

539 U.S. Route 15 Highway
P.O. Box 3485
Williamsport, PA 17701-0485
Phone: 570-326-1921
Fax: 570-326-1074
Website: http://www.littleleague.org

National Scholastic Surfing Association

P.O. Box 495
Huntington Beach, CA 92648
Phone: 714-378-0899
Fax: 714-964-5232
Website: http://www.nssa.org

NFL Rush

Website: http://www.nflrush.com

Pop Warner Football

586 Middletown Boulevard
Suite C-100
Langhorne, PA 19047
Phone: 215-752-2691
Fax: 215-752-2879
Website: http://www.popwarner.com

Surfrider Foundation

P.O. Box 6010
San Clemente, CA 92674-6010
Phone: 949-492-8170
Fax: 949-492-8142
Website: http://www.surfrider.org
E-mail: info@surfrider.org

USA Baseball

403 Blackwell Street
Durham, NC 27701
Phone: 919-474-8721
Fax: 919-474-8822
Website: http://web.usabaseball.com
E-mail: info@usabaseball.com

USA Cycling

210 USA Cycling Point, Suite 100
Colorado Springs, CO 80919-2215
Phone: 719-434-4200
Fax: 719-434-4300
Website: http://www.usacycling.org
E-mail: membership@usacycling.org

USA Diver

Website:
http://www.usadiver.com/diving_jr.htm

USA Gymnastics

132 East Washington Street, Suite 700
Indianapolis, IN 46204
Toll-Free: 800-345-4719
(Membership Services)
Phone: 317-237-5050
Fax: 317-237-5069 (National Office)
Fax: 317-692-5212 (Membership Services)
Website: http://usagym.org
E-mail: membership@usagym.org

USA Jump Rope

P.O. Box 569
Huntsville, TX 77342-0569
Toll-Free: 800-225-8820
Phone: 936-295-3332
Fax: 936-295-3309
Website: http://www.usajumprope.org
E-mail: info@usajumprope.org

USA Swimming

1 Olympic Plaza
Colorado Springs, CO 80909
Phone: 719-866-4578
Website: http://www.usaswimming.org

USA Ultimate

4730 Table Mesa Drive, Suite I-200C
Boulder, CO 80305
Toll-Free: 800-872-4384
Phone: 303-447-3472
Fax: 303-447-3483
Website:
http://www.usaultimate.org/index.html
E-mail: info@usaultimate.org

U.S.A. Water Ski

1251 Holy Cow Road
Polk City, FL 33868
Phone: 863-324-4341
Fax: 863-325-8259
Website: http://www.usawaterski.org
E-mail: memberservices@usawaterski.org

U.S. Figure Skating Association

20 First Street
Colorado Springs, CO 80906
Phone: 719-635-5200
Fax: 719-635-9548
Website: http://www.usfsa.org
E-mail: info@usfigureskating.org

U.S. Kids Golf

3040 Northwoods Parkway
Norcross, GA 30071
Toll-Free: 888-3-US KIDS
(888-387-5437)
Phone: 770-441-3077
Fax: 770-448-3069
Website: http://www.uskidsgolf.com
E-mail: customerservice@uskidsgolf.com

U.S. Ski and Snowboard Association

1 Victory Lane
Box 100
Park City, UT 84060
Phone: 435-649-9090
Fax: 435-649-3613
Website: http://usskiteam.com

U.S. Youth Soccer Association

9220 World Cup Way
Frisco, TX 75033
Toll-Free: 800-4SOCCER
(800-476-2237)
Fax: 972-334-9960
Website: http://www.usyouthsoccer.org

U.S. Youth Volleyball League

2771 Plaza Del Amo, Suite 808
Torrance, CA 90503
Toll-Free: 888-988-7985
Phone: 310-212-7008
Fax: 310-212-7182
Website: http://www.usyvl.org
E-mail: questions@usyvl.org

Varsity

6745 Lenox Center Court, Suite 300
Memphis, TN 38115
Website: http://www.varsity.com

Index

Index

Page numbers that appear in *Italics* refer to tables or illustrations. Page numbers that have a small 'n' after the page number refer to information shown as Notes at the beginning of each chapter. Page numbers that appear in **Bold** refer to information contained in boxes on that page (except Notes information at the beginning of each chapter).

A

"About" (President's Challenge) 357n
About.com, publications
 adverse weather exercise 281n
 cardiovascular exercise 129n
 disabilities, exercise 333n
Action for Health Kids,
 contact information 361
"Active at Any Size" (NIDDK) 303n
A.D.A.M., Inc., exercise-induced asthma
 publication 325n
Adaptive Adventures, website address **335**
aerobic activity
 described 10
 fitness guidelines 82
 guidelines 118
 intensity levels 84, 114–15, 132
 overview 114–15
aerobic exercise
 diabetes mellitus 329
 fitness guidelines *126, 127*
 weight management 8
Aerobics and Fitness Association of
 America, contact information 361

age factor, physical activity 83–84, *127*
AH-89-Xtreme 351
alcohol use, physical activity guidelines 121
Altena, Thomas 269n
alternating toe touches, described 140–41
Amateur Athlete Union, contact information 361
Amateur Athletic Union Basketball,
 contact information 369
Amateur Endurance, contact information 361
Amateur Softball Association of America,
 contact information 369
American Alliance for Health, Physical
 Education, Recreation, and Dance,
 contact information 362
American Athletic Institute, website address 362
American College of Sports Medicine (ACSM)
 contact information 362
 publications
  clothing 269n
  fitness facilities 103n
  hydration 289n
American Council on Exercise
 contact information 362

American Council on Exercise, *continued*
    publications
        asthma 323n
        indoor cycling 184n
American Diabetes Association,
    contact information 362
American Heart Association, contact
    information 362
American Hiking Society, contact information 369
American Lung Association, contact information 362
American Running Association,
    contact information 369
American Whitewater, contact information 370
American Youth Soccer Association,
    contact information 370
Amputee Coalition of America, website address **335**
anabolic steroids
        described **350**
        overview 349–53
        strength training 147
animal studies, brain circuit **16–17**
Ann and Robert H. Lurie
    Children's Hospital of Chicago
        contact information 362
        female athlete triad publication 345n
anorexia, over-exercising 254–55
anorexia athletica, overview 339–43
Aquatic Exercise Association,
    contact information 370
arm circles, described 140
asthma
        described 40
        exercise suggestions 323–26
AXIS Dance Company, website address 337

B

ballet, overview 208–10
"Ballet Activity Card" (BAM! Body and Mind) 205n
BAM! Body and Mind, publications
        ballet 205n
        baseball 187n
        basketball 191n
        canoeing 229n
        cheerleading 205n

BAM! Body and Mind, publications, *continued*
        diving 229n
        figure skating 241n
        fishing 229n
        football 197n
        Frisbee 199n
        golf 201n
        gymnastics 205n
        hiking 225n
        inline skating 213n
        kayaking 229n
        martial arts 211n
        safety helmets 263n
        skateboarding 213n
        snorkeling 229n
        snow skiing 241n
        soccer 217n
        softball 187n
        surfing 229n
        table tennis 219n
        tennis 219n
        volleyball 219n
        walking 225n
        water skiing 229n
        white-water rafting 229n
        see also Centers for Disease Control
                and Prevention
barre, defined 209
barriers
        exercise 72–73
        physical activity 303–10
        team sports 183–85
baseball
        injury prevention 279, 315
        overview 187–89
"Baseball Activity Card"
    (BAM! Body and Mind) 187n
basketball
        injury prevention 279, 314–15
        overview 191–92
"Basketball Activity Card"
    (BAM! Body and Mind) 191n
"Best Time of Day to Exercise"
    (Columbia University) 95n

Bicycle Helmet Safety Institute,
    contact information 370
bicycling
        injury prevention 279
        overview 193–96
        overweight 308
        stopping distance **195**
BlazeSports, website address **335**
blood glucose levels, tests **331**
blood vessels
        described 32–33
        lungs 36–37
body mass index (BMI), described 57
Body Works: A Toolkit for Healthy Teens and Strong
    Families (Office on Women's Health) 41n, 57n, 81n
Bone Builders, contact information 363
bone health, exercise 23–26
bone mineral density, described 253–54
bone-strengthening activity
        described 11, **26**, 114
        fitness guidelines 82, *126*, *127*
        guidelines 118
Borg Rating of Perceived Exertion 163–64, 196
bowling, disabilities 337
brain studies, exercise **16–17**
bronchial tree, depicted *36*

C

calcium, special importance 46–47
calisthenics, overview 137–43
Canadian Society for Exercise Physiology,
    contact information 363
cancer, physical activity 16–17
canoeing, overview 229–31
"Canoeing/Kayaking Activity Card"
    (BAM! Body and Mind) 229n
capillaries, described 32–33
"Cardio 101 - The Facts About Cardio"
    (About.com) 129n
cardiorespiratory endurance, described 128
cardiorespiratory health, physical activity 12–13
cardiovascular exercise, overview 129–32
CDC *see* Centers for Disease Control and
    Prevention

cell phones, emergencies 272
Centers for Disease Control and Prevention (CDC)
        contact information 363
        exercise intensity publication 163n
        see also BAM! Body and Mind
certification
        fitness facilities 106
        group indoor cycling instructors 196
        injury prevention 313
        safety helmets 263–64
"Chapter 3: Active Children and Adolescent"
    (DHHS) 81n
"Chapter 6: Safe and Active" (DHHS) 273n
cheerleading, overview 207–8
"Cheerleading Activity Card"
    (BAM! Body and Mind) 205n
"Childhood Sports Injuries and Their Prevention"
    (NIAMS) 311n
Children's Hospital of Chicago *see* Ann and Robert
    H. Lurie Children's Hospital of Chicago
"Choose A Challenge: Physical Fitness Test"
    (President's Challenge) 357n
"Choosing The Right Sport For You"
    (Nemours Foundation) 177n
chronic diseases, physical activity **307**
chronic obstructive pulmonary disease (COPD),
    described 40
circulatory system, described 32–33
clothing
        ballet 209–10
        basketball 192
        canoeing 230
        figure skating 242
        golf 203
        group indoor cycling 195
        gymnastics 205
        hypothermia 283
        kayaking 230
        martial arts 212
        overweight, exercise 310
        snowboarding 245–46
        summer exercise 272
        tennis 220
        volleyball 223

clothing, *continued*
    walking 226
    winter exercise 269–72
    see also protective gear
coaches
    cheerleading 208
    competition 184
    see also instructors
cold weather exercise, overview 281–85
College and Junior Tennis, contact information 370
Columbia University
    copyright information 166
    publications
        exercise intensity 163n
        workout timing 95n
    see also *Go Ask Alice!*
"Compulsive Exercise" (Nemours Foundation) 339b
compulsive exercise, overview 339–43
concussions, overview **265**
Consumer Product Safety Commission (CPSC)
    contact information 363
    safety helmets publication 263n
Cooke, David A. 41n, 57n, 81n, 109n, 137n, 163n, 263n, 281n
cooling down
    described 251
    injury prevention 313
    physical activity 304
    strength training **149**
    workout schedule 5
COPD *see* chronic obstructive pulmonary disease
coronary heart disease (CHD), physical activity 116–17
CPSC *see* Consumer Product Safety Commission
creativity, adequate sleep **66**
cross-training, described 181

D

Dance USA, contact information 370
dancing, overweight 306–7
Dank, Leonard 27n
Deaflympics, website address **335**
DEET, hiking 228
dehydration, described 291–92

Department of Health and Human Services
    see US Department of Health and Human Services
DHHS *see* US Department of Health and Human Services
diabetes mellitus, exercise suggestions 327–32
diary, physical activity 119
diet and nutrition
    mental health 61–62
    overview 41–55
    physical activity 121
Dietary Approaches to Stop Hypertension (DASH diet) 121
diets, weight management 59
disabilities
    exercise suggestions 333–37
    organizations **335**
Disabled Sports USA
    contact information 363
    website address **335**
diving, overview 231–32
"Diving Activity Card" (BAM! Body and Mind) 229n

E

eating disorders, female athlete triad 253–55, 346
EFIT acronym, described 92–93
electrical system, heart 33–34
electrolyte imbalance, dehydration 289
emotional concerns
    exercise **16–17**
    mental health 63–64
    weight management 58–59
ESTRO Xtreme 351
exercise
    asthma 323–26
    benefits overview 9–18
    bone health 23–26
    injury recovery 319–21
    safety tips 251–52
    time of day 95–97
    see also physical activity
"Exercise and Asthma" (American Council on Exercise) 323n
"Exercise for Your Bone Health" (NIAMS) 23n

"Exercise-Induced Asthma" (A.D.A.M., Inc.) 325n
exercise-induced asthma, overview 325–26
exercise-induced hyponatremia, described 287
exercises
    bone strength **26**
    calisthenics overview 137–43
    guidelines *126–27*
    muscle strength **22**
    overview 125–28
    stretching 151–53
"Exercising in Hot Weather" (Gaustad) 281n
exhalation, described 39

F

face muscles, described 21
fast foods, diet and nutrition 52–54
fats, diet and nutrition 51–52
Federal Trade Commission (FTC),
   fitness products cautions publication 109n
"Female Athlete Triad" (Ann and Robert H. Lurie
   Children's Hospital of Chicago) 345n
female athlete triad, overview 253–56, 345–47
figure skating, overview 241–42
"Figure Skating Activity Card"
   (BAM! Body and Mind) 241n
financial considerations, snack foods **54**
fishing
    fun facts **232**
    overview 232–33
"Fishing Activity Card" (BAM! Body and Mind) 229n
Fit Facts *see* American Council on Exercise
fitness
    overview 3–8
    self-assessment 75–80
"Fitness" (Office on Women's Health) 71n
"Fitness Basics" (Office on Women's Health) 125n
fitness facilities
    overview 103–8
    weight management **309**
    see also health clubs
"Fitness For Kids Who Don't Like Sports"
   (Nemours Foundation) 183n
fitness formula, overview 91–94
fitness friends, described 99–100

"Fitness Fundamentals: Guidelines for
   Personal Exercise Programs" (President's
   Council on Fitness, Sports, and Nutrition) 3n
fitness guidelines, overview 81–90
"Fitness: Keeping Safe and Injury-Free"
   (Office on Women's Health) 251n
fitness plan, described 71–73
"Fitness Self-Assessment" (NHS Choices) 75n
flexibility exercises, described 128
fluid balance
    hydration 290
    injury prevention 313
    overweight, exercise 310
football
    fun facts **198**
    injury prevention 279, 315
    overview 197–98
"Football Activity Card" (BAM! Body and
   Mind) 197n
"Formula for Fitness" (iEmily.com) 91n
fraud, filing complaints **112**
free-hand neck resistance, described 139–40
free play, described 186
free weights, described 145
Frisbee
    overview 199–200
    quick tips **200**
"Frisbee Activity Card" (BAM! Body and
   Mind) 199n
frostbite, described 281–82

G

Gaustad, Scott 281n
"General Physical Activities Defined by Level
   of Intensity" (CDC) 163n
goals
    motivation 297–301
    physical activity programs 332
Go Ask Alice!
    contact information 363
    publications
        exercise intensity 163n
        workout timing 95n
    see also Columbia University

golf, fun facts **202**
"Golf Activity Card" (BAM! Body and Mind) 201n
goofy-footed, described 235
Greene, Colleen 319–21
group indoor cycling, overview 194–96
growth plate injuries, described 312
guidelines
exercise *126–27*
fitness overview 81–90
physical activity 117–18
safety considerations **274**
gymnastics
fun facts **206**
injury prevention 316
overview 205–6
"Gymnastics Activity Card"
(BAM! Body and Mind) 205n

H

"Hard Facts about Helmets" (BAM! Body and Mind) 263n
health clubs
customer rights 109–11
described 100–101
see also fitness facilities
"Health Spas: Exercise Your Rights" (FTC) 109n
healthy eating, quick tips **6–7**
see also diet and nutrition
Healthy Women, contact information 363
hearing impairment, exercise suggestions 334–35
heart
depicted *28*
overview 27–35
physical activity 116–17
heart attack, physical activity **13**, 117
heart muscle, described 20
heart rate measurement
aerobic activities 6–8
cardiovascular exercise 129–30
moderate intensity 163
heart valves, depicted *29*
heat cramps, described 286
heat exhaustion, described 286
heat-related illnesses, described 312–13

heat stroke, described 286–87
heat syncope, described 286
helmets *see* safety helmets
Herkenham, Miles **17**
HHS *see* US Department of Health and Human Services
hiking
described 180
gear list **180**
overview 227–28
"Hiking Activity Card" (BAM! Body and Mind) 225n
HMG-Xtreme 351
home cooking, diet and nutrition 54–55
hot weather exercise, overview 284–88
"How Much Sleep Do I Need?" (Nemours Foundation) 65n
"How's That Work-Out Working Out? Tips on Buying Fitness Gear" (FTC) 109n
"How to Exercise Safely in Cold Weather" (About.com) 281n
hydration, overview 289–94
hydration status
color test *291*
heat illness 287–88
hyperthermia, described 286–87
hypoglycemia, exercise 330–31
hypothermia, described 282–83

I

ice hockey, injury prevention 279
IDEA Health and Fitness Association, contact information 363
iEmily.com
contact information 363
publications
fitness formula 91n
fitness friends 99n
health clubs 99n
infralimbic cortex, brain studies **17**
inhalation, described 38–39
injury prevention
overview 273–80
running 134

inline skating
fun facts **214**
injury prevention 280
overview 213–14
"Inline Skating Activity Card"
(BAM! Body and Mind) 213n
Inline Skating Resource Center,
contact information 370
The Inner Man (Dank) 27n
instructors
group indoor cycling 196
health clubs 104, 106, 110
martial arts 212
see also coaches
intensity
described 92, 114–15, 275
overview 163–73
International Fitness Association,
contact information 364
International Skateboarding Federation,
contact information 370

J

jogging, injury prevention 280
"Joining A Health Club: Is It For You?"
(iEmily.com) 99n
Jordan, Michael **192**
judo, described 211
jumping jacks, described 138
jump rope, described **138**

K

karate, described 211
kayaking, overview 229–31
Kidshealth.org *see* Nemours Foundation
knee injuries, described 255–56

L

lactose intolerance, calcium 47
leg raises, described 142
Lehmann, Michael **17**
Let's Move, website address **335**

life jackets
canoeing 230–31
kayaking 230–31
see also personal flotation devices
lifestyle activities
fitness 73–74
overweight 309
lifestyles
changes **94**
overview 113–22
lightning, safety tips **284–85**
Little League, contact information 370
LiveStrong, website address 364
lung diseases, described 40
lungs
depicted *36, 37*
overview 35–40
physical activity 116
Lurie Children's Hospital *see* Ann and Robert H.
Lurie Children's Hospital of Chicago

M

"Make a Fitness Friend" (iEmily.com) 99n
martial arts, overview 211–12
"Martial Arts Activity Card"
(BAM! Body and Mind) 211n
MASS Xtreme 351
medications
anabolic steroids overview 349–53
exercise-induced asthma 325–26
menstrual dysfunction, female athlete triad 253,
345–46
mental health
overview 61–64
physical activity 18
"Mental Health" (Office on Women's Health) 61n
metabolic equivalents (METS)
described 163–66
intensity level examples 166–173
metabolic health, physical activity 14
"Mind Over Matter: Anabolic Steroids"
(NIDA) 349n
MMA-3 Xtreme 351
moderate intensity, described 163–66

motivation, overview 297–301
"Motivation and the Power
   of Not Giving Up"
   (Nemours Foundation) 297n
muscles
      breathing 38
      overview 19–22
muscle-strengthening activity
      described 10–11, 114
      fitness guidelines 82, *127*
      guidelines 118
muscular endurance exercises, described 128
muscular strength exercises, described 128
musculoskeletal health, physical activity 15

N

Nadelen, Mary 269n
National Alliance for Youth Sports,
   contact information 364
National Association for Health and Fitness,
   contact information 364
National Center on Physical
   Activity and Disability
      contact information 364
      website address **335**
National Coalition for
   Promoting Physical Activity,
   contact information 364
National Collegiate Athletic Association,
   website address 364
National Heart, Lung, and Blood Institute
   (NHLBI)
      contact information 365
      publications
         heart 27n
         lungs 27n
         physical activity 113n
National Institute of Arthritis and
   Musculoskeletal and Skin Diseases (NIAMS)
      contact information 365
      publications
         bone health 23n
         sports injuries 311n

National Institute of Diabetes and
   Digestive and Kidney Diseases (NIDDK)
      contact information 365
      publications
         diabetes, exercise 327n
         physical activity 303n
National Institute on Drug Abuse (NIDA),
   anabolic steroids publication 349n
National Osteoporosis Foundation,
   contact information 365
National Recreation and Park Association,
   contact information 365
National Scholastic Surfing Association,
   contact information 371
National Sports Center for the Disabled,
   website address **335**
National Strength and Conditioning Association,
   contact information 365
National Wheelchair Basketball Association,
   website address **335**
National Women's Health Information Center
   (NWHIC), contact information 366
neck rolls, described 139
Nemours Foundation
      contact information 364
      publications
         alternate fitness activities 183n
         compulsive exercise 339b
         motivation 297n
         muscles 19n
         Pilates 155n
         running safety 257n
         sleep requirements 65n
         sports activities 177n
         strength training 145n
         yoga 155n
NFL Rush, website address 371
NHLBI *see* National Heart, Lung, and Blood Institute
NHS Choices, fitness self-assessment publication 75n
NIAMS *see* National Institute of Arthritis and
   Musculoskeletal and Skin Diseases
Nicklaus, Jack 201
NIDA *see* National Institute on Drug Abuse
NIDDK *see* National Institute of Diabetes and
   Digestive and Kidney Diseases

"No Limits - Exercising With A Disability"
    (About.com) 333n
North American Riding for the Handicapped
    Association, website address 337
nutrition *see* diet and nutrition
Nutrition Facts label
    depicted *44*
    described 43–44

O

obesity
    energy balance 14–15
    exercise 303–10
obligatory exercise, overview 339–43
Office on Women's Health, publications
    diet and nutrition 41n
    disabilities, exercise 333n
    fitness 71n
    fitness basics 125n
    fitness guidelines 81n
    mental health 61n
    safety tips 251n
    stretching exercises 151n
    weight management 57n
    see also US Department of Health
                and Human Services
Olson, Michelle 103n
osteoporosis
    exercise **24–25**
    female athlete triad 256, 346
    prevention program 25
overhydration, described 294
overload
    described **12**
    fitness formula 91–92
overweight
    energy balance 14–15
    exercise 303–10

P

PE Central, contact information 366
personal flotation devices, described 237
    see also life jackets

physical activity
    adverse effects **13**
    beneficial effects **12**
    benefits overview 9–18
    diabetes mellitus 327–32
    examples 84–85
    guidelines 117–18
    health benefits 115–17
    lifestyle overview 113–22
    longevity **107, 293**
    quick tips **6–7, 122**
    see also exercise
physical activity programs
    described **105, 290**
    diabetes mellitus 332
    disabilities 336
Physical Activity Readiness
    Questionnaire (PAR-Q) 105
physical education (PE) classes, described **83, 84**
physical examinations, fitness programs **184**
"Physical Fitness: A Guide for Individuals with
    Lower Limb Loss"
    (US Department of Veterans Affairs) 137n
Pilates
    beginner exercises **156**
    described 180
    overview 155–58
"Pilates" (Nemours Foundation) 155n
Pilates, Joseph H. 155–56
Ping-Pong *see* table tennis
Pointe, defined 209
Pop Warner Football, contact information 371
powerlifting, described 146
"Preparing for and Playing in the Heat"
    (Nadelen) 269n
President's Challenge
    contact information 364
    physical fitness test publication 357n
President's Council on Fitness, Sports, and Nutrition
    contact information 366
    publications
        exercise programs 3n
        snowboarding 241n
progression, described **12**
prone leg extension, described 142–43

protective gear
    baseball 188
    basketball 192
    bicycling 193–94
    football 198
    Frisbee 200
    injury prevention 276, 313
    overview 252–53
    quick tips 111–12, **254–55**
    running 258–59
    skateboarding 215
    snorkeling 234–35
    snowboarding 246
    snow skiing 243–44
    soccer 218
    softball 189–90
    surfing 236
    see also clothing; safety considerations
puberty, weight management 57–58
pulmonary circulation, described 33

R

repetitive motion injuries, described 312
resistance, described 145
resistance training, described 89–90
respiratory system, described 35–38
Responsibility Code for Skiers 244
RICE acronym, injury treatment 314, 316
Right to Play International, contact information 366
rock climbing, described 180
Rogers, Matt 133n
running
    injury prevention 280
    overview 133–36, 257–61

S

Safe Kids Canada, contact information 366
Safe Kids USA, contact information 366
safety considerations
    ballet 210
    baseball 188–89
    basketball 192
    canoeing 230–31

safety considerations, *continued*
    cheerleading 207–8
    diving 231–32
    figure skating 242
    fishing 233
    fitness facilities 104
    football 198
    Frisbee 200
    golf 203
    gymnastics 206
    hiking 228
    injury prevention 277
    inline skating 214
    jump rope **138**
    kayaking 230–31
    martial arts 212
    overview 251–56
    overweight, exercise 309–10
    physical activity 119–20
    physical activity guidelines **274**
    running 133, 260–61
    skateboarding 215
    snorkeling 235
    snow skiing 244
    soccer 218
    softball 190
    sports activities 317
    strength training 90
    surfing 236
    tennis 220–21
    volleyball 223
    walking 226–27
    water skiing 237–38
    white-water rafting 239
    see also protective gear
safety helmets
    baseball 188
    bicycling 193–94
    depicted *268*
    described 252
    football 198
    inline skating 214
    overview 263–68
    skateboarding 215

safety considerations, *continued*
    snow skiing 243
    types *267*
    white-water rafting 239
"Safety Tips: Running" (Nemours Foundation) 257n
"Selecting and Effectively Using A
   Health/Fitness Facility" (ACSM) 103n
"Selecting and Effectively Using
   Hydration for Fitness" (ACSM) 289n
Shape Up America, contact information 367
Sheppard, Alan **202**
skateboarding
    fun facts **214**
    injury prevention 280
    overview 214–15
"Skateboarding Activity Card"
   (BAM! Body and Mind) 213n
skating, overview 213–15
Skating Athletes Bold at Heart,
   website address 337
skeletal muscles, described 20–21
skiing, injury prevention 280
sleep
    mental health 62–63
    overview 65–68
    quick tips **76**
smooth muscles, described 19–20
snorkeling, overview 233–35
"Snorkeling Activity Card"
   (BAM! Body and Mind) 229n
snowboarding
    glossary **247**
    injury prevention 280
    overview 245–48
"Snowboarding" (President's Council on
   Fitness, Sports, and Nutrition) 241n
snowboarding glossary **247**
snow skiing, overview 242–44
"Snow Skiing Activity Card"
   (BAM! Body and Mind) 241n
soccer
    disabilities 336
    fun facts **218**
    injury prevention 280, 315
    overview 217–18

"Soccer Activity Card"
   (BAM! Body and Mind) 217n
soda, recommendations *50*
softball
    injury prevention 279, 315
    overview 189–90
"Softball Activity Card"
   (BAM! Body and Mind) 187n
Special Olympics, website address 337
specificity, described **12**
sports activities
    choices **179**
    choices overview 177–86
    fun facts **188**
"Sports and Recreation for Teens with Illnesses or
   Disabilities" (Office on Women's Health) 333n
sports beverages, described 292
sports calendar **178**
sports injuries
    overview 311–17
    prevention overview 278–80
spotters, strength training 146
sprains, described 312
standing one-legged toe raise, described 143
"Starting a Running Program" (Rogers) 133n
statistics
    physical activity injuries 273
    sports injuries 311
Steadman index 285
steroids *see* anabolic steroids
strains, described 312
strength training
    benefits **147**
    described 89–90, 181
    diabetes mellitus 329
    overview 145–49
"Strength Training" (Nemours Foundation) 145n
stress management, mental health 63–64
stretching
    described 114
    diabetes mellitus 330
    overview 151–53
"Stretching Exercises"
   (Office on Women's Health) 151n

students, tests scores **11**

summer exercise, clothing overview 272

supplements

    mental health 62

    overview 45–46

surfing

    overview 235–36

    wave ownership **236**

"Surfing Activity Card" (BAM! Body and Mind)
    229n

Surfrider Foundation, contact information 371

T

table tennis, overview 221–22

"Table Tennis Activity Card"
    (BAM! Body and Mind) 219n

tae kwon do, described 211

t'ai chi, described 181

team sports, *versus* other fitness activities 177–86

television, *versus* physical activity **83, 86**

tennis

    disabilities 337

    fun facts **220**

    overview 219–21

"Tennis Activity Card" (BAM! Body and Mind)
    219n

testosterone, described 349

"Test Your Fitness Flair" (iEmily.com) 91n

tobacco use

    physical activity guidelines 122

    weight management 59

track and field, injury prevention 315

trans fats, described **53**

TREN-Xtreme 351

trunk twists, described 141–42

TT-40-Xtreme 352

2008 Physical Activity Guidelines for Americans
    (DHHS) 9n, 81n, 273n

U

Ultimate Frisbee 200

United States Association of Blind Athletes,
    website address **335**

United States Handcycling Federation,
    website address **335**

University of Michigan, injuries,
    exercise publication 319n

USA Baseball, contact information 371

USA Cycling, contact information 371

USA Deaf Sports Federation, website address **335**

USA Diver, website address 371

USA Gymnastics, contact information 371

USA Jump Rope, contact information 371

USA Swimming, contact information 371

USA Ultimate, contact information 372

USA Water Ski, contact information 372

US Department of Health and Human Services
    (DHHS; HHS), publications

        fitness guidelines 81n

        physical activity guidelines 9n, 81n, 273n

        see also Office on Women's Health

US Department of Veterans Affairs,
    calisthenics publication 137n

US Figure Skating Association,
    contact information 372

US Food and Drug Administration (FDA),
    steroids publication 349n

US Kids Golf, contact information 372

US Ski and Snowboard Association,
    contact information 372

US Youth Soccer Association,
    contact information 372

US Youth Volleyball League,
    contact information 372

V

Varsity, contact information 372

vision impairment, exercise suggestions 334–35

vitamins

    mental health 62

    overview 45

VNS-9 Xtreme 352

volleyball

    disabilities 337

    overview 222–23

"Volleyball Activity Card" (BAM! Body and Mind)
    219n

W

walking
    described 89
    overview 225–27
    overweight 306
"Walking Activity Card" (BAM! Body and
    Mind) 225n
warming up
    described 251
    injury prevention 313
    physical activity 304
    workout schedule 4
    see also safety considerations
"Warning on Body Building Products Marketed as
    Containing Steroids or Steroid-Like Substances"
    (FDA) 349n
warning signs, compulsive exercise 341–42
water intoxication, described 294
water skiing, overview 236–38
"Water Skiing Activity Card"
    (BAM! Body and Mind) 229n
water sports
    described 180
    overview 229–39
    overweight 307
Weight-Control Information Network,
    contact information 367
weight machines, described 145
weight management
    exercise 8
    overview 57–60
    physical activity 86, 120–21
    see also eating disorders; obesity; overweight
weight training, overweight 307–8
"What Are the Lungs" (NHLBI) 27n

"What Exactly Does Moderate Intensity Mean?"
    (Columbia University) 163n
"What I Need to Know about Physical
    Activity and Diabetes" (NIDDK) 327n
"What Is Physical Activity?" (NHLBI) 113n
"What Is the Heart" (NHLBI) 27n
"What to Wear for Winter Exercise"
    (Altena) 269n
"What You Need To Know About
    Group Indoor Cycling" (American
    Council on Exercise) 184n
Wheelchair and Ambulatory Sports USA,
    website address **335**
wheelchair users, exercise suggestions 333–34
"Which Helmet for Which Activity" (CPSC) 263n
white-water rafting, overview 238–39
"White-Water Rafting Activity Card"
    (BAM! Body and Mind) 229n
"Who Can Participate" (President's Challenge) 357n
Williford, Hank 103n
winter exercise, clothing overview 269–72
Women's Sports Foundation,
    contact information 367
"Working out while injured"
    (University of Michigan) 319n

Y

yoga
    beginners **159**
    described 89, 180
    overview 158–61
    overweight 308
"Yoga" (Nemours Foundation) 155n
Yoga for the Special Child, website address 337
"Your Muscles" (Nemours Foundation) 19n